Introduction to
Podopaediatrics

To Margaret, Emma and Philip

Introduction to Podopaediatrics

edited by

Peter Thomson
Senior Chiropodist (Paediatrics)
Fife Health Board
Scotland, UK

W.B. Saunders Company Ltd
London · Philadelphia · Toronto
Sydney · Tokyo

W.B. Saunders 24–28 Oval Road
Company Ltd   London NW1 7DX, UK

Baillière Tindall

The Curtis Center
Independence Square West
Philadelphia, PA 19106–3399, USA

55 Horner Avenue
Toronto, Ontario M8Z 4X6, Canada

Harcourt Brace Jovanovich Group
(Australia) Pty Ltd
30–52 Smidmore Street
Marrickville, NSW 2204, Australia

Harcourt Brace (Japan) Inc.
Ichibancho Central Building,
22–1 Ichibancho
Chiyoda-ku, Tokyo 102, Japan

A catalogue record for this book is available from the
British Library

ISBN 0–7020–1584–9

This book is printed on acid-free paper

Typeset by Fakenham Photosetting Ltd, Fakenham,
Norfolk
Printed and bound in Great Britain by
The Bath Press, Avon

Contents

Contributors

Victor Cassar-Pullicino LRCP, MRCS, DMRD, MD, FRCP, Consultant Radiologist, Robert Jones & Agnes Hunt Orthopaedic Hospital, Oswestry, Shropshire SY10 7AG.

Fay Crawford D POD M, MChS, Teacher, London Foot Hospital, School of Podiatric Medicine, London W1P 6AY.

Brian Ellis FChS, Senior Lecturer, Department of Podiatry, Queen Margaret College, Clerwood Terrace, Edinburgh EH12 8TS.

Robin Grant MRCP, MD, Consultant Neurologist, Department of Clinical Neurosciences, Western General Hospital, Crewe Road, Edinburgh.

Edwin J. Harris DPM, Clinical Associate Professor of Orthopaedic Surgery, Department of Orthopaedic Surgery, Section of Pediatrics, Loyala University of Chicago, Stritch School of Medicine, Maywood, Illinois 60153, USA.

Sean P.F. Hughes MS, FRCS, Professor of Orthopaedic Surgery, Department of Orthopaedic Surgery, Royal Postgraduate Medical School, Hammersmith Hospital, London.

Alexandra M. John BSC, MSC (Clinical Psychology) Principal Clinical Psychologist, Department of Clinical Psychology, St George's Hospital, Tooting, London SW17 0QT.

Christopher Kelnar MA, MB, BChr, DCH (Edinburgh), MRCP (UK), FRCP (Edinburgh, MD Consultant Paediatric Endocrinologist, Royal Hospital for Sick Children, Sciennes Road, Edinburgh EH9 1LF.

Iain W. McCall MB, ChB, DMRD, FRCR, Consultant Radiologist, Robert Jones & Agnes Hunt Orthopaedic Hospital, Oswestry, Shropshire SY10 7AG.

Thomas M. Novella DPM, Attending Podiatrist, Kessler Institute, South Orange, New Jersey, USA. (Postal address: 124 East 71st Street, New York 10021, USA.)

Maureen O'Donnell FChS, Lecturer, Glasgow School of Podiatric Medicine, Queens College, 1 Park Drive, Glasgow G3 6LP.

Jill Pickard MCSP, certEd, Dip TD, Senior Physiotherapist, Northampton General Hospital, Northampton.

Caroline Pollacchi MSC, Aids Health Promoter, London. (Postal address: 15 Gorham Drive, Downswood, Maidstone, Kent ME15 8UU.)

George Rendall BSC, Teacher, Department of Podiatry, Queen Margaret College, Clerwood Terrace, Edinburgh EH12 8TS. (Postal address: Byfield, High Street, Gifford, East Lothian.)

Madeleine Rooney MD, MRCP, DCH, Consultant Paediatric Rheumatologist, Department of Molecular Rheumatology, Northwick Park Hospital, Watford Road, Harrow, Middlesex HA1 3UJ.

Christopher Steer BSC, MB ChB, DCH, FRCPE, Consultant Paediatrician, Victoria Hospital, Hayfield Road, Kirkcaldy, Fife KY2 5AH.

Heather Stirling BSC (Physio), MD, ChB, MRCP (UK), DCH, Lecturer in the Department of Child Life and Health, Royal Hospital for Sick Children, Sciennes Road, Edinburgh EH9 1LF.

Ian Stother MA, MB, BChir, FRCS (Edinburgh and Glasgow), Consultant Orthopaedic Surgeon, Glasgow Royal Infirmary, Glasgow G4 0SF.

Paul R. Stuart FRCS, Senior Orthopaedic Registrar, Department of Orthopaedics, Middlesborough General Hospital, Middlesborough, Cleveland.

John Thomson MD, FRCP (Edinburgh and Glasgow), DObst, RCOG, Consultant Dermatologist, The Royal Infirmary, Glasgow G4 0SF.

Peter Thomson D POD M, MChS, Podiatrist, Community Care Unit, Fife Health Board, Carnegie Clinic, Pilmuir Street, Dunfermline, Fife KY12 0QF.

Jennifer Tomes MA, MSC, ASPBS, Clinical Psychologist, Stratheden Hospital, Cupar, Fife KY15 5RR.

Ronald L. Valmassy DPM, Podiatrist, St Francis Memorial Hospital, 900 Hyde Street, San Francisco, California 94109, USA.

James Woodburn BSC, Senior Teacher, Huddersfield School of Podiatry, Department of Podiatry, University of Huddersfield, Queensgate, Huddersfield HD1 3DH.

Kit Woods MCSP, SRP, Physiotherapist to the Dance School of Scotland, Glasgow. In private practice. (Postal address: 11 Kingsford Court, Newtonmairns, Glasgow G77 6TS.)

Foreword

Approximately three and a half million years ago mankind descended from an arboreal habitat and hands that formerly grasped a branch confronted the formidable challenge of terrestrial weightbearing in an upright bipedal position. The modifications and structural engineering of the human foot associated with the changes in bodily structure necessary to accomplish this miraculous event can best be understood as one observes the evolutionary inheritance of the embryo, fetus and infant to prepare it for standing and walking in our present day environment.

In the study of Podopaediatrics one observes the progression and development of phylogenetic and ontogenetic changes that mirror the ancestral unfolding of the extremities from an aqueous environment to a terrestrial quadruped to an arboreal habitat and back to a terrestrial bipedal environment.

It is one of the major purposes of Podopaediatrics to explain the necessary modification and structural anatomical rearrangements of osseous and soft tissue that are intimately related to general bodily function for weight-bearing and locomotion and to be in position to recognise normal and abnormal situations. These studies coupled with a present day knowledge of medicine and physiology are essential to practising podiatrists who assume responsibility for lower extremity disorders in children.

The proper care of foot problems in infants and children runs the gamut of medicine since the health of the foot is closely associated with the general health of the child and nothing can substitute for a thoroughly well informed and knowledgeable professional.

Peter Thomson's *Introduction to Podopaediatrics* indicates that he is fully aware of the needs of the podiatrist specialising in this area. His text combines all of the elements of medicine necessary for a complete Podopaediatric practice.

This edition touches upon every aspect of juvenile footcare and should find a welcome place on every podiatric and medical practitioner's bookshelf.

Herman Tax

Preface

Although there are many excellent textbooks on paediatric dermatology, rheumatology, orthopaedics and other subjects covered in this book, *Introduction to Podopaediatrics* was compiled in order to try to satisfy the need for a comprehensive textbook which would provide the reader with not only a foundation for the medical topics discussed but also a much broader perspective to the general management of the young patient with a foot problem. This book should be seen as a text on paediatrics in its broadest sense and not one on orthopaedics/biomechanics per se.

Treatment of the child patient is often a matter of teamwork and this textbook aims to provide the podiatrist with a place in that team. Whilst most of the conditions mentioned have major clinical significance to podiatric care, certain conditions have been included where podiatric management is minimal There will also be found some conditions or some aspect of paediatrics where all that is required of the clinician is to be able to recognise, to acknowledge and thus to appreciate the implications for his management programme.

Therefore *Introduction to Podopaediatrics* should provide the clinician with access to information concerning the more common foot pathologies and also some background information to many of the primary medical conditions from which the child may be suffering. Thus not only should this book be a good base from which the student can approach the subject of podopaediatrics, it should also have sufficient depth in order to satisfy the needs of the experienced practitioner who now requires a work of reference.

Although orientated towards the podiatry/chiropody profession, because of the varied backgrounds of the many contributors, anyone dealing with lower limb problems in children ought to be able to find some aspect of this textbook useful. Whoever the reader may be, he or she will begin to appreciate the influence of other disciplines not only on the life of the patient but also on that patient's family. This appreciation should lead to the development of a greater and more knowledgeable dialogue between all relevant professions who have an input into the treatment and management of children (very often the same child). In this way we can all claim a degree of responsibility for improving the quality of life for those young people in our charge. It is hoped that this book provides the means for this to happen.

It is appreciated that the majority of topics referred to in the chapter headings merit complete texts and therefore in a textbook such as this only the essential core of a subject can be addressed. The reference and further reading sections will guide the user to more detailed works where appropriate.

Most chapters follow a standard and predictable course, mainly jointly written by: (i) a medical practitioner, who provides the reader with the scientific foundations to the subject, and (ii) a podiatrist, who provides the clinical aspect.

The remaining chapters are written either by medical practitioners or by podiatrists/physiotherapists alone.

Chapter 13 illustrates the effects of athletic activity on young bodies. This is not to say that, for example, ballet is considered detrimental to children but rather that it is a very popular pastime and one which ultimately leads the participant to pushing his/her body to its anatomical limits. The effects that this may have on the lower limb and the conditions which may then present will be true of any sport that is taken seriously by the child and which involves jumping and landing, twisting and turning.

Chapter 14 leaves the clinical arena and is a brief introduction to the social sciences in the guise of health education. This chapter indicates the problems which may be encountered when positive foot health to this particular patient group is promoted.

Acknowledgements

The success of any multi-author text relies entirely on the team spirit that exists from those who are contributing to the project. I have been extremely fortunate to have secured the services of many eminent people from a diversity of backgrounds, all willing to give up of their precious time in order to disseminate their knowledge to others. Therefore my first heartfelt thanks go to them.

However, there are two key players without whose help pen would never have touched paper. The first is Isobel Adams FChS who has generously shared with me her time and her extensive knowledge. The second is my wife whose encouragement and support inspired me to see the project through.

I would also like to thank Fife Health Board and in particular Dr Harry, Clinical Services Co-ordinator, and Mr J.B. Ivers MChS, retired Area Chief Chiropodist, for their help in the early days. Thanks also to the Pharmacy Department at Milesmark Hospital; to Isobel Walkingshaw, Area Health Education Officer and her team, in particular George Howie; and to the staff at the Dunfermline Maternity Hospital, especially Sister Beatrice Eskdale.

Special thanks to Sarah Carr for her impressive work in correcting and finalising the manuscripts and to Margaret Brown for undertaking to attend to most of my day-to-day paperwork. I would also like to thank the publishers, Baillière Tindall, and in particular Dr Steven Handley for his guidance and for his patience.

Mrs Alexandra John would like to thank Roger Bradford for his support and comments in preparing her contribution to Chapter 2.

Dr Edwin Harris (Chapter 9) would like to record his grateful thanks to Mr Patrick Carrico for his illustrations and to Linda Vlach for the typing and the preparation of his manuscript.

1 Embryology and the Neonate

Peter Thomson

This chapter will consider basic embryology and how nature achieves what is generally accepted as normal. It will also consider those factors, both environmental and genetic, which can influence the developmental process.

Embryo and Fetus

Human life begins with the fusion of the nuclei of the male sperm cell with that of the female ovum. These nuclei contain all the genetic material (stored on chromosomes) necessary for the creation of a new individual.

Spermatogenesis

Spermatozoa are produced in the seminiferous tubules of the testes. The germ cells or spermatogonia divide by mitosis to produce larger daughter cells with large nuclei. These daughter cells are called primary spermatocytes and since they are the product of mitotic division they contain the full complement or diploid number of chromosomes, i.e. 46.

If mitosis were the only method of cell division then the eventual fusion of the sperm and ovum would involve 92 chromosomes and not the 46, i.e. 23 pairs, necessary for human life. Therefore future cell division is by meiosis, a process of division which halves the chromosome number from the diploid 46 to the haploid 23.

Meiosis occurs at the primary spermatocyte stage and is a two phase process. The first stage is the reduction stage which reduces the chromosome number in half. The product of this division is the secondary spermatocyte. The second phase of meiosis is more like that of mitosis with each secondary spermatocyte

giving rise to two spermatids each containing the haploid number of chromosomes in their nuclei. These spermatids further differentiate into spermatozoa (Fig. 1.1).

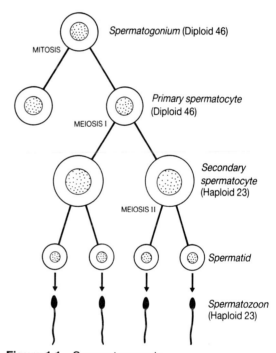

Figure 1.1 Spermatogenesis.

Although the production of spermatozoa takes place in the seminiferous tubules the sperms mature and are stored in the epididymis.

The mature sperm consists of three main parts:

1. The head: which comprises a condensed mass of nuclear material. The head is

almost completely covered by an enzyme cap, the *acrosome*, which aids in the penetration of the ovum.

2. The middle piece: consisting of a coil of mitochondria. Mitochondria supply adenosine triphosphate (ATP) in order to provide energy for the tail.

3. The tail: which by its wave-like movements drives the spermatozoon forward.

In a single ejaculation more than 300 million sperm are released yet only one will successfully fertilise the ovum.

Oogenesis

Within the ovary the oocyte is contained in a single layer of granulosa cells and together this is termed the primary follicle. Every month during her childbearing years a female will undergo ovulation whereby one of these follicles matures and will be expelled from the ovary and will travel to the uterus.

Maturation of the follicle begins in response to follicle stimulating hormone which causes the follicle to enlarge and the granulosa cells to proliferate. As this process continues a mucopolysaccharide is produced which separates the developing egg from its granulosa cells. This new outer layer is called the zona pellucida. As the follicle nears maturation a fluid filled cavity is seen to develop from within the follicle (the antrum). At this stage the follicle is known as the Graafian follicle and at ovulation the secondary oocyte (as the first stage of meiosis has by now taken place) is expelled from the ruptured Graafian follicle and the ovary into the peritoneal cavity close to the entry to the uterine tube.

As it matures the oocyte undergoes cell division similar to that of the spermatozoon and like that of the spermatozoon halves its diploid chromosome number from 46 to the haploid 23 (Fig. 1.2).

Phase II of meiosis only takes place after fertilisation. However, at each stage of meiosis one of the daughter cells can be seen to markedly differ in size to its partner. The smaller cell (polar body) eventually degenerates leaving only one cell to proceed to become a mature ovum. This should be compared to the process of spermatogenesis where for every

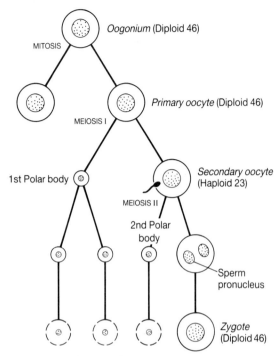

Figure 1.2   Oogenesis.

one mature ovum four mature spermatozoa are produced.

After the expulsion of the oocyte the lining of the Graafian follicle proliferates to produce the corpus luteum. The corpus luteum is responsible for producing oestrogen and a certain amount of progesterone for a further 10–12 days following ovulation. When fertilisation does not occur during this period the corpus luteum degenerates and menstruation occurs soon after. However, when fertilisation does take place the corpus luteum continues to produce its hormones, which are necessary for the maintenance and continuation of pregnancy, for another 12 weeks until the developing placenta is capable of taking over this task.

Fertilisation

This takes place in the upper fallopian tube. When a spermatozoon meets an egg the acrosome aids in penetration by producing enzymes which allow its entry through the zona pellucida. As it penetrates the outer cell wall of the ovum it is thought that other chemicals are released by the successful spermatozoon which change the biochemistry of the outer wall thereby preventing penetration by any other sperm.

On entry, the spermatozoon leaves its tail behind and the head greatly enlarges in size to become known as a pronucleus. A similar change takes place in the nucleus of the ovum. These two pronuclei, containing 23 unpaired chromosomes each, combine giving a fertilised ovum of 46 paired chromosomes in the one nucleus. Within a few hours these chromosomes duplicate and begin the first of many cell divisions termed cleavages.

During this period the zygote travels along the uterine tube towards the uterus and on to implantation by which time the mass of cells is called a morula (Latin, mulberry). Within this cluster of cells a fluid filled cavity is produced and the morula develops into a blastocyte which comprises an outer trophoblast layer of cells and an inner embryonic cell mass.

It is the trophoblast layer that produces enzymes which dissolve the lining of the uterus and so allow implantation to take place. The embryonic cell mass differentiates into:

1. Ectoderm which gives rise to the epidermis and nervous tissue.
2. Mesoderm from which originates skeletal, muscular, connective and blood tissue.
3. Endoderm which forms the lining of the digestive and respiratory tracts.

Lower limb development

In the human embryo, limb buds protrude at about the end of the fourth and beginning of the fifth week. The lower limb buds appear just distal to the base of the umbilical cord, at the level of the lumbar and upper sacral segments (L2–S3).

At six weeks the bud starts to divide into two distinct sections due to the formation of a ringlike constriction around the limb. The bud at this stage is classically described as 'paddle-shaped', as the proximal end remains cylindrical while distally it flattens out to form a foot plate, and it is at this distal end that the next visible change takes place with the appearance of five rays (Fig. 1.3). As the toes are forming,

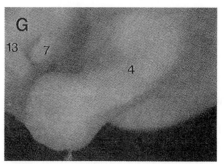

Figure 1.3 Fetus, days 38–40. Reproduced from England, *A Colour Atlas of Life before Birth*, with permission of Wolfe Publishing.

a second crease begins to divide the limb into two, giving the now recognisable main segments of the lower limb. This differentiation is similar to that which takes place in the upper limb. However, these changes lag behind those of the upper limb by a few days. As these changes are taking place, the mesenchyme in the limb bud has been condensing to form the hyaline cartilage templates on which bone will be laid down. The first of these templates is present by the sixth week.

By the 12th week small, well defined areas of ectoderm may be seen to form on the dorsum of the distal phalanges. These are rudimentary toe nails and initially such areas are seen only at the apices of the toes. The actual nails will not reach the free edge until week 36 and as yet, their keratinisation has not taken place.

On the skin, epidermal ridges will have formed on the soles of the feet by the 17th week. Unusual ridge patterns can be seen in some genetic anomalies such as Down's syndrome (syn. trisomy 21, mongolism).

Lower limb musculature

Muscles can be seen to be forming in the embryo around the seventh week, again as condensations of the fetal connective tissue, located near to the base of the bud.

Lower limb innervation

As the limb buds are forming, the spinal nerves simultaneously begin to penetrate the mesenchyme. As soon as the nerves have entered the bud they establish contact with the condensations and it is thought that this early contact between the nerves and the newly forming muscle cells is essential for their complete differentiation.

Bone formation

Ossification of the bones of the limbs usually begins at the end of the embryonic period (eight weeks gestation). The primary centre of ossification for the tibia appears on the seventh week.

Primary centres are present in all long bones by week 12 and it is from these centres in the diaphysis of the bone that the ossification process gradually inches towards the ends of the cartilage templates. At birth the whole of the shaft, except for the two epiphyses, is ossified. Secondary centres will eventually appear in these epiphyseal areas causing ossification to begin here as well. However, a plate of cartilage remains and this separates the diaphysis from the epiphysis – the epiphyseal plate. This gap will not close until maturity is reached and it is therefore important in the growth in length of bones. An epiphyseal plate is to be found at each end in the long bones whereas in the metatarsals it is found at one end only. In irregularly shaped bones such as the calcaneus, one or more primary centres of ossification may be found, as well as several secondary centres. At birth, primary ossification centres are seen in most of the bones of the foot with the exception of the three cuneiforms, the navicular and the distal and intermediate phalanges of the fifth toe.

Teratogenic effects of drugs

Women are well cautioned about the consumption of drugs during their pregnancies and certain existing drug regimens may have to be modified during this period. Especially in the first trimester, when cells are rapidly dividing, any drug has the potential to cause fetal abnormality since this is the time when organs and other structures are actively forming, and thus severe handicap is possible.

The following substances are examples of well known drugs and the effects that these may have on the developing child.

Cytotoxic drugs[1,2] (e.g. methotrexate, chlorambucil, cyclophosphamide)

In general this group of drugs cause growth retardation and malformation because of their metabolic effect. In particular, absence of digits on the feet has been reported. Methotrexate is a folic acid antagonist and has been shown to cause defects of the nervous system.

Thalidomide[3–5] (an antinausean and sleeping pill)

Thalidomide is possibly the best known teratogenic. In West Germany in the early 1960s it was noted that the incidence of amelia and phocomelia, which are rare hereditary occurrences, had suddenly increased. It was discovered that many mothers of children born with such handicaps had taken the drug thalidomide in the early part of their pregnancies. There are well documented incidences of amelia, phocomelia, apodia and adactylia as a result of this drug being ingested during pregnancy.

Anticonvulsants[6] (e.g. phenytoin, phenobarbitone)

These more traditional anticonvulsants have been shown to cause conditions such as talipes, polydactyly, metatarsus varus, hypoplasia of the distal phalanges and mental disorders. Phenytoin may exert its effects by its action on nucleic acid or folic acid metabolism or on collagen synthesis. None of these conditions mentioned have been recorded to date with the use of carbamazepine or sodium valproate, although some sources claim that this latter drug used alone or in conjunction with carbamazepine has shown an association with an increased incidence of spina bifida.

Drugs used in dermatology (e.g. etretinate, isotretinoin)

These are drugs used in the treatment of psoriasis and acne vulgaris respectively, and are becoming well known as teratogens. Etretinate has been shown to cause, on occasion, particular bony changes including epiphyseal closure, skeletal hyperostosis and extraosseous calcification.

Sulphonylureas[7,8]

First generation sulphonureas, e.g. chlorpropamide and tolbutamide which may be used in the treatment of diabetes mellitus, have caused sporadic reports of talipes and general foot abnormalities and may also cause damage to developing brain tissue.

Antibiotics[9]

Co-trimoxazole is a folic acid antagonist. Folic acid is necessary for DNA synthesis.

Miscellaneous

Povidone iodine. Sufficient iodine may be absorbed which will affect the fetal thyroid.

Podophyllum resin. Application is avoided on very large areas or in the treatment of anogenital warts as neonatal death and teratogenesis have been reported.

Griseofulvin. Fetotoxicity and teratogenicity have been found in animal studies.

Other drugs that have caused the occasional report of congenital malformation of the lower limb are: chlorpromazine (antipsychotic), phenylephrine (in hypotension) and disulfiram (used in the treatment of alcoholism). High dosages of vitamins A and D would fall into this category as well. Drugs which increase a baby's jaundice, especially when the baby is premature, may damage the brain. Examples of such drugs are promethazine, promazine hydrochloride and large doses of vitamin K.

In the 1950s several cases of cerebral palsy were notified along the shores of Minimata Bay in Kumamoto, Japan. These were traced to the eating of fish contaminated with alkyl mercury compounds which had been discharged from a factory into the sea.[10]

Smoking

Maternal smoking is a well established cause of retarded fetal growth.[11] In a heavy smoker (over 20 cigarettes a day) premature delivery is twice as frequent compared with mothers who do not smoke and also their infants weigh less than normal. These women also run the risk of a higher than normal incidence of stillbirth. Nicotine causes a decrease in uterine blood flow thereby lowering the supply of oxygen. The resultant deficit impairs cell growth and may also have an adverse effect on mental development.

Alcohol

Chronic alcoholism affects 1–2% of women of childbearing age. Excessive alcohol consumption will cause growth problems not only prenatally but postnatally as well. There is also an increased incidence of congenital dislocation of the hip and of mental defect in these children. Even moderate maternal alcohol consumption, e.g. 2–3 oz per day, may produce some symptoms of fetal alcohol syndrome. It is thought that the teratogenic agent is the acetaldehyde derived from the alcohol breakdown.[12–14]

Caffeine

There is no real evidence that caffeine per se is a teratogen in humans, but there is no positive assurance that excessive consumption is safe for the embryo either. A paper by Beaulac-Baillargeon in Canada suggests that there may be a relationship between cigarette smoking coupled with caffeine consumption and a reduction in placental circulation.[15]

Infectious agents causing malformation

Rubella

This may cause malformation of the eye, the internal ear and the heart, as well as poor fetal growth.

Cytomegalovirus

This virus causes mild disease in the adult. In early pregnancy this infection may bring about abortion or growth failure, microcephaly, mental retardation or epilepsy. It is considered that cytomegalovirus may figure significantly as a factor in mental handicap.

Toxoplasmosis

This is a protozoan parasite (*Toxoplasma gondii*), which has been shown to damage developing brain tissue.

Herpes (Type II – genital)

Infection may occur during delivery and the child has no natural immunity conferred on him from the mother. This infection may affect the eye, the central nervous system and the liver.

Syphilis

This is a spirochaete infection (*Treponema pallidum*), which is now rare in the UK as all pregnant women are screened and given serological tests (VDRL – Venereal Disease Research Laboratory) at their first antenatal visit. Signs of congenital syphilis include infections of the skin and of the nasal bones, eczema, hepatosplenomegaly and failure to thrive.

An estimation as to when a particular abnormality arose may be made by being familiar with the main stages of the embryonic period. For example:

Amelia: the incident must have affected the limb buds at or before the fifth week of gestation.

Absence of nails: this aberration would have taken place before the 12th week.

As the embryonic stage is the period when all bodily structures and systems are being developed (the period of organogenesis), so the fetal period (nine weeks gestation until birth) sees the maturation of these tissues and a rapid growth of the body. Since most cell differentiation has already taken place, few if any malformations can happen during this time. However, the child is not free from deformation nor from the effects of physical injury.

Intrauterine moulding

There is a direct relationship between load and the effect of that load on the rate of growth. During periods of rapid bone growth any abnormal or excessive load applied to that bone may result in its permanent deformation. Early fetal growth is very rapid. Dunn[16] described how a five year old required six years to double its weight whereas an embryo of only eight weeks gestation required just six days to do the same. Therefore the embryo is 365 times more vulnerable than the five year old child. In early fetal life the child is protected by amniotic fluid. The liquor amnii volume increases throughout the normal pregnancy from approximately 0.25 litres at 16 weeks to nearly 1 litre at 34 weeks. By the time the normal 40 week gestation period is completed this amount has decreased again by approximately 20%. When the pregnancy continues past term, this amount may be as little as 0.5 litres by 42 weeks. As the child grows and the amount of amniotic fluid decreases there is less fluid present to cushion the child, but because of a slowing growth rate the fetal skeleton is relatively less plastic. Some women may suffer from oligohydramnios, which results in a lack of amniotic fluid during their pregnancy. This also has the effect of reducing the cushioning benefit on the fetus.

The newborn

When it is time to leave the relatively safe aquatic world of the past nine months, the infant's entry into a bright, air-breathing environment can be quite traumatic. During the short journey down the birth canal the child is extremely vulnerable to injury. However, with the modern obstetric care available in this country this potential for damage is greatly minimised. Infant mortality in Britain, measured as deaths of infants under one year of age, per thousand births, has fallen steadily from 142 in the years 1900–02 to only 8.4 (provisional) in the year 1989.[17]

However, much may affect the child at this stage; e.g. when the child presents in the breech position then the necessary manipulation required for delivery may affect the hips, the spine or the arms. Dislocation of the hips is not uncommon in these babies, nor are palsies of the arms and legs. Erb's palsy is one of traumatic origin, and whilst its effects are normally transient, residual paresis may occur.

Damage to the face and head from a normal

vertex presentation is to be expected, despite the ability of the main bones of the skull to over-ride one another. Any resulting distortion usually subsides spontaneously within a short period of time. Two common deformations frequently seen arise from either (a) oedema, giving a *caput succedaneum*, which usually disappears within a few hours, or (b) haematoma, which is the result of haemorrhage between the skull bone and its periosteum, i.e. a *cephalhaematoma*, and this may not be noticed until the caput subsides.

The cephalhaematoma may take several weeks to subside and because of the subsequent breakdown of the blood cells involved, neonatal jaundice occurs. Neither condition results in any long-lasting effects.

Intracranial haemorrhage

Any type of injury that affects motor control is of interest to the podiatrist. The earlier the podiatrist can become involved as part of a team the better prospect there is for good foot function, within the limits of the condition. Intracranial haemorrhage is naturally of importance. Basically this may be divided into two main types.

1. *Intraventricular haemorrhage*: this is often found in premature babies. The haemorrhage is frequently minimal but it may be sufficient to result in cerebral palsy.
2. *Compression head injury*: this commonly results in a subarachnoid haemorrhage, caused either by a prolonged, difficult labour and/or by the baby being very large for its gestational age.

Frequently babies damaged in this way appear quite normal for some time but then they may become hypotonic and their reflex actions diminish. Muscle tone is a very good indicator of brain damaged infants as the legs can be seen to be held in marked extension. Gradually such children become very irritable, do not like to be handled and may fit.

Asphyxia

Another type of injury that may affect motor control is one due to asphyxia. During delivery the child is given many incentives to encourage breathing. The infant leaves an environment of a steady 37 °C to one of only 20–30 °C. Thus as the head presents itself to the outside world, the child experiences a cooling effect which stimulates the medulla in the brain. As the infant is being forced through the birth canal the thorax is compressed. This forces fluid out of the lungs; the arms are released and a recoil action takes place in the chest and air is sucked in. Any remaining fluid in the lungs is drained away by the pulmonary lymphatics.

The umbilical cord is then clamped, which has the effect of increasing blood pressure, and simultaneously decreasing arterial oxygen whilst increasing arterial carbon dioxide. However, there are instances when all of these stimuli may not produce a response as asphyxia may already have taken place in utero from compression of the cord or from the placenta peeling away prematurely.

Effects of asphyxia

Asphyxia will cause damage to brain cells and interfere with brain function through compromising the patency of the blood vessels and from oedema. This is true of the other organs as well and the kidneys and heart, in particular, are very susceptible to this type of injury.

Apgar scoring (Table 1.1)

The newborn baby is assessed initially one minute after delivery using a scoring system devised in the 1950s by Dr Virginia Apgar.[18] This system makes an appraisal of the need for resuscitation in the infant, depending upon its appearance and responses.

Table 1.1 Apgar scoring.

Points	2	1	0
Colour	Completely pink	Pink with blue extremities	Blue or white
Heart rate	Over 100/min	Below 100/min	Absent
Respiration	Crying lustily	Shallow and irregular	Absent
Muscle	Active movement	Some flexion of extremities	Flaccid
Reflex irritability	Cough	Grimace	Nil

A score of 0–3 = vigorous resuscitation procedures must be undertaken.

A score of 4–6 = indicates help is required.

A score of 7–10 = no intervention necessary.

This test is repeated five minutes after the child is born.

It is to be expected that the child who scores low on this scale at the second reading is in danger of some degree of handicap. There is also a relationship between babies who are premature or those with light birth weights and low Apgar scores and infant mortality.

Health education programmes directed towards showing pregnant women how they can best minimise the chances of fetal retardation or prematurity are therefore to be encouraged. Prematurity is often unavoidable as in gestational diabetes mellitus, and in multiple births. At least half of multiple birth babies weigh less than 2500 g (individual babies generally weigh less the more there are of them) compared to approximately 6% of singletons. In a study of twin pregnancies in Scotland it was shown that delivery occurred before the 37th week in 44% of the group involved compared with only 5.5% of single births.[19]

As well as the Apgar test the child is given an overall assessment, the main points of which are outlined below.

Cry. Is it normal, shrill, murmuring or high-pitched? A high-pitched cry is the sign of an irritable child and may indicate brain damage.

Muscle tone. Is it hypertonic or hypotonic?

Head and face. Is there any congenital cataract? Do the eyes show signs of jaundice? The tips of the ears should be level with the eye and the bases with the top lip. Low set ears may have an association with renal problems and with certain chromosomal abnormalities, e.g. Down's syndrome.

Neck and spine. The neck is checked for the presence of goitres and the spine for any obvious gaps or for evidence of spina bifida. Maternal thyroid stimulating hormone or thyroid replacement drugs pass over the placenta and will affect the fetus.

Arms and hands. The shape of the hands is important. Children suffering from Down's syndrome present with short stubby hands with fingers practically all of similar size and with the fifth finger curving inwards (clinodactyly). The hand of such children also has one main transverse crease. The position of the fingers is also an important indicator of genetic abnormality.

Hips. The hips are inspected for instability. A dislocation must be splinted and then followed up by orthopaedic management. The so-called 'clicking hip' is frequently treated by the wearing of a double thickness nappy to keep the hips in abduction. By the time the child has his final examination before leaving hospital such instabilities are no longer present.

Legs. Obvious fractures are sought and a normal length and position looked for. Breech babies tend to keep their legs up and still for a few days.

Feet. The feet are inspected for the required number of toes and for normal skin creases. Down's syndrome babies have an exaggerated space between the first and second toes and a marked creasing of the skin between the first and second metatarsals.

Edward's syndrome is associated with a rockerbottom foot. Talipes is looked for, the most common type being talipes equinovarus (TEV). When suspected it must be decided whether the condition is a true TEV, which may require surgical intervention, or whether it is simply a positional condition, which may only need manipulation. When a positional TEV presents it is possible to over-correct the foot physically by pushing up on the plantar surface.

Positional problems

Parents bring children to clinics for a wide range of positional problems, some trivial, some not so. Occasionally reassurance is all that is required, but at times it will be quite obvious that whatever the management it will have to be planned in the long term.

Included in the factors to be considered with positional problems is whether or not this is the first born, and the first born to a young

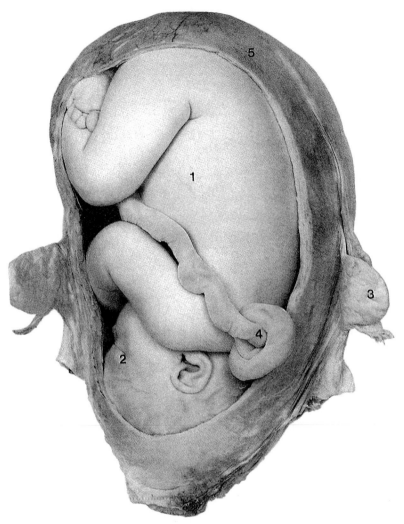

Figure 1.4 Fetus, week 28. Reproduced from England, *A Colour Atlas of Life before Birth*, with permission of Wolfe Publishing.

mother. Unstretched abdominal muscles will keep the uterus up and the fetus tight up against the mother's spine. As a result of the laying down of subcutaneous fat over the last two months the baby will have taken on a well rounded shape. This means that in a pregnancy that is going to term the child will fill its container much better and more fully than at any time before (Fig. 1.4). The size of that container will, to some extent, be determined by the size of the woman to whom it belongs. Therefore on examination an eye ought to be cast over the mother's stature for pointers to the possible aetiology of the presenting condition.

One of the most common conditions for which parents consult is undoubtedly the one concerning the child and his/her 'funny walk'. In clinical practice, many cases that present as gait problems are found to be singularly left sided, or it is found that the left side is worse than the right side. There is almost a ratio of 2 : 1 in favour of the left side.[16,20] This left-sided propensity may be due to the fact that most babies present with their backs to the mother's left side and therefore the child's left leg is abducted and overlies his right leg. It has also been postulated that when the leg is tightly abducted in this position it can result in an instability in the hip itself and this may be a

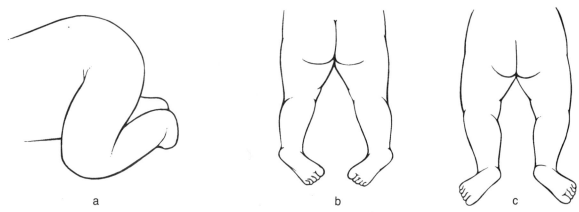

Figure 1.5   Typical sleeping positions giving rise to gait problems. a. Knee–chest position. b, Hips extended, internal rotation, ankle equinus. c, Hips extended and in external rotation and abduction of feet.

predisposing factor in congenital dislocation of the hip, where there is also a left sided bias.[16]

It does seem possible that many lower limb problems, perhaps not presenting themselves until the child begins to walk, may well have had their origins in fetal life and have gone undetected until now.

Extrinsic postnatal influences

It has been reported that the price to be paid for a larger and more mature infant at birth is a 2% incidence of congenital postural problems.[16] Intrauterine moulding lends itself naturally enough to characteristic sleeping positions which are adopted in infancy and which in turn can also help influence future gait patterns from delaying or accentuating normal developmental processes (Fig. 1.5a, b, c). Some babies when placed prone will automatically tuck their knees up to their chests and cross their feet over one another, in a manner very similar to their early fetal position (Fig. 1.5a). This encourages medial torsion on the tibia, puts the ankle into equinus and causes adduction at the forefoot. This will predispose to a pigeon-toed gait. Likewise when prone but with the hips in extension and the feet internally rotated, similar problems arise but probably with a leaning towards equinus at the ankle and this may contribute to persistent toe-walking later (Fig. 1.5b). An abducted gait can be encouraged when lying prone, with the hips in extension but the feet externally rotated, as this puts the hips into external

rotation with lateral torsions on the tibiae and a valgus position for the feet (Fig. 1.5c).

One of the major influences responsible for gait problems in otherwise healthy children is a persistent antetorsion on the femur or equally an increased anteversion where the forward drift of the leg has gone beyond the mature 12 degrees as the result of soft tissue contractions.

A common cause of persistent antetorsion is when the child repeatedly chooses to sit in the reversed tailor position (Fig. 1.6). This sitting habit is also linked to the child who has a generalised ligamentous laxity and is common in females. One hypothesis concerning the incidence of a temporary ligamentous laxity in children stems from the polypeptide hormone 'Relaxin' which is produced by the corpus luteum. This hormone is necessary for 'relaxing' normally taut ligamentous structures, e.g. around the sacro-iliac joint. When the mother is producing this hormone, which aids with the eventual birth, some may be passed on to the fetus where its effects persist. This may explain the female preponderance of hip instability in the neonate. On the other hand a permanent laxity appears to be genetically determined[16] (Fig. 1.7).

In the 1950s Sommerville described how the normally taut hip capsule ligaments mould away antetorsion. When the hip is extended the anterior capsule tightens, causing a torsional strain on the femoral neck, an area which grows rapidly and which is therefore malleable. It follows then that where there is a laxity in these ligaments the necessary forces

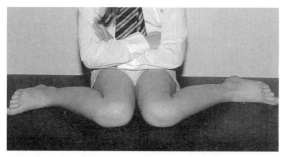

(a)

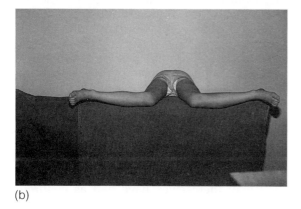

(b)

Figure 1.6   a, Reversed tailor position. b, Same child as in a, demonstrating 90 degrees internal rotation at hips.

will not be present to act on the femur at that part. In cases of persistent antetorsion there is almost always a joint laxity as well.[21]

With persistent antetorsion the child will be unable to exhibit much external rotation at the hip, the patellae will face inwards and he/she will intoe. The gait will be clumsy and the child will trip.[22] It may sometimes also be noted that they have complained of pain in their buttocks or hips. This pain is considered to be due to overuse of the external rotators of the hip in an effort to try to achieve a normal gait pattern. These young people can exhibit almost 90 degrees of internal rotation (Fig. 1.6b) at the hip with little or no external rotation. Since the child is unable to achieve the rotations at the hip he/she will try to obtain them at the level of the tibia. This rotation is also aided by sitting in the reversed tailor position, which forces the feet outwards and thus increases the external rotations on the tibiae. Some studies show that there will not be any significant change in the

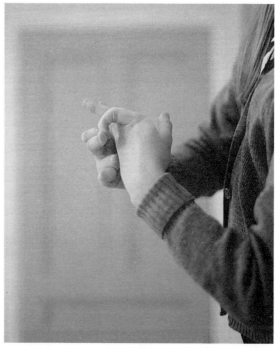

(a)

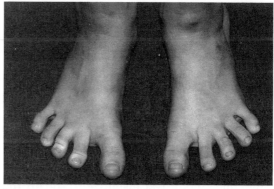

(b)

Figure 1.7   a, Gross generalised ligamentous laxity in an eight year old female. b, Feet of same child as in a – hypermobile unstable feet.

antetorsion beyond eight years of age. That is to say when a child aged eight has persistent antetorsion on the femur, further growth will not change this condition by any meaningful amount.[22, 23] There is a school of thought that suggests that correction may still occur up to the age of 12 and that all that has happened up to this point is that development has been delayed.[24]

In an attempt to have a near normal gait pattern the child will encourage any compensatory mechanism available to him, but such is the power of compensation that on walking there will now be lateral wear on the heel of the shoe, and the foot, just past midstance, will roll off rather than toe off. This action causes much subtalar pronation which in turn unlocks the bones in the forefoot causing it to become hypermobile and unstable.[25]

With this particular type of gait problem the pronatory effects should be cancelled out by placing the foot in a position where it can be made to operate at its most efficient when weightbearing. This should be the main objective when considering any treatment strategy.

Some children adopt a similar sitting position to the reversed tailor, and sit with the feet turned inwards. This results in internal rotations on the tibiae and an adducted and varus foot. In this position the talus is unable to rotate down and similarly the body of the calcaneus.

Knock knee

Excessive external tibial rotations may either bring about or exacerbate knock knee. With abnormal heel strike asymmetrical forces are produced at the epiphyses. There is an inverse relationship between the pressure across an epiphyseal plate and its rate of growth. This is the principle behind the procedure of stapling across an epiphysis in the treatment of gross genu valgum.

Along with stretching of structures on the medial side of the leg there will be a reciprocal slackening of structures on the lateral aspect. The child's body will eventually take up the slack and therefore the ilio-tibial tract will shorten and help to maintain the deformity (Davis' law). These secondary compensatory mechanisms can lead to an increased Q-angle. This is the angle occurring between the anterior superior iliac spine and the ipsilateral patella, and a perpendicular line drawn up from that same patella. The greater this angle, the more the patella will be predisposed to lateral tracking and to potential chondromalacia.

With any degree of knock knee the line of body weight is going to shift and to be medial to the foot instead of bisecting through the second toe, thus contributing to greater pronation. When deformity is sufficiently severe, pronation will also be encouraged from pull from the lateral hamstrings and this will cause more external rotation on the tibia.

This chapter has reviewed the delicate beginnings of human life and has tried to put them into the context of problems for which parents may seek advice and help. Such problems may have arisen from failures in early cell life, from environmental hazards for the yet unborn child, or from extrauterine postural problems as the result of intrauterine moulding.

Therefore on examination of children it is necessary to obtain as comprehensive a background history as possible. It is quite in order to question the parents on the pregnancy itself, the actual birth and the position of that child in the family. It is essential to assess the child's age, height, posture, and the finesse of his/her motor control. It is important that the parents are asked about similar problems that they may themselves have had as children. How effective was any previous treatment for either the child or for the parent as a child? Do they, the parents, have any resultant problems?

The practitioner must be familiar with the natural history of the condition presented to him and also with its natural variations, and must never forget the crucial importance of the growth factor itself.

References

1 Milunski A *et al*. Methotrexate induced congenital malformations. *J Paediatr* 1968; 72: 790–5.
2 Greenberg LH *et al*. Congenital abnormalities probably caused by cyclophosphamide. *JAMA* 1964; 188: 423–6.
3 Taussig H. A study of the German outbreak of phocomelia; The thalidomide syndrome. *JAMA* 1962, 180: 1106–14.
4 Smithwells RW. Defects and disabilities of thalidomide children. *Br Med J* 1973; 1: 269.
5 Deformities Caused by Thalidomide. Report on Public Health and Medical Subjects. No. 112, London, HMSO, 1964. (Survey of deformed children born in England and Wales.)
6 Loughnan PM *et al*. Phenytoin teratogenicity in man. *Lancet* 1973; i: 70–2.

7 Campbell GD. Chlorpropamide and foetal damage. *Br Med J* 163; 1: 59, 60.

8 Soler NG *et al*. Congenital malformations in infants of diabetic mothers. *QJ Med* 1976; 45: 303–13.

9 Warkany J. Teratogenicity of folic acid antagonists. *Cancer Bull* 1981; 33: 76–7.

10 Matsumoto H, Koya G, Takeuchi T. Fetal Minimata disease: A neuropathological study of two cases of intrauterine intoxication by methyl mercury compound. *J Neuropathol Exp Neurol* 1965; 24: 563.

11 Butler NP, Goldstein H, Ross EM. Cigarette smoking in pregnancy: its influence on birthweight and perinatal mortality. *Br Med J* 1972; ii: 127–30.

12 McKnight A *et al*. Alcoholic consumption during pregnancy; a health education problem. *J R Coll Gen Pract* 1987; 37(295): 73–6.

13 Wright JT, Barrison I. Alcohol and the fetus. *Br J Hosp Med* 1983; March: 260–6.

14 Jones KL *et al*. Problems of malformation in offspring of chronic alcoholic women. *Lancet* 1973; 1267–71.

15 Beaulac-Baillargeon L, Desrosiers C. Caffeine/cigarette interaction on fetal growth. *Am J Obstet Gynecol* 1987; November: 1236–1240.

16 Dunn P. Congenital postural deformities: further perinatal associations. *Proc R Soc Med* 1974; 67: 1174–1178.

17 *Annual Abstract of Statistics 1991. Infant and Maternal Mortality*. Central Statistics Officer, HMSO.

18 Apgar V. Proposal for a new method of evaluation of newborn infants. *Anesth Analg* 1953; 32: 260–7.

19 Patel N, Barrie W *et al*. Scottish Twin Survey 1983, Preliminary Report. Social Paediatric Research Unit/University of Glasgow.

20 Tax H. *Podopaediatrics* 2nd ed. Williams and Wilkins, 1985.

21 Sommerville EW. Persistent foetal alignment of the hip. *J Bone Joint Surg* 1957; **39B**(1): 106–113.

22 Kling J, Hensinger R. Angular and torsional deformities of the lower limb in children. *Clin Orthopaed Rel Res* 1983; No. 176, June: 136–147.

23 Fabry G, MacEwan GD, Shands AR. Torsion in the femur: a follow-up study in normal and abnormal conditions. *J Bone Joint Surg* 1973; **55A**(8): 1738–1758. December.

24 Yngve D. Gait problems in children – a matter of rotation. *Post Grad Med* 1984; 76(4): 56–64. 15 September.

25 Root ML, Weed JH, Orien WD. *Normal and Abnormal Function of the Foot*, Vol II. Los Angeles, Clinical Biomechanics Corporation, 1977.

Further Reading

Sadler TW. *Langman's Medical Embryology*, 5th edn. Williams and Wilkins, 1988.

Whitfield JC. *Dewhurst's Textbook of Obstetrics and Gynaecology for Postgraduates*, 4th Ed. Blackwell Scientific Publications, 1985.

Williams and Warwick. *Gray's Anatomy*, 36th Edn. Churchill Livingstone.

2
Psychological Considerations in the Child Patient

Jennifer Tomes and Alexandra M. John

Building relationships

The location of this chapter near the beginning of this textbook reflects the view that specific podiatric interventions, however essential and skilfully applied, may be important in the absence of a positive, collaborative working relationship between the podiatrist and his young patient. There is extensive literature which documents the need to attend to this working partnership prior to and during treatment, if progress both in the clinic and in the longer term is to be achieved.

In order to establish and facilitate this partnership, there are a number of specific psychological techniques available, but more importantly perhaps is the inventive and caring use to which these techniques are put. The podiatrist's experience, understanding, concern and ways of relating to other people all have a bearing on the success or otherwise of a consultation.

Expectations

At a first meeting between any patient and therapist, the patient is likely to maintain a precarious balance between hope of improvement and fear of the process involved or, in the case of children, fear and curiosity. For children fear may predominate as they do not have the experience by which to understand and to measure this new situation. Expectation of help and improvement is a critical emotion at the onset of treatment and, if fostered, can be a crucial element in subsequent behaviour change and compliance. Most expectations are set at the first meeting and it has been shown

that these expectations are related more to the personal qualities of the therapist than to the clinical content of the consultation.[1] Working with children and their parents, therefore, requires an appropriate therapeutic style to facilitate treatment and to ensure satisfaction and compliance with the process on the part of the family.

Therapeutic style

The important elements in an effective therapeutic style are those associated with healing in its widest sense. One element which has been noted by many researchers to predominate is perceived friendliness and, although it is difficult to define this in terms of its component parts, it appears to consist of an active interest in the child, genuineness, respect, acceptance, warmth and empathy with his/her difficulties. This 'personal' approach leads to greater trust and to more consistent application of advice.[2] In specific terms, the developing relationship may be enhanced by sitting reasonably close to the patient, listening carefully while maintaining good eye contact and nodding to indicate interest and understanding. Non-verbal aspects of communication are just as important as what is actually said, and indeed are believed by some to convey more than four times as much information as the verbal message.[3] Taking and reading notes during the meeting can therefore mean that crucial signs are missed. In delivering information, it is important to ensure that the message conveyed by expression, tone of voice, posture and eye contact is congruent with the verbal aspect of the exchange. A dislocation between the two breeds confusion and misunderstanding. Work with children requires a particular emphasis on the non-verbal elements since a young child may understand little of the discussion taking place between the adults and will respond only to the podiatrist's manner and appearance. Notice, too, the patient's non-verbal expression of symptoms which may be more telling than what is actually said.

Sharing information

In the effort to build a relationship, the avoidance of jargon is to be recommended[4] as child, and possibly parent, may fail to understand and they may consequently feel intimidated. Instead, speak simply and directly but avoid the use of patronising language which might reinforce the power imbalance that is inherent in the relationship. Research has shown that patients appreciate being given honest information although they do not always like to ask for it, as they fear that such an enquiry may indicate a lack of trust in the clinician's judgement,[5] and they may wait for him to take the initiative in the consultation. Sharing information pertinent to the presenting problem reduces drop-out from treatment, although care should be taken not to alarm a child with worrying details at too early a stage. Any important messages or advice should be delivered in a specific rather than a general way and they are best understood and remembered when they are presented in a logical sequence in explicit categories. Such messages or advice should be repeated more than once. Ley[6] found that a great deal of information given by clinicians is promptly forgotten after the consultation. To aid recall, patients should be encouraged to repeat instructions, and this repetition should lead to greater satisfaction and compliance with the recommended treatment.[7] Supplying the family with written instructions is to be highly recommended.

Context of treatment

A further point to note in developing a relationship is to consider with child and parent how the advised treatment will affect their daily lives, and an attempt should be made to tailor treatment to that context. By doing this a degree of concern and care for the patient is shown and this is likely to be rewarded with successful outcomes.[8]

Translating these points into practice with children, it is evident that considerable patience, warmth and friendliness are required to establish a good working relationship and to respond appropriately to the child. While it is possible to analyse some of the elements involved in achieving this, much of the success in working with children and their parents depends on instinctive, personal qualities inherent in the podiatrist. The child may be handicapped by his parents' expectations and come burdened with fears and misapprehensions about treatment. These factors will require all the therapist's personal skills to overcome. Alternatively, depending on previous experience in clinical settings, the child may be unconcerned about the treatment or his environment and such a state may be used positively in the therapeutic endeavour.

Problems encountered in consultation

The waiting room

Prior to meeting the family, the tone of the consultation may be set by ensuring that the waiting room is well equipped with toys, books and drawing materials appropriate to children of all ages. These will serve to amuse, interest and distract children from any apprehensions while a start is made to establish a friendly atmosphere. However, this may be difficult to achieve for the peripatetic podiatrist who is reliant on general waiting rooms which are often sparsely furnished.

On first meeting the family in the waiting room, the podiatrist should greet them by name and introduce himself, and this introduction should be addressed to both child and parent. While proceeding to the consulting room, some comments that show an interest in personal aspects of the child's daily life and preoccupations should be made. A simple enquiry about mode of transport to the clinic, or whether children have missed school in order to attend, are possible openings. These questions may also help to judge the state of anxiety of the child and they may reassure him. Korsche and Negrete[4] found that there was a direct relationship between the amount of conversation and the patient's reported satisfaction with the encounter and although this particular study investigated the feelings of adults it may be appropriate when also dealing with children.

Stranger anxiety

Babies up to the age of approximately six months tend to be pleased to engage with strangers, but from six months to approximately three years they may show a specific fear of unknown people and they may cling to their parents for reassurance. Do not attempt to prise the child of this age from his carer. During discussion of the problem with parents, children may gradually make little forays away from 'base' in order to explore the room, particularly when there are interesting toys around. Any subsequent treatment for children of this age should be carried out with the child sitting on a parent's knee. Primary age children will be less affected by stranger anxiety although they may still possibly be somewhat wary, whereas adolescents may participate fully in the consultation. Any uncommunicativeness by adolescents may be due to either moodiness, characteristic of this age, or a desire for privacy about the body. Whatever the age of the children they should be included in the discussion provided that they are able to take an active part. As with adults, children vary in their degree of comfort or discomfort with strangers.

White coats

Unless it is necessary to wear a white coat for the protection of clothing during certain treatments, then do not do so. For both children and parents, who may be somewhat fearful, the white coat can be an intimidating sign of authority and this may have been associated with hospital visits and with painful treatments in the past. It should not be necessary to proclaim status by wearing a white coat; instead try to engage the family's respect by more honest means such as empathy and consideration.

Instruments

The sight of certain podiatric instruments and equipment may well be daunting to those unfamiliar to a clinic. When the child shows an inclination to explore of his own volition then encourage this in so far as it is safe so to do. Some children may be interested to be shown how things work, and this may serve to take the fear and mystique out of the situation, and even the preschool child can be given something to hold and to look at in order to engage his interest and to give him a sense of involvement in the proceedings. A child should never be approached with any fearful-looking instrument without first allowing him to see, to investigate and to understand it.

Surgeries

Where possible, clinics should be held on familiar territory for children, either in school or at health centres. This may not be possible other than for the initial consultation, but it will help to put the child at ease. Wherever the clinic is held, it will help considerably if the room is welcoming: warm, bright and supplied with toys and with technical equipment kept to a minimum.

Physical contact

Touching can have significance in various ways depending upon the context in which it occurs. Little children are familiar with their basic care which involves touching by known adults, and indeed physical contact is one of the most primitive and reassuring forms of comfort. It can make patients feel more relaxed, comforted and supported.[9] Touch may, however, be very threatening. The literature on 'body space' suggests that people develop a boundary around themselves through which no-one may pass without feelings of violation being engendered. There are certain exceptions to this, notably that doctors and other clinicians are exempted from observing the boundaries for the purpose of examination and treatment. It should be borne in mind, however, that children, and especially adolescents, may find touching threatening when they do not either understand these exemptions or appreciate the ultimate intent to help. Small children are taught not to have anything to do with strangers and such children may therefore be very wary. Throughout the teenage years, there is a growing awareness of how the body appears to others and a developing sense of self-identity may make the adolescent's boundaries more prickly than at other times in life. This may lead to particular problems when examining the adolescent.

With recent increased concern about child sexual abuse and the resultant widespread teaching in schools and homes about the nature of touch, particular care should be taken by podiatrists. It is vital to explain to children the reason for touching and to describe to them where they will be touched, what it will feel like and, especially important, to ask the child's permission before an approach is made.

Involving the child in treatment

There are many ways in which the child may be involved in treatment and it is essential that every effort is made to do this not only to ensure a successful outcome in the clinic but also to ensure compliance with any treatment regime that may be necessary between visits. Specific techniques for enhancing the relationship between podiatrist and child will now be discussed and they will include planning treatment; ensuring cooperation; use of reward; goal setting; recording progress; modelling appropriate behaviour and use of relaxation.

Planning

When taking the history and subsequently discussing treatment options and their possible advantages or disadvantages, it is important to include the children and to listen to their opinions. It is helpful to ask them why they think they have come, and how the problem affects them. When there are choices to be made, children may have a view about how each option will affect their daily lives, and they should therefore be consulted about how the alternatives could be managed in practice. Consider the social context into which the treatment must fit.[10] For example, a treatment strategy which will cause embarrassment to the child, by his having to wear an unfashion-able shoe, or an intervention which relies on a teenager's memory in the middle of an exam period at school, will be doomed to failure. Try to consider the practicalities of the recommended treatment as a team with the child and his parents and try to foresee any likely difficulties. However, there are occasions when no options are available, but even so, involve everyone in discussions and explanation. Review all the implications of treatment, the required number of clinic visits and the prognosis so that the family has appropriate expectations to aid, rather than to hinder, success.

Ensuring cooperation

An anxious or distressed child will not cooperate with treatment and it is both insensitive and counterproductive to force him to undergo possibly painful procedures while he is in this state. Even if he does return for further clinic appointments, he will not make intervention easy. In the interests of success in the long term, it is worthwhile taking one or more sessions in order to establish a friendship and trust and no intervention at all should be made at this stage. To many, this seems an unnecessarily protracted procedure and also wasteful of time, but experience has shown this not to be. Indeed Ley[11] found that extra clinic visits increased the patient's understanding and compliance, and therefore facilitated a positive outcome. Initial visits can be kept short and cheerful. To familiarise children with the surroundings and any instruments to be used, allow them to explore: to sit on the couch; to smell the soaps and ointments; to hold the instruments and to test the light. When the visit is interesting and free from anxiety and pain, children are more likely to trust 'their' podiatrist and when the time comes for them to undergo treatment they may better tolerate pain and discomfort if this friendship is maintained.

When the moment is judged to be appropriate to begin treatment and this may not be until several sessions have elapsed, a full explanation should be given in language that the child will understand. It is particularly helpful to give a 'running commentary' on what is happening at each stage telling the child what sensations will be experienced and how long each will last. This may be done in a positive and encouraging manner. The perception of pain may be modified by redefining the sensation as something other than pain: for example, a 'tingling' or 'numb' feeling may be easier to tolerate than 'pain'. This helps many children to cope with such situations. When appropriate during treatment, allow children to help in any suitable way, and in general the podiatrist should be patient and gentle.

Use of reward

The most potent tool in our repertoire for encouraging children, and indeed adults too, to behave in a certain way, is to use reward effectively. In its technical sense reward, or positive reinforcement, means any event or object which follows a behaviour and increases the likelihood of that behaviour occurring again in the future. Thus it is only possible in retrospect to tell whether the offered reward was in fact rewarding to the child, although an informed guess can be made as to possible reinforcers. Information from parents and children is invaluable in this respect. Rewards may either be material such as small toys or pencils or in a less tangible form such as praise, encouragement, hugs or privileges. Naturally occurring rewards in the child's life are more effective in the long run. Adults and older children develop self-satisfaction in achieving a goal, thus providing rewarding consequences for themselves from within. For the younger age group, however, a combination of praise and material reward is most effective, the exact balance being determined in consultation with the family.

Many adults ignore children when they are either behaving well or are using well established skills and pay attention to them only when there are difficulties. Under this contingency, the good behaviour is likely to vanish. The most effective way of ensuring continued good behaviour is to acknowledge it in some way. During a consultation, this means not taking compliance for granted, but being liberal with praise or allowing small 'prizes' for cooperation. Parents should be encouraged to continue this practice between clinic visits. Small, frequent rewards are more effective than the occasional grander ones and these rewards should be given as soon as poss-

ible after the behaviour to which they refer. When it is impractical to use reward with any regularity, a bridge can be created between behaviour and reinforcement by supplying a token which may later be traded for a reward at a mutually-agreed exchange rate. Such a system is known as a token economy. For example, to encourage a child not to tamper with a dressing, home-made tokens could be awarded for intervals during which the child did not touch his foot and, contingent on a target number of tokens being earned, the reward allocated at bedtime.

The only limit to the variation in use of reward is the ability to imagine interesting and novel ways of applying it.

Goal setting

When planning an intervention, a number of small, easily attainable goals should be specified. By doing this, it is clear both to parent and to child what is expected and there is opportunity for success and frequent reward and also any progress may be assessed. Setting the goal too high encourages failure and disillusionment. Children's concepts of time are variable and a long-term goal may seem so remote as to be irrelevant to the young child. Children should be involved in discussion and selection of appropriate goals and these goals should be based upon a blend of what is required clinically and what the children feel they can achieve. When targets are agreed in an atmosphere of trust and friendliness the child's enthusiasm and compliance are likely to be engaged. Targets should be reviewed at each session and modified where necessary. When such targets have proved too difficult to attain, they may be revised to a lower level but the child's efforts should nevertheless be acknowledged. On the other hand, if the targets have been found to be easy, the requirements can be extended with the child's agreement and praise should be given for the successful completion of each particular stage of treatment.

Recording

Recording progress either in or outside the clinic session has a number of benefits in ensuring compliance. For the podiatrist, an accurate daily record informs as to the adherence or otherwise to the recommended treatment. In addition, achievement of goals is accorded a status by their being noted in writing, and this gives the podiatrist further opportunity to add praise to any reward previously given by parents. For the child, discussion of a suitable recording method, designing appropriate charts and monitoring progress towards an agreed goal is an effective way for the child to be involved fully in treatment on a continuing basis during and between clinic visits.

Modelling

As a teaching strategy, modelling the desired behaviour is extremely effective. That is, rather than explaining to child and parent what is required, demonstration will enable better understanding and retention of the information. It has been shown that children who viewed videotapes of models undergoing medical procedures, and who successfully used coping strategies, showed subsequently reduced levels of anxiety.[12] Watching a demonstration then imitating the model has the added advantage of creating a practice situation for the child; for example, telling a child how to change a dressing will be much less effective than showing and encouraging him to practise in the clinic.

Relaxation

When a child is extremely anxious, it may be useful to employ relaxation techniques. These techniques are intended to ease muscle tension, slow breathing and decrease production of adrenaline by bringing into play the parasympathetic nervous system. As a result, a calmer frame of mind can be achieved. Children may be taught exercises which are designed to tense then relax related muscle groups. These exercises encourage children to note the contrasting feelings. The instructions for these exercises may be tape-recorded for daily practice at home. Very young children may be coached into 'being floppy', 'like a rag doll' and appropriate praise should be given for the child's attempts. Expert help with relaxation techniques can be sought from clinical psychologists.

Medication

In cases of severe anxiety, it is worth discussing with the child's general practitioner the possibility of using a once-only dose of medication to allow treatment to be carried out. This course of action should only be considered where other strategies have been tried unsuccessfully, and would arise very rarely when proper care and attention is devoted to methods of building trust and to promoting cooperation.

Involving the parent in treatment

For the treatment to be a success, and in particular for children in the younger age group, the podiatrist is reliant on the parent to bring the child to the clinic and to supervise treatment between sessions. However, it is equally important to involve the parent in discussion and planning so that efforts with the child are not sabotaged. Parents too need praise and encouragement from the podiatrist for playing their part, although such praise and encouragement will naturally be delivered in a different manner from that used when dealing directly with children.

It is not possible to categorise adequately parents who are encountered in the clinic. However, there are two types who pose particular problems for the podiatrist in his assessment and treatment.

Firstly, there are some parents who minimise their child's foot problem. They possibly do not appreciate the importance of appropriate treatment through their lack of knowledge, or they simply do not cooperate with the podiatrist. This situation may occur in the context of a poor relationship between clinician and parent, or where there are multiple family problems of a practical and emotional nature. Where this is the case, the child's footcare may have little priority. This may lead to only a token involvement with the treatment process or, at worst, non-attendance. Those with low self-esteem are less likely to act on advice given about treatment.[13] It is important in this case to explain carefully the long-term prognosis if treatment is not followed. Achieving a productive working relationship with such parents may require empathic concern for their difficulties, acknowledgement of their stresses, and a degree of praise for their commitment this far in attending the clinic. In order to help the child, it may be necessary to nurture the parent.

The other type of parent encountered in the clinic is the one who magnifies the significance of a minor foot problem, thus imposing unnecessary restrictions on the child and encouraging invalid status. Such parents are over-involved with their children and achieve some satisfaction from the closely dependent relationship. The podiatrist's duty here is to put the problem into perspective, although this is not always an easy task. Involving the child more than the parent in treatment in such cases may help to maintain a healthier balance.

Engaging parents at an appropriate level is therefore an important and varied task. The best chance of success lies in judging the parents' concerns, beliefs and expectations, and using these as the starting point for work. The art of treatment lies in assessing the whole patient, and indeed the whole family, and then moulding one's manner and advice to suit.

The psychological effect of chronic illness on children and their families

Chronic illness refers to a disorder with a protracted course, which may be progressive and fatal, or the child may have a relatively normal life span despite impaired physical and/or mental functioning. It has been estimated that an approximate 10% prevalence rate of chronic illness is to be expected in the child population.

Early research on the psychological effects of chronic illness emphasised the negative consequences. Studies suggested that chronically ill children were at increased risk of emotional and behavioural problems and that the family in general suffered profound disruption to its normal functioning, resulting in significant psychological problems for its members.

Whilst it is clear that chronic illness can have such effects, not all research has demonstrated that the negative sequelae are inevitable. The impact of chronic illness is clearly not a single event, but a process that varies with the course of the illness. The risk factors for the children and their families experiencing particular difficulties or becoming caught up in the process of adjustment is poorly understood, although the evidence does suggest that the parental access to information and to emotional support plays a crucial role in helping to reduce difficulties.

This part of the chapter focuses on the psychological challenges that confront these families and the factors that help influence eventual adjustment.

The first stage: diagnosis

The family's reaction to this will be affected by previous experiences of serious illness as well as the pre-morbid psychological adjustment of the individual family members. Separation from family and friends and the pain and anxiety associated with the diagnostic procedures make large demands on the coping skills of the patient and those of his family. The initial emotional reactions which are similar to those associated with bereavement should be accepted and should not be labelled pathological. Kubler-Ross's (1969) five stage model[14] is useful to consider in understanding the tasks parents have to face in adjusting to the diagnosis of chronic illness. Firstly there is denial and isolation; this stage shields the individual from the shock of the news and allows them to incorporate the news at their own pace. The second stage, anger, is frequently displayed erratically and results from a lack of control over the situation. Bargaining is the third stage. Illness is viewed as being a punishment and the family may try to strike a bargain in order to prolong life. The fourth stage, depression, occurs when there is a realisation that bargaining cannot occur and that the child's condition has to be accepted. The final stage of acceptance occurs when the family has been able to acknowledge the implications of the chronic illness yet not allow this to interfere with family life. Acceptance is very important in the process of bonding between the child and his carers. The child with a congenital handicap may have poor attachment behaviours, e.g. a poor suck response, does not fixate or smile easily. He may have an unusual facial appearance. All these factors may contribute to the carer having doubts about the child's viability and may result in the carer remaining consciously unattached to the child. Parents at such times need information, support and counselling in order to appreciate the potential positive relationship that could be established with the child.

At one time it was considered that individuals passed through each of these stages in a fixed and time limited fashion and were then able to move on in their lives. Today adjustment to loss is considered to be a varying process which is much like a wavy line with peaks and troughs with the peak occurring at times of transition in the family life cycle: e.g. birth of another child, attendance at nursery, school for the first time or leaving home. In the family life cycle each of these points creates new challenges for them. A child with Down's syndrome will require special schooling provision in order to enable him to reach his potential. To ensure this, parents have to seek professional help from educational psychologists and others and in so doing reawaken their feelings about the discrepancy between the expectations they held for their child and the reality.

It is therefore important not to view these stages as fixed since parents and siblings may be oscillating between any of the stages depending upon what is happening in the family life cycle. It is at such times families may require some professional support.

Adjustment can be promoted by the way in which parents are told, when they are told, and finally what they are told. On occasions diagnosis may be made at birth but for others it is an evolving situation when there is no definitive time that the parents can be given a diagnosis. In a number of studies parents have indicated that they wished to be told the truth early. The research also highlighted the importance of being told the truth in a sensitive manner rather than simply being given reassurance.

In the case of the child and family being the patient, further complications arise as the child needs to be spoken to at the appropriate cognitive level. This is important both at the time of initial diagnosis (when age appropriate) and at follow-up and review. Medical staff and professions allied to medicine may be misled about the child's ability by just listening to his use of language and therefore may talk to him in an inappropriate way. The mismatch between the manner in which the child speaks and his real abilities may be attributable to several factors: e.g. the unfamiliar setting or his own anxieties about what is happening. When a child is very anxious he may regress both in the way in which he talks and how he behaves. Another factor may be the child's own physical limitations. Some children with cerebral palsy have great difficulty expressing their thoughts verbally due to their motor difficulties but may well understand everything that is being said. It is therefore important to establish the child's level of understanding from those who know him well before communicating with him. Frequently young children will not talk to strangers (and in fact are positively discouraged to do so in nursery and school settings) and they will look to the parent to respond. Staff awareness of these issues will enable them to understand that the child is not 'being difficult' and unresponsive but rather that he requires reassurance and help to settle into the new situation.

Talking to parents about their child will facilitate better communication and thus better adherence and compliance to medical regimes. In addition it is important to address the child patient: with the preschool child, reassurance about the reason for the admission or hospital appointment is appropriate. However, older children may well want to ask questions and therefore an open discussion is appropriate. Whatever the age the child initially learns about his condition he will require more sophisticated explanations as he matures. As such, parents, carers and professionals have to be prepared to provide varying amounts of information depending upon the child's maturity and his express wishes for further information.

The second stage: treatment

Frequently the commencement of treatment is perceived by parents as a time of relief and optimism with the focus being on the concrete tasks at hand such as daily injections, physiotherapy, speech therapy and other medication schedules. Despite this, the illness may require repeated admission to hospital, resulting in separation from the family and disruption in schooling and peer relationships. A parent may have to give up work to look after the child, suffer extra expenses involved in living in hospital, travel and special diets. This focus on the 'here and now' enables the family not to consider the long-term implications of the illness or disability but rather to pace the integration of the information associated with diagnosis and treatment.

A number of factors have been identified which affect the psychological adjustment in children and their families. Age at onset of the illness has been highlighted as being important for psychological adjustment. A follow-up study of children with cancer noted that those children who had been diagnosed and treated in early life were less likely to experience adjustment problems in later life, when compared with those whose diagnosis occurred in middle childhood or adolescence.[15]

The developmental stage of the child is also important. A clear knowledge of the developmental milestones of childhood and adolescence is essential as this allows the health professional to help the child. Young children are, for example, developmentally frightened of strangers and of the dark and of loud noises. Staff should be aware that children may not be frightened of issues directly related to their illness but rather of those which are associated with it and such children will require help to cope with their change of circumstances. For example, a child who has to come into hospital for urodynamic studies due to poor bladder function may not be frightened of the examination, but rather frightened of being separated from his parents for some time. Discussions with the child about the positive and negative aspects of coming into hospital will hopefully help to uncover the child's anxieties and help to alleviate his concerns. The same principle is important for outpatient appointments, as a child may have all kinds of thoughts about why he is having to come to the hospital. A young child may think that it is to punish him for being naughty. A slightly older child (7–10 years) knows that the purpose of the treatment is to make him better. Adolescents may experience a difficult time as they may have concerns about their physical appearance, their sexuality and enforced dependency. Although children with handicapping conditions are familiar with the procedure for examination by the

time they reach adolescence they also express similar concerns to their able-bodied peers.

Research has demonstrated that children who are older than six months recognise their carer well and need them to develop appropriately. Bowlby[16] described three stages of acute distress that children experience when they are separated from their carers. These are protest, despair and detachment. It is therefore important to enable carers to stay with their child. In addition repeated admissions to hospital for children under the age of four are associated with marked adjustment problems in the longer term, specifically in terms of behavioural problems and reading problems at adolescence. In the light of this research it is important to admit children to hospital only when it is absolutely necessary and to ensure primary care is always available to the child and family later.

It is possible that a child with a handicapping condition shall have an inpatient stay in hospital, either for observation, medical or surgical treatment, and therefore attention has to be paid to ensure that the child does not develop psychological problems, On occasion a child or his parents may elect to come into hospital; for example, to loosen a tendon to facilitate more functional motor control. Although the child and family are in more control of the situation it does not protect them from becoming stressed by being in hospital and by having to adjust to what is happening and why.

The child's cognitive ability is also important since with increasing maturity the child develops a greater understanding of the implications of the illness and the potential restrictions that these will place on his life. A child with diabetes quickly becomes aware of the daily routines of insulin injections, of measuring blood sugar levels and of dietary restrictions. The difference between himself and his peer group also gradually emerges. Cognitively more mature children can begin to understand the underlying cause for the diabetes mellitus and how the insulin injections prevent hyperglycaemia. It is at this time that children should be helped to find ways of incorporating such routines into their lives so that the level of intrusion is minimised. It is important that children and their families find the right balance between spending time on therapy and other age appropriate activities, as it is very easy for families to become preoccupied with only one aspect of a child's development. Realistic goals should be set and emphasis placed on ensuring that the child continues to be involved in activities which are appropriate to his age.

Children who were severely affected with haemophilia, have been shown to be less affected than children with a milder form of the disease. The same trend also occurs in children who have juvenile arthritis, thalidomide, partial hearing or partial sight. In attempting to understand these results it has been proposed that children who are severely affected recognise their limitations and do not attempt to compete with their able-bodied peers, whilst the mildly affected children try to compete in both worlds. The child's constant failure in the able-bodied world results in a poor self-image and poor adjustment.

The condition itself can also have a variable effect on stress levels: Donovan[17] studied families of adolescents 10–21 years who had a diagnosis of autism or undifferentiated mental retardation. Mothers of children with autism reported higher stress levels especially where behavioural difficulties were concerned than the mothers of children with mental retardation.

The issue of dependency/independency is a crucial one for all children but for those with a chronic illness the issue has heightened significance. Initially the child with diabetes is dependent upon his parents to give him his injections. However, it is possible to promote independence by ensuring that the child takes responsibility for knowing about the disorder and for being able to give injections himself as early as possible. Dependency does not have to be an invariable accompanyment of chronic illness, but depends upon the nature of the illness. Hoare[18] found epileptic children were more dependent than diabetic children who were no different to healthy controls.

Children who have mental or physical handicaps also have to negotiate the issue of dependency. Parents have to provide a secure base for much longer and have to provide appropriate learning experiences for the child in order to foster his independence. In certain circumstances the young person will never be able to attain full independence from adults.

However, this should not prevent him from gaining some privacy and independence from his parents by living in sheltered accommodation if this is what he and his parents wish.

The child's understanding of illness is also important to acknowledge and to use in the work situation. The studies into children's concepts of illness and health were pioneered by Nagy in the late 1940s. The subsequent research has focused on delineating ages and developmental stages at which children acquire health beliefs and knowledge. Bibace and Walsh[19] using a Piagetian model described six stages in the children's understanding about illness aetiology. Under the age of four the children pass through the stages of incomprehension and phenomenism. The latter stage refers to the fact that children think that illness is due to some magical, global or circular response, e.g.

Adult: 'How do people get a cough?'
Child: 'From the wind.'
Adult: 'How does the wind give you a cough?'
Child: 'It just does.'

Between the ages of four and seven children pass through the stages of contagion and contamination. Children believe that illness in the contagion phase is due to objects or people being near them but not touching them. They then progress in their understanding by being able to distinguish the cause of the illness and how it is effective. The child perceives that the harmful object is outside the body but that illness is contracted by bodies touching.

Children between the ages of seven and eleven will pass through the stages of internalisation thereby gaining an understanding that illness is located in the body but that the cause may be external. The child becomes aware that the illness may be contracted from another individual and he is likely to believe that illness is contracted by touching another person or animal. He is also likely to believe that non-contagious illnesses may be contracted.

At the ages of eleven and older, psychological and psychophysiological are the two relevant stages of explanation. Children understand illness is due to a malfunctioning organ e.g. bronchospasm, where the bronchioles and bronchi experience spasm due to an allergen. In the most mature conceptions, children understand that illness is due to internal physiological processes but in addition they also perceive that there could be a psychological explanation for the illness. A knowledge and an awareness of the concepts of illness is important in talking to children so that appropriate explanations can be provided and so that the child is informed appropriately.

Whilst most research has focused understandably on the child patient's reaction to chronic illness and his treatment, it is important not to forget the impact on the siblings. It has been recognised that they are particularly vulnerable to developing emotional and behavioural problems. A number of factors have been identified, namely the residual effects of parental distress due to the care of the child with a handicap, an increased responsibility at home and decreased parental attention and resources, and finally a pathological identification with the sibling with the handicap. However, the research literature produced a variety of positive and negative outcomes when considering this question. The conflicting results are partly attributable to the methodological weakness of the studies, for example no control groups, indirect measures based on parental interview which may well be biased and a reliance on single measures, such as the current psychological state of the child. This last issue may easily misrepresent how the sibling is adjusting, as adjustment will inevitably vary over time as different demands are placed on the child.

One study found that brothers and sisters were not embarrassed by having a sibling with a handicap but by having to cope with problem behaviour in a public place, especially when they were in charge and when they felt unsure as to how to cope.[20]

Factors such as a small family, a small age gap between the sibling and the child with the handicap, younger siblings and a handicapping condition that is not obvious have been associated with greater problems for the siblings.[21]

Dyson[22] compared 55 older siblings in Canada (aged 7.5–15 years) of younger children with a handicap (aged 1–7 years) with 55 matched siblings of children without a handicap. Dyson found that there was no difference in level of self-concept, behaviour problems and social competence between the two groups. The study also supported previous

studies showing that there was no higher incidence of psychopathological behaviour.

Dyson also looked at the personal attributes that related to adjustment in siblings of handicapped children. Siblings of children with a mental handicap in general showed better behavioural adjustment and a higher social competence than siblings of children with a sensory, physical handicap or milder handicapping conditions. The author felt that the discrepancy was due to differential social consequences. It was thought that a mental delay may encourage an earlier social and family acceptance than other disabilities such as sensory or physical handicaps, speech disorders or learning disabilities. It is possible that some of the conditions are ill defined and therefore will produce a sense of frustration in the family which could affect sibling adjustment.

Suelzle and Keenan[23] considered that families of children with a handicap became more isolated as the children became older. Dyson also reported that there was an increase in behavioural problems in the siblings as the child with the handicap became older. Such changes may occur because there are a number of clubs and organised activities for younger children with a handicap, as well as the school acting as a social network for the family, but as the children outgrow these there are very few new networks to replace them in the adolescent and adult worlds. This may result in the families becoming more internally dependent upon one another for care and entertainment than their able-bodied counterparts.

Siblings have also reported that their parents are being overly involved with protecting the ill child. The research also noted that siblings were reluctant to express their feelings of dissatisfaction as well as their negative feelings to the family. Other studies have noted that adjustment was poorest when the patient's health was deteriorating but that their needs were also unmet when the patients were feeling well.

The third stage: illness remission

Illness remission occurs for most children. This may be either a favourable response to treatment or a remission of the illness when the symptoms are in abeyance. Such periods may continue for days, months or years. It is at such times that the illness and related matters may retreat into the background and other age appropriate activities may take precedence. Frequently parents report concerns about their child's health and also worry about the recurrence of the illness. At these times parents require much support in order to foster adjustment.

Returning to normal routines such as school and other pre-illness activities, as soon as treatment permits, contributes to psychological adjustment and self-esteem. In addition it is important to re-establish the old family routines and appropriate disciplines as, paradoxically, poor adjustment is likely to result where parents maintain a permissive attitude with poor limit setting as far as the children's behaviour is concerned.

Although children with a handicapping condition do become ill and have these adjustment problems, they do not experience a remission in their condition whether it be cerebral palsy, developmental delay or diabetes. Instead parents have to come to terms with visits to other professionals, e.g. physiotherapists, occupational therapists, podiatrists in order to enhance their child's development and quality of life. They will have to confront the issue of mainstream or special needs schooling. Later in adolescence the issue of leaving home becomes more complex depending upon the child's level of dependency.

The fourth stage: discharge

A variety of ambivalent feelings may be produced once the treatment is completed; relief that the discomfort and inconvenience has ended but also concern that the protective element has also finished. Families require support at this time in order to foster their own self-reliance and independence of the medical team. It is important at this time to help the child return to his normal pattern of life. Of particular concern to both the parents and children are the problems associated with losing contact with the peer group, falling behind with school work and the types of restrictions that may be placed on recreation.

Parents of children with a handicap do not experience discharge from the medical team in the same way. Once the young person has reached 16–19 years of age, depending upon the area they live in, they have to be transferred to the adult services. When they have a physical or mental handicap they will be transferred to the appropriate community team. This transfer may be difficult as the family lose a set of professionals that they have come to trust. At the same time the family has to be making new decisions about the young person's future.

The fifth stage: terminal illness

This is a major area and due to space constraints will not be discussed here. There is a large body of literature available on this area. Two papers by Pettle-Michael and Lansdown[24] and Mulhern et al[25] have been quoted in the references for those who may be interested.

Conclusion

In focusing on the challenges that families have to confront when they have a child with a chronic illness it is clear that many families adjust and cope well using their own support networks. However, there are some children and families who require positive help in order to find the appropriate strategies to support themselves and each other. It is at this point that mental health professionals have a major role to play. They have to be sensitive to each family's differing coping styles and such professionals must be able to offer help and support without undermining the family's own strengths in this area. To be able to do this requires training and time with the families to gain an understanding of their individual needs.

References

1 Stimson GV, Webb B. *Going to See the Doctor: the Consultation Process in General Practice.* London, Routledge and Kegan Paul. 1975.
2 Geersten HR, Gray RM, Ward JR. Patient non-compliance within the context of seeking medical care for arthritis. *J Chron Dis* 1973; 26: 689–98.
3 Argyle M, Salter V, Nicholson H, Williams M., Burgess P. The communication of inferior and superior attitudes by verbal and non-verbal signals. *Br J Soc Clin Psychol* 1970; 9: 222–31.

4 Korsche B, Negrete V. Doctor/Patient communication. *Sci Am* 1972; 227: (Aug) 66.

5 Coe RM. *Sociology of Medicine*. New York, McGraw Hill, 1970.

6 Ley P. *Proceedings of British Association for Advancement of Science*. 1974.

7 Bertakis KD. The communication of information from physician to patient: a method for increasing patient retention and satisfaction. *J Fam Pract* 1977; 5(2): 217–22.

8 Wooley FR, Kane RL, Hughes CC, Wright DD. The effects of doctor/patient communication on satisfaction and outcome of care. *Soc Sci Med* 1978; 12(24): 123–8.

9 Montagu A. *Touching*. New York, Harper and Row, 1978.

10 Stimson GV. Doctor/Patient interaction and some problems for prescribing. *J Roy Coll Gen Pract* 1976; 26 Suppl. 1: 88–96.

11 Ley P. A method for increasing patient's recall of information presented by doctors. *Psychol Med* 1973; 3: 217.

12 Melamed BG, Siegel LJ. Reduction of anxiety in children facing hospitalization and surgery by use of filmed modelling. *J Con Clin Psychol* 1975; 43: 511–21.

13 Rachman SJ, Phillips C. *Psychology and Medicine*. Pelican, 1978.

14 Kubler-Ross E. *On Death and Dying*. New York, McMillan, 1969.

15 Koocher GP, O'Malley JE, Gogan JL, Foster DJ. Psychological adjustment among paediatric cancer survivors. *J Child Psychol Psychiatry* 1980; 21: 163–73.

16 Bowlby J. *Attachment and Loss, Volume 2. Separation, Anxiety and Anger*. London, Hogarth Press, 1973.

17 Donovan AM. Family stress and ways of coping with adolescents who have handicaps: maternal perceptions. *Am J Ment Defic* 1988; 92: 502–9.

18 Hoare P. 'Does illness foster dependency?'. A study of epileptic and diabetic children. *Dev Med Child Neurol* 1984; 26: 20–4.

19 Bibace R, Walsh H. Development of children's concepts of illness. *Pediatrics* 1980; 66: 912–17.

20 Hart D, Walters J. Brothers and sisters of menally handicapped children, Unpublished manuscript. 1979.

21 Howlin P. Living with Impairment: the effects on children of having an autistic sibling. *Child: Care, Health Dev* 1988; 14: 395–408.

22 Dyson L. Adjustment of siblings of handicapped children. A comparison. *J Paediatr Psychol* 1989; 14(2): 215–29.

23 Suelzle M, Keenan V. Changes in family support networks over the life cycle of mentally retarded persons. *Am J Ment Defic* 1981; 83(3): 267–74.

24 Pettle-Michael SA, Lansdown RG. Adjustment to the death of a sibling. *Arch Dis Child* 1986; 61: 278–83.

25 Mulhern RK, Lauer ME, Hoffmann RG. Death of a child at home or in hospital: subsequent adjustment of the family. *Pediatrics* 1983; 71: 743–7.

3
Torsional and Frontal Plane Conditions of the Lower Extremity

Ronald L. Valmassy

When it is realised that the developing child is not merely a small adult, and that structural and positional developmental changes occur in a continuous and dynamic fashion, then the satisfactory treatment results which all hope to achieve with a paediatric patient population are obtained. Knowledge of all the developmental changes that may occur in the growing child's lower extremity should result in a successful diagnosis and treatment of a paediatric gait problem. As many have stated, the early years of development represent the golden years of treatment, when the practitioner may favourably influence development so that normal gait patterns are achieved by adolescence. When that philosophy is embraced, while cautiously advising that some problems will be outgrown, while others warrant treatment, then success will be attained in this most rewarding segment of patient care.

Although a practitioner will at times be called upon to treat traumatic, dermatological or neurological problems, the vast majority of cases involve a flatfooted condition, associated with either an intoed or an out-toed gait pattern. When a patient, whose parents are concerned regarding their child's foot problem, presents for treatment it must be realised that the true aetiology of that problem may often lie outside the foot. It is the purpose, then, of this chapter to present the transverse and frontal plane developmental changes which occur in the growing child's leg, and how these will often influence the development of that child's foot and resultant gait pattern. Additionally

the ability to evaluate and treat other common pathological conditions such as metatarsus adductus, equinus and talipes calcaneovalgus will also be discussed.

Femoral component

In reviewing articles dealing with developmental changes occurring in the transverse plane of the femur, antetorsion/anteversion and similarly retrotorsion/retroversion are often used interchangeably. In an attempt to clarify and simplify the process for practitioners and for the purposes of this chapter, torsional versus positional changes allows the developmental process to be understood and utilised clinically in a more efficient fashion.

At birth an angle exists between the condyles and the head and neck of femur of approximately 30°. As normal development of this segment occurs there is a gradual 'unwinding' of this relationship so that by the age of five or six a 20° external change has occurred on the transverse plane, thereby leading to an average angle of antetorsion of 8–12°.[1-3] When this change does not occur, or occurs slowly, then an intoed type of gait will be precipitated. In certain cases, this bony unwinding will be delayed up until the age of 13 or 14. This certainly explains why some youngsters who appear pigeon-toed for such a long period of time will ultimately appear 'normal' when they become teenagers. It appears that approximately 90% of those youngsters possessing an internal femoral torsion will outgrow the pathology by this age, unless of course, there was a significant familial tendency towards this deformity. In these cases, there is little likelihood of the torsional component improving spontaneously over time.[4] Additionally, it has been reported clinically, that youngsters being treated for torsional problems of the femur often demonstrate readily observable angle of gait changes which seem to correspond to overall growth spurts and increases in height.[1] It is postulated that 'growth spurts' not only affect the length of the long bones, but may also contribute in part to transverse plane alterations. In other instances, there may be excessive 'unwinding' of the femoral segment which may result in an external femoral torsion. As this represents an over-growth, there is generally no treatment which can be easily provided to reverse this problem, which is often reported as retrotorsion.[2,5] Caution must be exercised when informing parents which problems are most likely to resolve with time, as an external femoral torsion or position may potentially appear worse at age 13 to 14 depending upon subsequent rotational tendencies.

The other component of the transverse plane development of the femur is associated with the soft tissue or positional changes which occur over the first few years of life. This soft tissue change involves an internal positioning of this femoral component relative to its position on the acetabulum. As this gradual internal rotation of the entire femoral segment occurs, the long axis of the femur is externally rotating or – 'unwinding'. The overall net effect is to have the patella placed on the frontal plane, generally by the age of five to six.[3, 5–7] This positional change is associated with the soft tissue structures affecting the hip joint including the capsule, ligaments and muscles. This positional adaptation is generally attributed to the child's intrauterine position wherein he/she was held in an abducted and externally rotated position in utero.[5, 8] At birth, the ratio of external to internal rotation is normally three to one, with a total range of motion approaching 100°.[7–9] As normal development occurs, the overall range of motion, as well as this external position, gradually reduces. Although a tendency towards an externally rotated position persists throughout

the first few years of life, this should reduce by age five to six, at which time the patellae will typically be functioning on the frontal plane in gait. Interestingly, as the child develops into an adult, there is a gradual return to a slightly greater degree of external rotation.

The muscles responsible for externally rotating the femur include the following: gluteus maximus, obturator externus, obturator internus, gemelli, quadratus femoris, piriformis, sartorius, adductor magnus, adductor longus and adductor brevis. The ischiofemoral ligament will assist in limiting internal rotation. Internal rotation of the femur is accomplished via contraction of the iliopsoas, tensor fasciae latae, gluteus medius and gluteus minimus. The iliofemoral and pubofemoral ligaments tend to limit lateral rotation.[2, 3]

An additional component that may contribute to leg rotation is the position of the acetabulum. Although the normal position of the acetabulum is located so as to place the head of the femur on the sagittal plane, there may certainly be skeletal variations.[2, 8, 10] The most common variation and certainly a normal variant is one where the acetabulum is more externally rotated, which complements the overall externally rotated position present in the infant. However, when the acetabulum is significantly internally placed, then this would contribute to an internally positioned limb, a factor which some authors feel is significant, yet commonly overlooked, in the overall development of the angle of gait.[2, 5, 10]

Frontal plane conditions of the femur

With regard to frontal plane changes associated with the femur, the development of coxa vara or coxa valga is the most clinically significant. Although marked changes associated with frontal plane alterations of the head and neck of the femoral segment are rare, it is still appropriate to discuss them.

The angle of femoral inclination is the angle formed in the frontal plane between the long axis of the head and neck of the femur and the long axis of the femoral shaft. In neonates, this angle is 140–150° and reduces to 120–132° (average 128°) in the first six years of development.[3, 11]

Coxa valga

When the angle of femoral inclination has not reduced to 128°, the condition of coxa valga is said to exist. The aetiology may be due to a lack of development of the head and neck of the femur relative to the shaft of the femur from dysplasia (usually bilateral) or from some type of trauma (typically unilateral). There is an awkward gait and frequently a degree of hip dislocation is present in this rare, usually congenital condition. A clinical result of this may be a concomitant genu varum.

Coxa vara

Coxa vara occurs when the angle of femoral inclination has reduced past 128°. Typically this represents an overgrowth and may sometimes be seen with a slipped capital femoral epiphysis. It may be caused by trauma or may be developmental in nature. Coxa vara is difficult to evaluate in radiographs of very young infants and is usually first noticed when the child begins to walk. The leg is shorter on the affected side and adduction of the leg is restricted as well as internal rotation. Coxa vara may result in genu valgum.

Clinical evaluation of the hip

Although radiographic studies may be obtained in order to measure some of the torsional parameters previously discussed, this is not a common practice when routinely determining the range of motion available at the hip. Typically, a combination of off-weight-bearing measurements, coupled with gait analysis, where applicable, is generally sufficient in determining whether the problem involves soft tissue or bone. When the primary aetiology based on clinical evaluation can be determined, an appropriate treatment plan may more readily be instigated.

Prior to measuring any range of motion, the child, when ambulatory, should be allowed to walk around the office or clinic, without his/her hand being held, in order that an overall evaluation of gait may be appreciated. Even in the youngest of children, the position of the head, shoulders and pelvis should be observed in order to determine if a limb length discrepancy is present. Visualisation of the patellae will provide the examiner with a general idea as to where the lower limb is functioning. Up until the child is five to six years of age the normal clinical presentation generally places the patellae in an externally located position. This would be expected in a child who had normal torsional and positional development of the femoral segment.

When the child walks in a fairly adducted manner, with each patella on the frontal plane, then the presence of a pseudolack of malleolar torsion, an internal tibial torsion, a metatarsus adductus, a rigid forefoot valgus, or a rigid plantarflexed first ray deformity would be suspected. If one or both patellae function in an internally deflected position then it may be assumed that at least a portion of the deformity lies within the femoral segment. It is clinically difficult to determine the extent of the involvement from other levels, solely by visualising the patellar positions. It is also difficult to determine whether an intoed gait associated with internally facing patellae (often reported as the squinting patellae syndrome)[10, 12] is due to a soft tissue or osseous anomaly. However, in internal femoral torsion as the patient walks towards the examiner, the adducted gait pattern is typically consistent in nature; i.e. there is little deviation in the angle and base of gait noted from step to step. However, when there is an actual movement of adduction noted as the patient is ambulating, then this motion may be attributed to tight medial musculature, which, in tightening during the swing and contact phases of gait, initiates the adduction noted. Most typically this motion is caused by a tight medial hamstring. The movement is quite distinct from the marked adduction noted in children with spastic adductors or hamstrings associated with various types of neurological deficits.

Documentation of the angle and base of gait, patellar position and extent of calcaneal eversion should all be recorded at the conclusion of this portion of the examination.

Once the gait evaluation portion of the examination has been completed the non-weightbearing range of motions should now be assessed. Although it is not in the scope of this chapter to present all the diagnostic parameters which are useful in determining the presence of a dislocated or dislocatable hip, suffice it to say that no opportunity should be missed to evaluate hip stability and congruency in the developing child. The importance of this is magnified whenever the opportunity of evaluating the stability of the hips in children under 12 months of age arises. As the status of the hips may possibly change spontaneously, it is essential to evaluate that segment's stability even when recent examinations by other practitioners have been performed and found to be normal.[12, 13]

Clinical signs indicative of a possible dislocated hip include redundant skin folds of the thigh associated with an apparently shortened limb, and a positive anchor sign which is represented by asymmetrical gluteal folds (Fig. 3.1). A Trendelenburg gait with associated

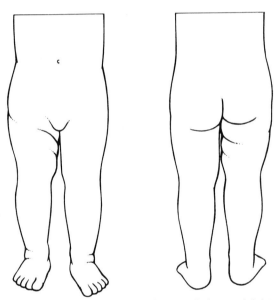

Figure 3.1   Abnormal skin folds and elevated right buttock, indicating positive anchor sign.

mild shoulder and hip drop, along with a unilateral external leg position, are often noted in the ambulatory child with frank hip dislocation. Clinical tests for a dislocatable hip, which may occur in as many as 1 : 100 live births, often become inappropriate after the first few months of life. This is due to tightening of soft tissue structures in and about the hip. Spontaneous resolution of this problem is a common phenomenon.[12, 13]

Although Barlow's manoeuvre has been uti-

lised for many years,[14] it has recently been felt to be an ineffective manoeuvre for eliciting stability of the femoral head within the acetabulum.[13] Additionally there is some concern that inappropriate application of the manual forces performed via this examination may actually lead to some disruption of normal femoral–acetabulum development. Barlow's manoeuvre as presented in the classical description is most appropriately initiated within the first few months after birth, and is accomplished with the child lying flat on his back with the hips and knees maintained in a flexed position. The middle finger of each hand of the examiner is placed over the greater trochanter and the thumb of each hand is applied to the inner side of the thigh at the level of the lesser trochanter. The thighs are carried into mid-adduction with the test consisting of the application of pressure backwards and outwards with the thumb.[12]

When the hip is dislocatable, or unstable, this pressure will allow the femoral head to slide posteriorly over the posterior acetabular rim. Release of the pressure allows re-entry into the acetabulum. The test is limited and becomes less useful as the child becomes older. Although it may be attempted up to the seventh month the test is most reliable at birth to four weeks.

Of greater importance is the ability to actually diagnose the presence of a frankly dislocated hip which occurs in approximately 8–10 per 10 000 (0.1%) live births with females involved from four to six times as often as males.[12] Familiarisation with the more common and reliable tests for a congenital dislocation of the hip is essential so that appropriate radiographs may be taken when necessary.

There are three clinical methods which seem to be most reliable in assisting the clinician to determine whether or not a congenitally dislocated hip is actually present or not. All clinicians involved in the evaluation and treatment of lower extremity disorders in the paediatric population should be capable of effectively performing the following tests.

1. Ortolani's sign (reducing test for congenital dislocation of the hip). With the infant supine, the hips and knees are flexed to 90°. The hips are examined one at a time by grasping the baby's thigh with the middle finger over the greater trochanter and then simultaneously lifting and abducting the thigh to be examined while stabilising the opposite thigh and pelvis. When the hip is dislocated, the femoral head will move from a posterior dislocated position to a more inferior and distal position within the acetabulum. The examiner can feel the head relocate which is described as a 'palpable click', not an 'audible click'. This test is most reliable in the early months of postnatal life. It must be remembered that there are other structures around the hip such as ligaments that may also cause a clicking and thus although this is a very useful test, it is not pathognomonic for a congenitally dislocated hip.

2. Abduction test. With the child supine and the hips and knees flexed the hip is gently abducted. There will be restriction of abduction on the dislocated side caused by shortened and contracted hip adductor muscles. This is easily seen in unilateral dislocation, while in bilateral dislocations, abduction will be symmetrical but limited. The test is most reliable after two months of age. As newborns are generally flexible it is not uncommon to perceive false negatives.[5, 12, 15]

3. Galeazzi's sign (Allis' sign). The child is placed supine with his knees and hips flexed and the level of the knees is observed. With a dislocation, the affected side will be lower. This test is most reliable after the age of 18 months. A bilateral dislocated hip deformity will be missed if reliance is placed upon this examination alone.

The last two tests are reliable for quite some time and may be positive even when a dislocated hip has gone undetected for several years. Due to the ease of performing these tests they should be carried out immediately prior to the tests preferred in order to determine the status of internal and external hip rotation.

There are numerous methods of determining the ranges of motion of the hips in the transverse plane. The child may be prone or supine, seated or lying down, with the knees either extended or flexed. All the tests are capable of reflecting the information that is necessary in order to reach a correct diagnosis and to fashion an appropriate treatment plan.

One effective method of determining the transverse plane range of motion of the hip involves measuring the internal and external rotation available at the hip, with the child in both a hip flexed and hip extended position. Although it may be necessary to perform the examination on the lap of one of the parents, it is generally preferable to obtain the information with the child directly on the examination table. Initially the range of motion should be assessed first externally and then internally by placing the hips through the range of motion in the transverse plane. This may be performed without instrumentation in order to allow the examiner to orient himself with the overall positioning of the limbs. A general impression of the actual available ranges of motion may be achieved at this time if the examiner can imagine the face of a clock placed proximal to the patella with an 'hour hand' rising perpendicularly from the centre of the patella. When the patella is lying parallel to the supporting surface the 'hour hand' would reflect a position of 12 o'clock or zero degrees. Thus each 'hour' position would equate with a 30° change. Therefore, on examining the left extremity of a youngster whose patella approached a 'two o'clock' position with external rotation this would be documented as an approximate external deviation of 60°. This is only a cursory form of examination and is most useful in screening examinations or at times of initial assessment prior to performing a more complete examination.[2, 5, 7]

With regard to a specific examination, the examiner should utilise whichever of the commonly available measuring devices that he feels is most accurate and reproducible in his hands. Initially, the child is seated in a hip flexed position with the amount of external and internal hip position recorded for each limb (Fig. 3.2). When measuring external rotation of a limb care should be taken to ensure that the contralateral buttock does not rise from the couch as this would indicate that excessive force was being generated with the examination technique. This would make it appear that there was a greater degree of external rotation available than was actually present. Conversely, when measuring internal hip rotation care should be taken not to elevate

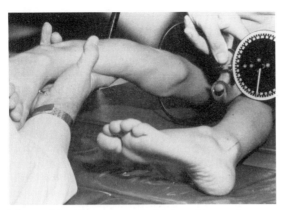

Figure 3.2   Measurement of internal femoral rotation.

the buttock of the side being rested as this would erroneously increase the amount of internal rotation present.

The tests should be repeated with the child in a hip extended position. Following the recording of the actual degrees of external and internal rotation elicited it must also be noted whether the ends of the ranges of motion were soft and spongy or abrupt and bony in nature. Children should demonstrate greater external than internal rotation of the femoral segment up until the age of six or seven, with anywhere from two to three times as much external rotation being present in relation to internal rotation at that age. The total range of motion available on the transverse plane may be anywhere from 100–120° at birth.[1, 3] Over the following years the general tendency is for internal and external rotations to equalise themselves with the total range of motion generally decreasing to approximately 80°. Any significant alterations relative to these values are generally measured in children with lower extremity gait disturbances.[3, 5, 7]

When performing the range of motion examination of the hips, certain specific clinical observations must be noted. These are extremely useful in establishing a diagnosis for marked internal or external femoral rotation problems.

As previously mentioned the quality of the end of the range of hip motion should be recorded, e.g. a measurement of 80° of internal hip rotation and 30° of external hip rotation in both the hip extended and hip flexed position, and the end of the range of motion was abrupt

or 'bony' in nature, then that patient's clinical presentation would be consistent with an internal femoral torsion. Conversely, 90° of external rotation with 10° of internal rotation in both the hip extended and hip flexed position, with that same bony feel to the end of the range of motion, would be consistent with an external femoral torsion.[3, 5]

However, in cases where there was a marked difference in the measured rotations, and the examiner felt that the ends of the range of motion were generally 'spongy' or 'yielding' in nature, then muscle or ligamentous involvement would be the suspected aetiology of the problem. A clinical example of the preceding situation would be the following[3, 5]: when examination reveals 60° of internal rotation and 30° of external rotation with the hip extended, and then a similar amount of internal rotation with 60° of external rotation while the hips are flexed, then soft tissue involvement is likely. Specifically the pubofemoral ligament, the ileofemoral ligament or the ligamentous teres should be suspected of limiting the external rotation as these structures, if contracted, would limit external rotation with the hip extended. However, once the hip is flexed and the structures become relaxed the increased available external rotation can be recorded.

If there was the same apparent change elicited in external versus internal rotation produced by examining the child first in the hip flexed and then in the hip extended position, the hamstrings should be suspected of being involved in restricting external rotation. In this instance, specific evaluation of the hamstrings would be necessary in order to complete the examination.[7]

With femoral rotation problems the following clinical possibilities should be noted:

1. An external hip position will be present when the internal rotation available increases with the hip moving from an extended to flexed position, or vice versa. Specifically when a limited amount of internal rotation is noted only with the hip flexed and knee extended then there is a tight or shortened lateral hamstring. When the limitation of internal rotation is only present with the hip in an extended position then a contracture of the iliopsoas

must be suspected and this can then be tested on an individual basis.[2, 3]

2. A measured range of motion, which remains essentially unchanged regardless of the hip position and which is accompanied by a bony or abrupt feeling at the end of the range of motion, is typically a femoral torsion problem (internal or external). Conversely a range of motion which is obviously altered in its external or internal measurement, depending upon the flexed or extended nature of the hip, and accompanied by a spongy feel at its end of the range of motion, typically reflects a femoral position problem (internal or external).[3, 5, 7]

3. Although a soft tissue problem will typically present and remain as a soft tissue problem throughout the child's development and treatment, the same may not hold true for a problem which was originally torsional in nature. An internal or external femoral torsion would most likely lead to a degree of internal or external femoral position as well. As the soft tissue structures crossing the hip joint will most likely contract and adapt to an externally or internally deviated femoral segment they will often add to the overall deformity.

4. Ranges of motion may vary significantly from individual to individual over a period of years. Regardless of what our off-weight-bearing measurements tell us, the most important factor is evaluating the overall gait presentation, and any subsequent compensatory changes generated by the alteration of that gait.

Following evaluation of the femoral segment the knee should next be evaluated.

Transverse plane evaluation of the knee

With regard to evaluating the rotations of the knee in the transverse plane, it must be appreciated that the overall available range of motion of this joint is capable of changing a great deal over the first few years of life. As in most major joints of the upper and lower extremity, the rotation present in the knee will be quite large at birth and throughout infancy, with a rapid tightening of the structures noted

over the first few years of life. The total range of motion in the transverse plane with the knee extended may be anywhere from zero to 15–20°.[2, 3] As has been pointed out by various authors it is generally difficult to fully extend the knee in a young infant due to the retention of the in-utero hip flexed, knee flexed attitude. Because of this the available motion noted is most likely visualised with the knee in a slight degree of flexion. Conversely, evaluation of the transverse plane range of motion with the knee in a fully flexed attitude may exceed 35–45° total range of motion.[3]

When the development of the knee joint as well as its surrounding ligamentous and muscular attachments proceeds in a normal fashion, then there will be no interruption in the development of a normal angle of gait. However, when there is a tightening of the medial structures due to retention of the in-utero position accompanied by weak lateral musculature or increased intervention of the medial structures, then a developmental and functional asymmetry of the internal versus external range of motion at the knee will exist. In such cases, the tibia will develop and then function in an internally rotated position. Just as it is possible to differentiate between an internal femoral position and an internal femoral torsion it should be possible to diagnose the presence of an internal tibial position versus an internal tibial torsion. Referred to in the past as a pseudolack of malleolar torsion, and classically described as an increase in the overall range of knee rotation, the deformity should be evaluated and considered in a different clinical perspective.[3] All authors agree that if there was an intoed gait present in the early walker and that the child's knee functioned in the frontal plane, then the deformity would always lie distal to the femoral segment. In cases where there was a measured normal tibial torsion and no other pathology noted in the foot (see previous discussion), then the problem would typically lie within the knee joint itself. Again, this condition was referred to as a pseudomalleolar torsion or pseudo-lack of malleolar torsion, a rather confusing term at first, but an accurate description of the clinical presentation which was observed: that of an adducted foot in a child whose knee functioned on the frontal plane, giving the clinical impression of a low or internal tibial torsion.

However, in cases where a normal tibial torsion was present, the resultant deformity was attributed to a hypermobile or loose knee which appeared clinically as being due to a torsional problem. Such observations led to the description of a pseudo-lack of tibial torsion.[3, 12, 13]

Upon clinical examination of a youngster with this presenting problem, the examiner will note that besides the child's gait pattern being adducted, the affected foot will appear to strike in a different position with alternating steps, an effect precipitated via the soft tissue contractures. Additionally, there will be a greater tendency towards tripping and instability in gait due to this gait disturbance.[13]

When performing the non-weightbearing examination for this particular segment, it is generally unnecessary to utilise any of the commonly used measuring devices. Clinical interpretation of the amount and extent of rotation will be sufficient, particularly when considered in light of the presenting complaint and initial gait evaluation.

In a normally developing infant and child, up to the age of three to four years it would be expected that there would be little rotation noted in the child's knee with full extension as the knee would be locked in this position. However, upon flexion of the knee, even to a minimal degree, a marked increase in the overall total amount of transverse plane rotation available would be noted. Examination of the knee in this position should normally yield close to equal amounts of internal and external rotation of the proximal to distal aspect of the femur. However, when upon examination of the tibia in this 'resting' position, a greater amount of external than internal rotation was observed, then it would be realised that tight medial musculature had placed the resting position of the tibia in an internal position. Subsequent attempts at eliciting internal rotation of the tibia relative to the femur would not yield much movement as the tibia would already be in its abnormal, internally located position.[3, 13]

The overall range of motion of the knee would generally remain unaffected, with the actual deformity representing an excessive degree of internal rotation of the tibia. Although the literature cites a variety of effective methods of examining this, the pathology

as it should be understood indicates excessive internal rotation of the tibia relative to the femur leading to an adducted gait pattern.[1-3]

Further examination of the child's knee in both hip flexed and hip extended position is also beneficial, as is evaluation of hip range of motion in both extended and flexed positions. When the rotation of the tibia changes with hip extension and flexion, the musculature crossing the knee is the primary deforming force. However, when the tibial rotation remains essentially unchanged with hip extension and flexion, then it may be suspected that the primary aetiological problem is ligamentous in nature. Some secondary muscular involvement would also be expected in those instances much in the same manner as there is some musculature contracture at the hip with internal femoral torsion problems.

Appreciation of this fact and an understanding of the biomechanical changes of the knee over the first few years of life will clarify why the deformity is only found in the early walker and is often considered to be a self-limiting process. It should be remembered that the early walker's gait pattern is one of knee flexion with whole foot contact at 'heel strike'. Knee extension occurs much later than at heel contact and for a brief period of time only. Thus when the knee remains flexed for a prolonged period of time in the early walker, especially at heel contact, and when the medial structures are tight, then it is easily seen why the foot becomes adducted with this specific deformity.[2, 5, 7]

It is important to remember that as the child matures and develops, a more normal type of gait pattern will develop between three and four years of age and that more of an actual heel contact with full knee extension as the foot approaches the supporting surface will be noticed.

Development of the knee

Genu varum

The normal amount of bowing at the level of the knee is a result of a lateral curvature of either the tibia or of the tibia and femur and is often found with normal coxa valga. This varus attitude is a normal developmental finding and typically is present in the infant and early walker. Developmental genu varum is present from birth and may be present up until four years of age.[5, 16]

Normal genu varum may be exaggerated by either an internal rotation of the femoral segment or by an internal tibial torsion, both of which will externally rotate the lateral aspect of the posterior calf musculature. This will tend to emphasise the overall clinical appearance of a normal frontal plane bowing of the knee.[7] The clinical aspect of this condition which it is important to recall is that certain disease processes can mimic or aggravate this deformity. These must be considered as possible differentials when there is either excessive bowing present or a failure of a varus attitude to reduce significantly by the age of four. The differential diagnosis must be made between rickets, Blount's disease and an asymmetrical development of the epiphyses (see discussion under tibial varum, below).[2, 5, 9]

Genu valgum

A genu valgum or knock-kneed appearance is a normal physiological position noted during a child's development. Frequently associated with coxa vara, the position generally develops normally following the normal genu varum position previously discussed. Generally it is first noticed between three and five years of age, and will persist for several years before it is eventually outgrown by age eight.[5] Some authors note that a second physiologically normal episode of genu valgum may occur in the 12 to 14 year old, depending upon other rotational factors influencing the femoral component at that time.[1]

As a child develops, the normal genu valgum attitude appears due to the obliquity at the femur, wherein the medial femoral condyle is lower than the lateral femoral condyle. When the position persists the lateral femoral condyle will bear more weight than the medial femoral condyle. This, combined with varying rates of development of the medial and lateral aspects of the tibial epiphyses, will lead to varying degrees of a valgus position, according to Tax,[5] and may be associated with a curvature of the femoral or tibial shaft. Normal epiphyseal plate development, affected by either

infection or trauma, may also lead to a significant genu valgum.

In measuring genu varum and genu valgum, the child should lie supine on the examination table.

1. Genu varum: the malleoli are brought together and the distance between the medial femoral condyles is measured.
2. Genu valgum: the knees are first allowed to come into contact with each other and the distance between the two medial malleoli is then measured.

In the classic presentation and study of the deformity (Morely, 1957),[5] a helpful grading system was introduced for clinical reference.

Grade I: where intermalleolar distance ≤ 2.5 cm.
Grade II: where intermalleolar distance = 2.5–5.0 cm.
Grade III: where intermalleolar distance = 5.0–7.5 cm.
Grade IV: where intermalleolar distance ≥ 7.5 cm.

Genu recurvatum

While in the stance position the child should be examined for pathologic genu recurvatum. This posterior deflection of the femur on the tibia may normally be present, measuring approximately 5–10° until the age of five years. Any amount greater than that in children under five, or any amount at all after the age of five, may be indicative of some lower extremity pathology.[2, 3]

A congenital gastrocnemius equinus may cause this deformity to occur when there is an inability to compensate at the level of the subtalar and midtarsal joints. The genu recurvatum position allows the foot to function in an attitude that is somewhat plantarflexed to the tibia, thereby decreasing the abnormal pull on the posterior musculature. When this type of compensation is allowed to continue, the abnormal deflection of the posterior surface of the knee will become progressively worse and most likely symptomatic. Identification of this condition is essential if future problems are to be avoided.

Consistent monitoring is particularly important when utilising functional foot orthoses in the treatment of a pes planus deformity associated with a suspected congenital equinus.

When the orthotic device successfully inhibits abnormal subtalar and midtarsal joint compensation, then the Achilles tendon will be placed under constant tension. If in fact there is an accommodative contracture of the posterior musculature, then the Achilles tendon will lengthen and a measurable increase in ankle motion may be appreciated. No change in the original angle of genu recurvatum should be noted during treatment. If on the other hand it is observed that the original angle of genu recurvatum is being increased through the use of the functional foot orthoses then this indicates the likelihood of a congenital equinus. In such instances the orthotic devices should be discontinued and surgical lengthening considered.[3, 7]

Tibia

Transverse plane

Evaluation of the transverse plane rotation of the tibia will allow a full appreciation of all the components leading to the overall development of a patient's angle of gait to be obtained. Along with the previously discussed soft tissue and osseous changes affecting the femur and knee, the twisting or torsion which occurs in the tibia will contribute to the placement of the foot during gait. Most authors agree that there is very little, if any, external rotation noted of the tibia relative to the fibula at birth. However, as the tibia undergoes a gradual 'unwinding' process, in which it will externally rotate relative to the fibula, clinical documentation can be made of the gradual development of this segment and of its effect on the eventual angle of gait.[17, 18]

The amount of true tibial torsion which occurs during development of the tibia on the transverse plane is between 18 and 23°.[1, 3, 19] This torsion can be measured radiographically, or with computerised axial tomography. However, as it is impossible to measure true tibial torsion clinically, the malleolar position is measured and that is the position of a bisection of the tibial malleolus relative to a bisection of the fibular malleolus.[3]

Malleolar position, or tibio-fibular rotation as it has been termed by various authors, changes in a slow, gradual fashion from year to year, with approximately 13 to 18° of external malleolar position being noted by the age of seven to eight. Whereas external femoral rotation may occur up to 13 to 14 years of age, external rotation of the tibial component is generally completed by this earlier age.[18–20]

Additionally distinction should be made between a low tibial or malleolar torsion and an internal tibial or malleolar torsion (Fig. 3.3). When the clinical measurement of the tibial

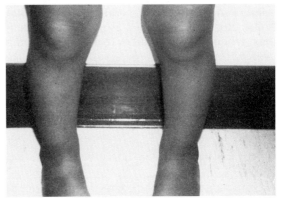

Figure 3.3 Adducted gait secondary to low tibial torsion. Note each patella is on the frontal plane, indicating normal femoral rotation.

position is less than zero, e.g. −8°, then this is a fairly significant deformity which will be difficult to be 'outgrown' as the tibia has not even attained the position which should be present at birth. On the other hand, a less significant deformity would be present if 5° of external malleolar torsion was measured in a four year old who should possess approximately 8° of tibial torsion by this time. A recent study of 281 children between one and a half years and six years of age documented what was felt to be true by other authors, viz. that there is a gradual external positioning of the tibia relative to the fibula. The data demonstrated a steady increase in external malleolar position from 5.5° at 18 months of age to 11.2° at six years of age. The data reported was consistent with the values reported by other authors that a normal adult position of 13–18° of the transmalleolar position would be achieved by seven to eight years of age.[18]

Measurement of tibial or malleolar torsion is

accomplished with the child lying on his back or seated, with his knee maintained in as extended a position as is possible. When the measurement is performed with the knee flexed to 90° and when there is an element of internal tibial position present, then the measurement of true tibial or malleolar torsion may be altered. The femoral condyles are placed equidistant from the supporting surface with the patella laying in the frontal plane. By placing his thumbs and index fingers anterior and posterior to each malleolus the examiner will be able to determine when there is an internal or external tibial torsion present by interpreting his finger position. Each malleolus is then bisected with the position mapped in relationship to the bisection of the fibular malleolus. This examination is carried out with the subtalar joint in its neutral position and the foot held at a 90° angle to the leg. Then, visualising the angle of the transmalleolar axis relative to the frontal plane, a tractograph or goniometer may be used to document the actual amount of either internal or external tibial torsion which is present (Fig. 3.4).

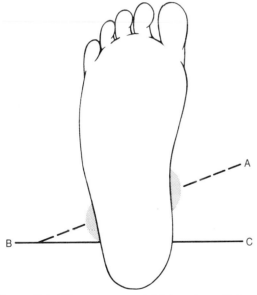

Figure 3.4 Measurement of tibial torsion utilising bisection of the malleoli.

It is important to remember that when this measurement is obtained, a closed kinetic chain situation is promoted by virtue of the examining technique. Therefore it is essential to maintain the foot in its neutral position. Inadvertent pronation of the foot will internally rotate the tibial segment and this will cause the examiner to record a lower tibial torsion than is actually present. Conversely, inadvertent supination of the foot may mask an actual low tibial torsion by externally rotating the tibial segment during examination.[21]

Tibial varum

Tibial varum may exist along with genu varum and is often considered as a portion of the overall bowing process of the distal leg. Physiologic bowing of the lower extremity is normal from birth to two to four years of age, with as much as 5–10° of normal frontal plane bowing present at birth. This bowing gradually reduces to 2–3° at approximately age two to four, and represents the normal adult value.[3, 19] When there is greater than 5° of tibial bowing present, a measure of compensation will be required from the subtalar joint in order to allow the calcaneus to assume a vertical position to the ground. In cases where tibial varum exceeds the subtalar joint range of pronation, the individual will compensate in a varus attitude throughout the gait cycle. This may lead to chronic lateral instability or to the development of a retrocalcaneal exostosis, or 'pump bump'.

In completing the differential diagnosis for severe bowing of the tibial segment, rickets and Blount's disease must be included. Although rickets is not commonly seen, the possibility of this process occurring must be borne in mind when evaluating the infant with marked genicular bowing. Causes of rickets can all be associated with a vitamin D deficiency which may be secondary to renal disease, malabsorption problems or to a general lack of the vitamin due to malnutrition.[5, 12] Any concern regarding the presence of this condition may best be diagnosed via radiographs which will determine an abnormal widening or flaring of the metaphyses.

Blount's disease, on the other hand, is due to a growth disturbance of the medial aspect of the proximal tibial epiphysis and is typically associated with a failure of epiphyseal growth followed by changes in the stress forces affecting the area. This may be manifested in two forms, viz. in the infant and in the adolescent.

The infant form is seen in the one to three year old and is most classically associated with a chubby, active child who was an early walker – prior to nine months of age. The adolescent type will be manifested somewhere between eight and thirteen years of age and is generally not as common as the infant type.

Tibial valgum

This is not a common presentation in the lower extremity. However, when present, it is generally the result of an epiphyseal injury or a malunion of a tibial fracture. In evaluating the various aetiologies for a flexible flatfoot deformity, an anteroposterior view of the ankle is necessary in order to rule out any abnormal force generated by a valgus ankle joint, with or without tibial valgum.

Ankle joint dorsiflexion

At birth there is unrestricted ankle joint dorsiflexion present so that the dorsum of the foot may approach the anterior aspect of the tibia, an angle of approximately 75°. This amount of dorsiflexion rapidly reduces to approximately 20–25° by the age of 3, 15° by age 10 and 10° by age 15 (Fig. 3.5).[3, 7] This latter value represents

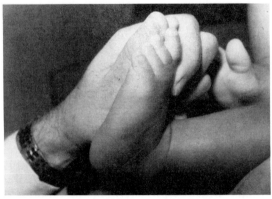

Figure 3.5   Normal ankle joint dorsiflexion in a two year old child.

the average adult norm. When a congenital tightness is present there is a consistent lack of dorsiflexion present from birth, with virtually no or minimal measurable dorsiflexion noted. When obtaining this measurement, certain

guidelines should be followed in order to ensure accurate and reproducible figures.

Generally it is best to perform this manoeuvre with the patient supine. The hip may be either flexed or extended. The foot is then maximally dorsiflexed to the leg with the subtalar joint maintained in the neutral position. This is essential as a pronated subtalar joint will cause the midtarsal joint to unlock, thereby introducing additional forefoot dorsiflexion (Fig. 3.6).[3]

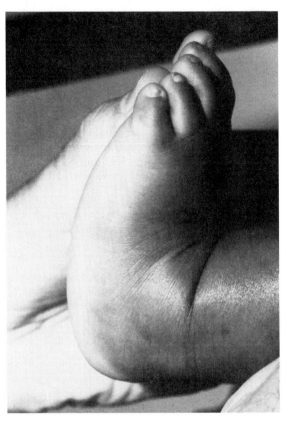

Figure 3.6   Excessive dorsiflexion of the forefoot on the hindfoot during incorrect casting of a congenital equinus has led to a rockerbottom type flatfoot. Surgical correction was required to effectively increase ankle joint motion.

Occasionally certain children may plantarflex their foot as an attempt is made to passively dorsiflex it. In these cases the plantar surface of the foot may be stroked and then the foot maximally dorsiflexed as the child is withdrawing. If this is unsuccessful the problem may be overcome by initially flexing the knee in order to dorsiflex the foot with the gastro-cnemius now relaxed and then slowly extend-ing the knee again. When recording the actual measurement, care must be taken in placing the tractograph so that one arm extends along the lateral aspect of the foot and the other accurately bisects the lower leg. When this measurement is within normal limits for the child's age, it is not necessary to retake the measurement with the knee flexed. However, when there is a marked lack of dorsiflexion, it is necessary to determine to what extent if at all the soleus is implicated. When ankle dorsi-flexion is limited with the knee extended but greater than 15° with the knee flexed, the child has a gastrocnemius equinus. When the limi-tation is present in both the knee flexed and knee extended positions then a gastrocnemius-soleus equinus is most likely responsible; an osseus ankle block would be uncommon in this age group.

When the child is being examined because he is a toe walker, extreme care must be exer-cised in measuring dorsiflexion. Although most children who exhibit tendencies towards toe walking have no lower extremity pathol-ogy, the practitioner must be able to rule out musculoskeletal as well as possible neurologi-cal conditions. When there is a true lack of dorsiflexion or brisk reflexes present upon examination, further evaluation is manda-tory.[2, 5]

The practitioner should be aware than an abnormally pronating foot may also cause an apparent equinus condition. In the older child, the pronated foot will unlock the midtarsal joint and initiate dorsiflexion of the forefoot relative to the hindfoot in gait. Over time, foot-to-leg dorsiflexion occurs at the level of the midtarsal joint rather than at the ankle joint. Subsequently, accommodative contracture of the posterior musculature gives rise to a clini-cally apparent equinus. It is this type of 'func-tional' equinus which responds well to orth-oses and stretching exercises; a true congenital equinus does not change through the use of either modality.

Subtalar joint range of motion

A functional orthosis is only appropriate for use in a paediatric patient after the child has initiated a heel–toe type of gait, a situation which generally occurs at age three to three and a half years. Prior to that time there is generally full foot contact and the gait is essen-tially apropulsive. Therefore an accurate assessment of subtalar joint motion is not an essential part of the examination until func-tional orthoses are used. Then the calcaneus is bisected and full inversion and eversion of the subtalar joint (in the same fashion employed in the adult foot) is measured. However, one im-portant difference is the range of both inver-sion and eversion that is present in the devel-oping child's foot. Just as in the other major joints of the lower extremity, the ranges of motion of the subtalar joint are much greater than the standard adult values. Therefore measurements upward of 45 to 50° of total sub-talar joint motion as compared with 20 to 30° present in the adolescent or adult foot should be expected.[3, 19]

In assessing the subtalar joint range of motion in the child's foot the borders of the posterior surface of the calcaneus should be established prior to bisecting the calcaneus. Next, the full amount of inversion and ever-sion of the foot relative to the distal one-third of the leg should be measured. Care should be taken to maintain the foot in a dorsiflexed pos-ition relative to the leg when performing this portion of the examination; a plantarflexed foot will reflect extraneous frontal plane ankle joint motion.

Midtarsal joint range of motion

A significant varus or valgus deformity, which is often related to the adult foot only, will present in the child's foot. Therefore it is essential for the practitioner to fully assess the position of the child's forefoot to hindfoot re-lationships.

This portion of the examination is the same as for the adult's foot. The child is placed in the prone position with the calcaneus properly bisected as a reference point. The subtalar joint is placed in the neutral position and the mid-tarsal joint is locked. This is accomplished by placing a dorsiflexionary force on the plantar surface of the fifth metatarsal, just proximal to the metatarsal head.[22] In this fashion, the two axes of the midtarsal joint (the oblique and the longitudinal) cross each other and limit extraneous midtarsal joint mobility upon examination. In sighting down the hindfoot towards the forefoot, a measurable varus or valgus deformity will become apparent. In no instance should the forefoot be 'loaded' with pressure directed upwards onto the first metatarsal. Such an action would unlock the midtarsal joint and supinate the longitudinal axis of the midtarsal joint, thereby initiating a false degree of forefoot varus. A forefoot varus or valgus deformity present upon examination will not be outgrown as the child develops and should be addressed. Any degree of forefoot deformity should be supported to prevent abnormal compensation during development or in later years.

Metatarsus adductus

One of the most common paediatric abnormalities which responds well to early conservative treatment is metatarsus adductus, a transverse plane deformity occurring at Lisfranc's joint, which is reflected by adduction of the metatarsals towards the midline of the body. There are several factors involved in the aetiology of this pathology, the most significant being abnormal intrauterine position with increased uterine wall compression. Other factors are a congenitally tight or malinserted abductor hallucis tendon or a tight malpositioned anterior tibial tendon. Metatarsus adductus occurs in approximately 1 : 1000 births with no sexual distinction; there is a 4–5% transmission rate to the second child regardless of the aetiology of the initial problem.[5]

The clinical picture is best visualised by placing the child's foot into a 'V' formed by the second and third fingers. The following signs are then evident:

– concave medial border,
– convex lateral border,
– prominent styloid process,
– increased metatarsus primus adductus.

There is no abnormal subtalar joint range of motion present non-weightbearing. Clinically the deformity may be classified into mild (flexible), moderate, or severe (rigid). By far, the mild to moderate forms are most prevalent,

and thereby very amenable to conservative therapy. The practitioner must also consider the possibility of a functional type of metatarsus adductus which is commonly associated with a tight or malinserted abductor hallucis tendon. As this form of metatarsus adductus often goes unnoticed until the child initiates weightbearing, it is essential for the practitioner to pull the infant into a weightbearing attitude in order to determine the presence of such pathology. The resultant loading of the forefoot which occurs is sufficient to cause the tight abductor hallucis to pull the hallux into an adducted position.

Radiography is useful in treating this deformity for two reasons. First, it allows the practitioner to determine the extent of the metatarsus adductus by measuring the specific amount of adductus present and, secondly, it provides a baseline radiograph of the pathology. The latter reason is most important as it will allow the practitioner to determine if any subluxatory changes are being initiated with over-aggressive use of serial plaster immobilisation.

The radiographic angle measured is determined utilising a bisection of the second metatarsal shaft relative to a perpendicular bisection of the lesser tarsus. The following values are acceptable during normal development:[3]

Birth	15–30°
Early walker (9–16 months)	20°
4 years	15°
Adult	15°

Positive radiographic findings associated with a metatarsus adductus are:

– an increase in the metatarsus angle,
– an apparent decrease of the adductus laterally,
– increased metatarsal base superimposition laterally,
– hypoplasia of the medial cuneiform,
– an associated metatarsus primus adductus.

A metatarsus adductus is a significant lower extremity congenital abnormality. A failure either to arrive at an early diagnosis or to initiate appropriate treatment may result in any of the following in the older child:

1. Painful styloid process.

2. Difficulty with shoe fitting in the more rigid deformity.
3. Retrograde pronatory influences into the hindfoot as the flexible type accommodates itself to footwear.
4. Early bunion formation.[2, 3]

The first line of defence in the mild to moderate form of metatarsus adductus which is diagnosed within the first few months of life is passive stretching by the parents. This form of treatment serves two purposes. It may correct a very mild metatarsus adductus, or minimally, it will increase flexibility prior to the initiation of serial plaster immobilisation.

In the moderate to severe deformity, serial plaster immobilisation is the most effective method for treating a metatarsus adductus. Whenever serial plaster immobilisation is utilised, it is best to initiate it prior to ambulation as the deformity will generally be less rigid and the casts will not hamper the child's initial attempts at walking.

A below-knee cast is most appropriate in treating the non-ambulatory child. However, when the child is ambulating, it is usual to utilise an above-knee cast for the last two applications. This is recommended as the ambulatory child will otherwise tend to circumduct the below-knee cast, leading to excessive transverse plane motion at the knee which will later cause an internally deviated limb position in gait.

Serial plaster immobilisation becomes less appropriate as the child becomes older, with only minimal positive results obtained in the child between 24 and 36 months of age. When correction becomes clinically apparent, serial plaster immobilisation should be continued for half as many times again in order to decrease the likelihood of recurrence. When too much motion is achieved too quickly, a radiograph should be taken to rule out midtarsal or subtalar joint subluxation. These are common problems created by overzealous abduction of the forefoot during casting and are to be avoided. This type of subluxation will persist into later life and actually present the patient with more potential pathology than the original complaint.

Following successful treatment with plaster, the practitioner must maintain the correction with night splints. The Ganley splint is most appropriate for this as it maintains the forefoot in a corrected position relative to the hindfoot. The splint should be utilised for approximately twice as long as the casting period in order to provide the best possible results.

In conjunction with the splint the child will have to wear straight last shoes for two to three years post casting. Reverse last shoes, or Tarsopronator shoes, should generally be avoided at any stage as these may place a constant subluxing force on the developing child's foot. Although they provide apparent cosmetic changes, these types of shoes are not acceptable from a functional point of view. In cases where there is a residual amount of metatarsus adductus present after treatment, and the child's foot exhibits some excessive pronation, rigid functional orthoses should be employed.

In cases where the child's problem is resistant to the preceding conservative therapy or initially diagnosed at a later age, surgical correction is the treatment of choice. Surgical considerations may range from soft tissue release to osteotomies depending upon the child's age and the severity of the condition.

Talipes calcaneovalgus

This condition is a positional deformity which clinically presents in a dorsiflexed, abducted and everted position of the forefoot and heel relative to the leg. In many respects, this condition represents a deformity which is the clinical antithesis of a talipes equinovarus. Talipes calcaneovalgus may be either flexible or rigid in nature and is specifically attributed to abnormal intrauterine position and compression. Typically this positional deformity is found in the first born child of a young mother who would be most likely to demonstrate tight uterine musculature thereby decreasing available space for the developing fetus.[2, 22]

Although this apparent valgus attitude of the foot relative to the leg is a common positional variation noted at birth, it generally reduces spontaneously. However, when there is a marked tightening of the peroneal musculature combined with prolonged positioning of the forefoot in an abducted and dorsiflexed position, this may require treatment. When the deformity does not spontaneously resolve in the first three to four months, then certain characteristic clinical findings other than the abnormal foot position may become evident, e.g. a marked redundancy of the lateral skin folds of the foot and ankle, an apparent tightening of the peroneal musculature and a decreased ability to move the foot into a corrected adducted, inverted and plantarflexed position. A hallmark of a more severe deformity is that when the examiner moves the foot into a corrected position, and then allows the foot to hang freely it immediately returns to its abnormal position. However, when the foot remains for several seconds in the corrected position, and then slowly moves back into the valgus attitude, then a more flexible, less severe problem exists. Additionally if the child is noted to intermittently and actively adduct and plantarflex the foot then this also indicates a more flexible deformity which may reduce spontaneously or following minimal treatment.

When the deformity is left untreated, the child will typically be a late walker. When accompanied by an external position of the femoral or tibial component, this combination makes the initial attempts at ambulation an extremely difficult undertaking. When the child finally is able to stand and walk, often as late as 16 to 20 months, the deformity generally will not spontaneously resolve due to the abducted positioning of the foot. The child's foot then proceeds to develop in a markedly pronated and abducted fashion.

It is for this reason that early treatment ranging from parental manipulative exercises and shoe therapy in the more flexible cases to serial plaster immobilisation in the more significant cases is warranted.

It must be noted that even when a more severe presentation is successfully treated via serial plaster immobilisation, night splints and shoes, prolonged treatment by means of functional foot orthoses, often for life, becomes an appropriate adjunctive treatment.[23]

Treatment considerations

The most common sequelae of abnormal transverse and frontal plane development of the lower extremities will generally be reflected in the function of the child's foot. Any significant frontal or transverse plane deviation from the norm will place an abnormal pronatory effect on the developing child's foot and will either precipitate or aggravate an existing abnormally pronated foot. It must be remembered that the child's foot undergoes constant developmental changes over the first seven to eight years. When a child first stands and initiates ambulation, his feet are 'fat, flat and floppy', with no discernible arch and an apropulsive type of gait. This appearance and function is the result of an everted calcaneus and an increased medial fat pad, along with a prerequisite to place the entire foot on to the supporting surface with each step in order to attain some degree of stability. The developing child's foot may be everted by as much as 5–10° with the initiation of weightbearing, with an average of approximately 7–8° being the norm. As the child matures and develops, the everted position of the calcaneus generally reduces to a perpendicular attitude by the age of seven to eight years. However, if the child demonstrates calcaneal eversion in excess of this degree, then it should be suspected that there is an abnormal pronatory force present which is maintaining the foot in this abnormal position (Fig. 3.7). Additionally the fat pad will

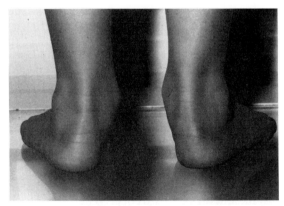

Figure 3.7 Abnormal degree of calcaneal eversion.

generally disappear and the foot will take on the overall anatomical characteristics of the adult foot. At approximately three to four years of age, the child's proprioceptive capabilities will have improved to the point where he will develop a heel-to-toe type of gait, as opposed to the full foot contact type of gait associated with the early walker.[7, 19] This is best visualised by noting when the child can manoeuvre safely up and down stairs without having to stand on a single step with both feet prior to moving on to the next step.

When a frontal or transverse plane deformity is diagnosed, then some form of treatment must be directed to the foot in order to minimise the pronatory effects of the leg. An internal femoral torsion or position, and an internal or low tibial torsion, will generally lead to adduction of the talus. The internal position of the leg and talus precipitates a closed chain pronatory effect on the developing child's foot which will maintain or aggravate the already pronated and everted attitude. This pronated foot position and function is typically increased when the child reaches the age of self-awareness at four to five years of age when he will attempt to improve the cosmetic appearance of his feet by actively abducting and pronating them to a greater extent.[1, 2]

Conversely, an external femoral torsion or position, or external tibial torsion, may also aggravate or precipitate a significant pes planus (Fig. 3.8). This occurs due to the fact that a

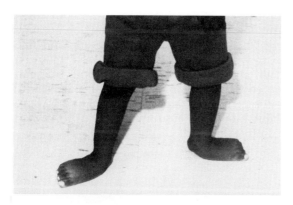

Figure 3.8 Marked external femoral and tibial torsion aggravating a bilateral talipes calcaneovalgus.

markedly abducted gait will maintain the centre of gravity in an exaggerated position medial to the subtalar joint axis. When this happens the foot is constantly maintained in an abducted and everted position with little ability for normal development. A significant genu valgum will also lead to the same type of abnormal pronatory forces being generated into the child's foot. However, this will be due

to the valgus forces being transmitted through the frontal plane displacement of the tibia. Again the centre of gravity becomes shifted to a more medial position relative to the axis of the subtalar joint, which in turn maintains the foot in its pronated and everted attitude.[21]

When the lower extremity evaluation reveals that there is abnormal compensation occurring within a child's foot or when there is a history of unsteadiness or fatigue with normal activities, then some form of functional foot orthosis will have to be employed. Although a Root type of functional foot orthosis may be prescribed in these cases, the degree of calcaneal eversion and subtalar joint pronation may be so excessive that a more aggressive type of control may become necessary. A UCBL orthosis has proved effective in controlling the abnormal pronation associated with compensated transverse plane abnormalities. With regard to heel stabilisers, there are two types which are most successfully utilised with this type of problem. A type B heel stabiliser is useful when the foot is mildly or moderately pronated. A type C heel stabiliser, which has a more aggressive medial and lateral flange, is appropriate when the foot demonstrates a greater degree of pes planus, with or without a torsional component.[2, 5] Perhaps the most successful device for use with the pronated foot associated with a compensated transverse plane deformity is a Blake type of inverted orthosis. This relies upon a cast modification in which the calcaneus is markedly inverted relative to the forefoot, thereby relying primarily on control of the calcaneus in gait.[24] Typically constructed with a deep heel cup of 20–25 mm and a hindfoot post, this device encompasses the finer points of both a Root type of orthosis and a heel stabiliser to improve function and to disallow abnormal pronation.

In cases where a child functions with an internal femoral position and an adducted gait either a gait plate or a type D heel stabiliser may be used. Both devices will promote a more abducted gait. However, they may accomplish this while simultaneously introducing some degree of increased pronation into the hindfoot. For that reason they should be used with caution. In addition, since these devices are constructed in a significantly different fashion from the previously described orthoses, they generally require replacement more frequently if they are to remain effective. Such devices are fabricated with an extension distal to the fourth and fifth metatarsophalangeal joints. This rigid lever arm effect will alter propulsion so that the child will be forced to pronate and to abduct his foot in gait.[7] Not only does this improve the cosmetic appearance of the foot, but it will also dynamically assist in stretching whatever tight medial musculature might be associated with an internal femoral or tibial position. Additionally, the devices are appropriate for use in the older child who has a torsional component as the aetiology of their adducted gait; who may function more efficiently in a more abducted position. Again, due to the fact that these devices are ineffective once their lateral aspects become proximal to the fourth and fifth metatarsophalangeal joints, they require close monitoring.

When one of the functional foot orthoses is chosen to restrict the abnormal pronation associated with a compensated transverse plane deformity, parents should be made aware of the two specific aspects of the devices. First, the orthoses are likely to worsen the overall cosmetic appearance of the child. When, for example, the child is adducted in gait and demonstrates 5° of calcaneal eversion during gait, there will be an increase in the adducted position of the foot by approximately 5° when the heel is controlled in a vertical position. Although this increased adducted position may appear worse to the parents, it typically improves the function of the foot in gait and will greatly reduce any concomitant instability or fatigue. Second, parents should be made aware of the fact that the devices will typically be effective for a period of approximately two years. Once the distal aspect of the orthosis reaches the midshaft portion of the metatarsals or the heel cup becomes too narrow, it has significantly lost its effectiveness. The child may complain of symptoms at that time as well, as the device will place excess pressure in the heel cups, arch or forefoot area.

With regard to the use of night splints for treatment of the transverse plane deformities discussed in this chapter it must be appreciated that there are as many different opinions as to the effectiveness of the splints as there are splints available. Many agree that although a splint may be effective in cases of internal tibial position or internal tibial torsion, there does not seem to be any indication for the use of splints for femoral rotation problems. In response to this the fact that most children with a transverse plane deformity assume sitting and sleeping attitudes that tend to reflect a position of comfort or reinforcement of their rotational problems should be remembered. Although a parent may admonish a child to stop sitting with their legs tucked in underneath their buttocks and to encourage cross-legged or straight-legged position while playing, altering an abnormal sleeping position cannot be easily encouraged. It is this author's feeling that night splints do have at least some degree of a corrective influence on the developing child's limbs in these cases. When a child with an internal transverse plane deformity can be kept from sleeping on his stomach, with the lateral aspect of his feet against the mattress, some positive change will be anticipated. Conversely, a child with an externally rotated limb will also typically sleep on his stomach, but generally with the medial aspect of his feet against the mattress. Again, a splint utilised for this pathology should precipitate a positive change. In both cases, the described position of comfort, maintained for 10 to 14 hours of daily sleeping and napping will not only reinforce the deformity, but will also decrease the likelihood of spontaneous resolution. The use of a splint will alter the child's sleeping position and will prohibit him from assuming such a position of comfort (Fig. 3.9).

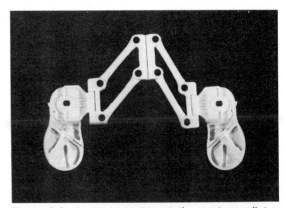

Figure 3.9 Langer counter rotation system splint.

In cases where there is an internal tibial position or an internal tibial torsion, a night splint may be successfully utilised to improve the situation. Although there are varied opinions as to whether or not the correction actually occurs within the long axis of the tibia or within the soft tissues surrounding the knee, the fact remains that generally a measurable clinical difference following completion of therapy will be maintained.[2, 5, 25]

Regardless of which of the available splints is chosen there are a few general guidelines which apply to all devices. In treating internally rotated problems subluxation of the child's foot must be avoided. This is one of the common abnormal sequelae of long-term splint use. When the foot is markedly abducted by means of a night splint, the first area to be affected is the midtarsal and subtalar joints. Excessive, prolonged abduction will potentially lead to a severe flatfoot deformity unless certain precautions are maintained. This is easily accomplished in the more rigid splints by placing a varus wedge in the child's shoes or by introducing a 10–15° varus bend into the bar itself. Additionally the available amount of external rotation which is present should not be vigorously exceeded. Setting a splint at an extremely deviated position which is greatly in excess of the total amount of external rotation present will not only make the use of the bar an uncomfortable proposition for the child but may well lead to avascular necrosis of the head of the femur. Carefully assessing the total degree of external positioning available at the hip, knee and tibia and then slowly approaching that combined external position will generally yield a satisfactory result.[12]

Conversely, marked adduction of an externally deviated hip, knee or tibia via a night splint may precipitate a dislocated hip in infants and children with a dislocatable hip. Due to the fact that a dislocatable hip cannot be seen on radiographs and that the clinical tests for this condition are questionable at best, even in the neonate, extreme caution must be exercised. Adduction of the feet past midline may generate sufficient pressure to dislocate an unstable hip.

When the decision is made to utilise a splint, parents should be aware of the protracted nature of the treatment plan and they should be prepared to use the splint for a period of at least one year in some instances. When marked measurable change is not evident after one year's use of the splint, the decision to alter the type of splint being used or to abandon that method of treatment should be considered. In any event, night splint therapy can be a useful adjunct in the overall management of the child with transverse plane pathology. The initial decision as to whether or not to utilise a splint should be based on the child's age, the extent and level of the deformity, and the degree of compensation in gait.

When the child is adducted, yet relatively stable and not demonstrating any signs consistent with abnormal pronation of the foot, treatment may not be necessary at all. However, when signs of moderate to severe compensation are present, treatment combining both night splints and custom foot orthoses should be employed in order to provide the child with the best chance of eventually developing a normal gait pattern.

Early recognition and treatment of the common transverse and frontal plane deformities outlined in this chapter will hopefully lead to a child whose lower extremities are mechanically sound and efficient and capable of carrying him into adolescence and then adulthood in a comfortable and efficient fashion. The ability to identify those children who require treatment, as well as the ability to identify the type and the extent of the treatment eventually employed, is dependent upon the individual practitioner's ability to accurately assess the lower limb development of the young child and to appropriately identify those children requiring treatment.

References

1 LaPorta G. Torsional abnormalities. *Arch Podiatr Med Foot Surg* 1973; 1: 47–61.
2 McCrea JD. *Pediatric Orthopedics of the Lower Extremity*. Mount Kisco, NY, Futura Publishing Company, 1985.
3 Sgarlato TE. *A Compendium of Podiatric Biomechanics*. San Francisco, California College of Podiatric Medicine, 1971.
4 Crane L. Femoral torsion and its relation to toeing-in and toeing-out. *J Bone Joint Surg* 1959; 41A: 255.
5 Tax H. *Podopediatrics*. Baltimore, Williams and Wilkins, 1980.

6 Elffman H. Torsion of the lower extremity. *Am J Phys Anthropol* 1945; 3: 255.

7 Valmassy RL. Biomechanical evaluation of the child. *Clin Podiatry, Podopediatr* 1984; 1(3): 563–79.

8 Shands AR, Steele MK. Torsion of the femur. *J Bone Joint Surg*, 1958; 40A: 47–61.

9 Staheli LT, Engel GM. Tibial torsion, a new method of assessment and a survey of normal children. *Clin Orthoped Rel Res* 1977; Number 86.

10 Weseley MS, Berenfeld PA, Einstein AL. Thoughts on in-toeing and out-toeing: Twenty years experience with over 5,000 cases and a review of the literature. *Foot Ankle* 1981; 2 (1): 41–46.

11 Schuster RD. In-toe and out-toe and its implications. *Arch Podiatr Med Foot Surg* 1976; 3 (4).

12 Tachdjian MO. *Pediatric Orthopedics*. Philadelphia, WB Saunders Company, 1972.

13 Valmassy RL, Day S. Congenital dislocation of the hip. *J Am Podiatr Med Assoc* 1985; 75 (9): 466–471.

14 Barlow TG. Early diagnosis and treatment of congenital dislocation of the hip. *J Bone Joint Surg* 1967; 44B: 292.

15 VonRosen, S. Treatment of congenital dislocation of the hip in the newborn. *Proc Roy Soc Med* 1963; 56; 801.

16 Kite J. Torsion of the legs in young children. *Clinical Orthopedics*, Number 16. Philadelphia PA, JB Lippincott, 1960.

17 Hutter CG Jr, Scott W. Tibial torsion. *J Bone Joint Surg* 1949; 31: 511.

18 Rosen H, Sandwick H. The measurement of tibiofibular torsion. *J Bone Joint Surg* 1955; 37A: 847.

19 Root ML. A discussion of biomechanical considerations for treatment of the infant foot. *Arch Podiatr Med Foot Surg* 1973; 1: 41–46.

20 Swanson AB, Greene PW, Allis HD. Rotational deformities of the lower extremity in children and their significance. *Clin Orthoped Rel Res* 1963; Vol. 27.

21 Valmassy RL, Stanton B. Tibial torsion, normal values in children. *J Am Podiatr Med Assoc* 1989; 79 (9): 432–435.

22 Root ML, Orien WD, Weed JH. *Normal and Abnormal Function of the Foot*. Los Angeles, Clinical Biomechanics Corporation, 1977.

23 Ganley JV. Lower extremity examination of the infant. *J Am Podiatr Assoc* 1981; 71 (2): 92–98.

24 Blake RL. Inverted Orthotic Technique, *J Am Podiatr Med Assoc* 1986; (5) May, p. 801.

25 Schoenhaus HD, Poss KD. The clinical and practical aspects in treating torsional problems in children. *J Am Podiatry Assoc* 1977; 67 (9): September.

4

Radiological Examination of the Child's Foot

Iain McCall and Victor Cassar-Pullicino

The standard radiograph has provided an easy and cost-effective method for assessing the foot. Most bone conditions may be diagnosed and the structural alignment and dynamics of the foot easily analysed with these techniques. In recent years there have been a number of technological advances which have increased the scope of investigation but which have not replaced the radiograph. Techniques such as computed tomography and magnetic resonance have increased the range of structures that can be imaged and in particular can allow visualisation of muscles, tendons, nerves and arteries without the use of contrast agents. The gamma camera with emission computed tomography using Tc99 labelled bone seeking compounds such as methylene diphosphonate (MDP) has provided a means of assessing the dynamics of bone turnover, which is sensitive if non-specific and enables the identification of early lesions. However, the continued importance of the plain radiograph makes it pertinent that the first consideration should be the radiological investigation of the feet and assessment of the normal development and anatomical variants of development which have no pathological importance save to avoid the mistaken diagnosis of disease.

Radiological technique

The radiological examination of the ankle and foot requires a few standard views in order to demonstrate the major areas of interest, due to the overlapping structures and multiplicity of normal variants. Routine views of the ankle include an anteroposterior (AP) and a lateral

(see Figs. 4.4 and 4.5), the former being undertaken with slight dorsiflexion of the ankle and pronation of the foot. In order to evaluate the entire ankle joint space and distal talofibular articulation, the ankle must be internally rotated by 15–20°. The talofibular joint is well demonstrated in this view. Oblique views taken at 45° of external and internal rotation may demonstrate the medial malleolus more clearly but the value is limited. Stress views of the ankle in the AP projection may occasionally demonstrate ligament laxity but comparison with the normal side is essential as the range of normal is wide. Angulation over 20° or a difference of more than 5° between the two ankles is, however, invariably abnormal and some centres undertake injection of local anaesthetic in the ligaments prior to stress views in order to obliterate any guarding effect due to pain.

The exposure must be adequate to penetrate bone but not too great to blacken out the soft tissues. Demonstration of displacement of the soft tissue outline is of great importance in injury. The pre Achilles tendon fat pad may be obliterated or displaced by haemorrhage following tears to the ligament or from calcaneal fractures. An ankle effusion is demonstrated by a bulging soft tissue mass displacing the fat line anteriorly and posteriorly.

Routine views of the foot include AP, lateral and oblique projections. The anteroposterior view requires two different exposures and centring points for the forefoot and hindfoot. The central beam is perpendicular to the plate for the forefoot but is angled 17° cephalad for the midfoot. The oblique view is performed with the patient supine, the knee flexed and internally rotated and the lateral aspect of the foot elevated 30° from the cassette. The central beam is perpendicular to the cassette and centred over the base of the third metatarsal. The lateral view is usually taken with the lateral aspect of the foot placed against the cassette. Both AP and lateral views may be obtained weightbearing which enhances structural changes that may not be detected on the non-weightbearing films (see Fig. 4.10). Axial views of the calcaneus involve the beam being angled 40° cranially to the cassette with the back of the heel resting on the cassette. This may also be undertaken with the patient weightbearing, standing on the cassette with the tube angled 45° axially, centred on the posterior ankle joint (see Fig. 4.19A, B). The subtalar joints require specialised views due to their individual angle. The lateral oblique is performed with the limb rotated 60° from the lateral and on a 17° board wedge. The foot is dorsiflexed and the beam is centred one inch below the medial malleolus and angled 25° to the foot. This view shows the posterior and anterior joints well. The third view is the medial oblique, which has the lower limb rotated medially through 60° and placed on a 30° wedge. The beam is centred on the lateral malleolus and angled 10° cephalad. The sinus tarsus is best demonstrated on these views. The sesamoid bones may be seen on the AP and lateral views but tangential views may also be performed with the patient prone, the toes pushed upwards against the cassette and the beam tangential to the first metatarsal. Weightbearing tangential views of the hindfoot may be obtained with the patient standing in special radiolucent blocks (Coby's views). This demonstrates the line of weightbearing through the talus and calcaneus.

Linear tomography

Linear tomography provides an image in a selected plane, while blurring out structures above and below that plane. It has proved highly valuable in the past but has been largely superseded by computed tomography but it remains of value in defining the extent of tethering injury. Injuries and necrosis of the talus may also be well demonstrated and any subtle fracture may be evaluated by this method. This is the best method of evaluating bone when metal is present in the foot. Tomograms in both the AP and lateral planes may be required.

Computed tomography

The anatomy of the foot in the axial plane may now be demonstrated in great detail by computed tomography (CT) which will also image sagittally and coronally (frontal plane) (see Figs. 4.13B, 4.19D). The technique involves a rotating X-ray source with an arc of X-ray detectors. The whole system rotates about the foot and the X-ray absorption over multiple projections is measured. The multitude of numbers translated into a grey scale are built up to produce an image which may be manipulated by varying the level and the grey scale, thus allowing both the bone and the soft tissue to be clearly delineated. The acquisition time is now fast and the detail excellent. The angle and position of the slice may be chosen from the scout film and the foot is positioned within the gantry according to the plane of the scan. The technique is particularly good for evaluating the subtalar joints and hindfeet.[1]

Skeletal scintigraphy

Radioactive isotopes, which are used in imaging, produce gamma rays during their decay process. Technetium-99(m) is such an isotope and is particularly useful as the energy of the gamma rays are ideal for imaging in a gamma camera. It has a relatively short half-life and is easily produced. It also combines well with phosphonate compounds, which act as a transportation system to bone. Following intravenous injection of the Tc MDP, the foot can be imaged immediately to identify the isotope in the blood vessels and within three minutes of the injection to demonstrate any increase in activity in the extracellular fluid which may indicate increased vascularity. After three hours the isotope will have cleared from the soft tissue while remaining in bone (see Fig. 4.6). Thus any area that has localised increased blood flow or increased bone activity will show a higher uptake of isotope than the normal surrounding bone. This feature is highly sensitive and a normal bone scan will largely rule out a pathological bone abnormality. However, it does not identify specific disorders and tumours, fractures, arthritis and infection may all be manifested by increased activity on both phases of the scans. Isotope scanning is particularly valuable in identifying the early lesions shortly after the onset of symptoms but before radiographic changes have manifested themselves. However, normal variations do occur in children and in particular there is increased uptake at the normal growth plates (see Fig. 4.6). Greater specificity for the diagnosis of infection may be achieved using other isotopes such as gallium 67 or by labelling white blood cells with indium III. More recently techniques to label white cells with technetium-99(m) have also been developed. The cell labelling studies are particularly valuable when infection is superimposed over trauma or after surgery.

Ultrasound

When a sonic beam is applied to a structure the strength of the echo at the boundary of two substances is related to their different acoustic impedance. Bone and soft tissue have widely differing acoustic impedance so that almost all the sound is reflected. However, in the foot the soft tissues are easily accessible and are superficial to the bone (see Fig. 4.24B). Sonography will therefore demonstrate tendons, muscles and ligaments[2] and peritendinous fluid accumulation may be detected in cases of tendinitis. Fluid collections in abscesses may also be clearly defined and the ability to visualise structures in real time permits tendon movements to be studied. Its role in relation to magnetic resonance has yet to be fully evaluated but it has a major advantage in its low cost, ease of access and rapid examination time.

Arthrography

The cartilage outline in joints cannot be visualised on plain radiographs without the injection of water soluble contrast medium, air or both. The injections into the joint are simple to perform and have been particularly valuable in assessing the ankle joint (see Fig. 4.15). Ligamentous injury around the joint may be demonstrated by leakage of contrast but should be performed as soon after injury as possible.[3] Injury to the lateral complex may also be confirmed by injecting contrast into the peroneal tendon sheath, which will flow into the joint. Connections from the ankle to the posterior subtalar joint and the flexor tendons are a normal variant and occur in 10% and 20% respectively.[4]

Arthrography of the subtalar joints by injecting the talonavicular joint may be valuable in differentiating normal from fibrous or cartilaginous coalition.

Magnetic resonance imagining

This new technique depends upon the intrinsic magnetism of the hydrogen proton and its response when affected by various magnetic fields. The hydrogen proton will alter its magnetic alignment when given energy in the form of a radiowave and will give back this energy in a similar way after removal of the stimulus. This is called relaxation and the density of the hydrogen protons and their differing speeds of relaxation with different tissues enable a detailed tissue image to be produced when analysed by computer. Two types of relaxation are usually used in imaging. These are the spin–lattice or T1 relaxation and the spin–spin or T2 relaxation. The use of different pulse sequences which vary the time of pulse repetition and echo measurement, i.e. T1 or T2 weighting, will enable differing tissues to be highlighted (Fig. 4.1).

The advantage of magnetic resonance is its ability to demonstrate tissues such as cartilage, ligaments and synovium which are not visible on X-rays and to identify tissue types and fluids more precisely. It is presently used for diagnosis of avascular necrosis and cartilage disorders, particularly of the talus, for tumours and vascular lesions of the foot and for ligament and tendon injuries. However, its role is constantly being evaluated and developed.

Developmental skeletal anatomy

The bony skeleton develops from a cartilage template by means of enchondral ossification

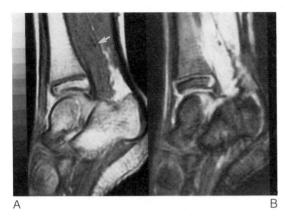

A   B

Figure 4.1 Haemangioma – magnetic resonance scan. A, T1 weighted image, showing the bright signal of marrow and subcutaneous fat, the slow signal of ligaments, cortical bone and tendons and the intermediate signal of muscle. The low signal of phleboliths are demonstrated (arrow) and there is an accessory soleus in the pre-Achilles triangle. B, T2 weighted image showing the intermediate signal of marrow and muscle and the relatively higher signal of articular cartilage, due to its increased water content. The very bright signal of the haemangioma is seen involving the soleus and accessory muscles.

in primary diaphyseal centres with secondary centres appearing later at the bone ends in the epiphyses. Ossification of the diaphyses occurs early in fetal life but some primary and most secondary epiphyseal centres appear after birth. Fusion of these secondary centres occurs in the second decade.

The only tarsal bones consistently ossified at birth are the talus and calcaneus. The remainder begin to ossify early in the first decade (Fig. 4.2A,B,C,D). Initially most of the bones are cartilage so that lucent spaces on the radiograph between the ossification centres are wide. The cartilage matrix of the partially ossified bone may, however, be demonstrated on magnetic resonance. The development of the ossification centres follows a reasonably predictable format and ageing of the skeleton may be achieved by comparing the appearance against standard references (Fig. 4.2).[5]

Growth of the epiphyses and ossification centres in the tarsal bones may not always be sharply defined. Irregularity of the distal tibial and fibular growth plates is common and may contain small areas of ossification. These should not be confused with fractures or areas of infection. The rate of ossification may be irregular and this enhances the appearance of the abnormality.

The epiphysis of the calcaneus can often be irregular, fragmented and sclerotic, despite the fact that this is a normal finding. The calcaneus may develop from two ossification centres, sometimes mimicking a fracture, while overlap of epiphyseal lines or other adjacent bones may also cause confusion in cases of trauma. All tarsal bones may ossify in a very irregular fashion and this may appear rather sclerotic, which in the case of the navicular may mimic osteonecrosis or Kohler's disease.

Conical epiphyseal ossification centres may be seen in the phalanges of asymptomatic children. These changes have been noted in 4–26% of children 4–15 years old and are usually bilateral and may fuse earlier than the normal epiphysis. Dysplastic splitting of the epiphysis or metaphyseal margin is not uncommon and has been noted more commonly in the distal phalanx of the great toe.[6] The epiphyses at the base of the proximal phalanx of the first toe may divide, also be sclerotic and develop as a single ossification centre and then develop a cleft (Fig. 4.3).[7] Incomplete developmental fissures may also be seen through the proximal phalanx of the first toe, distally and laterally. Similar fissures are seen in other toes.

Accessory ossification centres are common in the ankle and foot. Both medial and lateral malleoli may have centres at the distal tip and these must not be confused with avulsion fractures. These centres occur medially in 17–24% of females and up to 47% of males. Most are bilateral and commonly ossify between 6 and 12 years. The well defined cortical margins and the lack of a sharp line between the two bones should enable an accurate diagnosis (Fig. 4.4).

The secondary ossification centre of the talus is located posteriorly. It appears at 8–11 years and normally fuses at 16–20 years. It is the posterior part of the talar tubercle and is located lateral to the flexor hallucis longus tendon. When it does not fuse, it is called the os trigonum and may separate in forced plantar flexion (Fig. 4.5). A small anterior os supratalare may also cause confusion with a fracture.

On the medial aspect of the navicular an accessory ossicle develops in the tendon of tibialis posterior. It is usually situated slightly proximal to the main body of the navicular and may affect tendon function when growth is

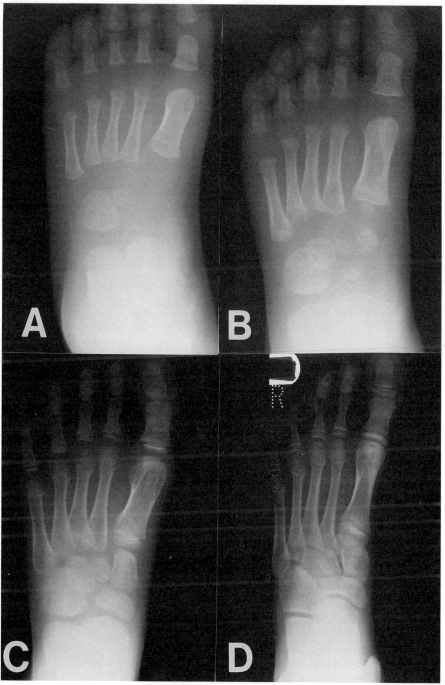

Figure 4.2   Normal development of the ossification centres of the foot at ages 18 months (A), 3 years (B), 6 years (C) and 10 years (D).

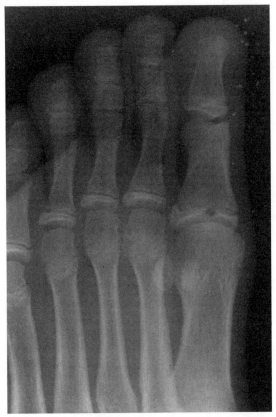

Figure 4.3 The ossification centre of the base of the first proximal phalanx of the great toe is divided in the centre. This may be misinterpreted as a fracture.

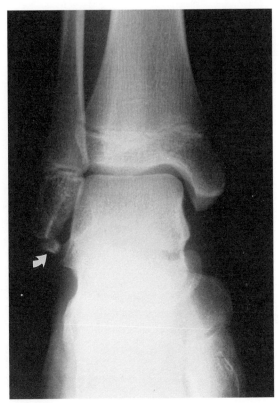

Figure 4.4 Os subfibulare. This AP view of the ankle shows the os subfibulare below the fibula (arrow) and is differentiated from a fracture by its complete cortication.

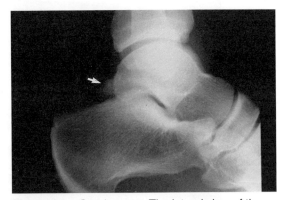

Figure 4.5 Os trigonum. The lateral view of the talus shows the persistent separation of the posterior talar ossification centre (arrow).

accelerated during puberty (Fig. 4.6A,B).[8] The os supranaviculare is located on the dorsal margin of the navicular, distal to the joint space. It may cause a substantial lump and pain may ensue. On isotope scanning, increased activity may be seen in cases of pain. This suggests a stress phenomenon and they must not be confused with an avulsion fracture (Fig. 4.6B). Accessory ossification centres are also found at the distal end of the first metatarsals, while duplication of ossification centres of metatarsal heads may occur. Os intermetatarsum is variable in size and shape, lying between the base of the first and second metatarsal. It may be bilateral, separate or attached.

Multiple sesamoid bones are present in the foot. The os peroneum is commonly seen on the inferolateral aspect of the cuboid, lying in the tendon of the peroneus longus, and may be multicentric and very large (Fig. 4.7). All the metatarsal heads may have sesamoids but the two of the first metatarsals are always present.

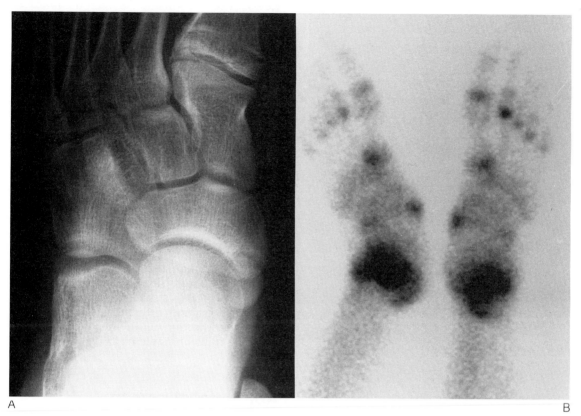

Figure 4.6 Accessory naviculi. A, The well defined ossicle is situated promixal and medial to the navicular. B, The increased isotope activity is seen at the site of the accessory navicular. Normal activity is also seen at the ossifying epiphyseal plates. Abnormal activity is seen in the head of the right second metatarsal consistent with Frieberg's disease.

However, these appearances may vary and bipartite or multipartite bones, some of which are sclerotic, are not uncommon.

The accessory ossification centres and sesamoids are summarised in Fig. 4.8.

Other important lesions include the talar beak, which is a developmental variant and may be very large; projections of cortical bone from the surface may be seen in some tarsal bones.

Developmental calcaneal spurs may be seen in infants and will disappear by the age of one.

Calcaneal cysts may be simulated by the normal arrangement of the trabecular pattern in the body of the calcaneus.

Finally spur-like enlargements of the distal phalanx of the great toe may mimic an osteochondroma but are a normal finding and of no clinical significance.

Alignment of the foot

The talocalcaneal joints are the basis of the alignment of the hindfoot. In young children the anatomic relationship of the talus and calcaneus is demonstrated on the AP and lateral views. Lines drawn along the longitudinal axis of these bones serve to identify their relationship. The lines are usually constructed through the mid axis of each hindfoot bone but when delineation of the bones is poor on the AP view, the medial cortex of the talus and the lateral cortex of the calcaneus may be utilised. The accuracy of these lines is also lost in the very young when the amount of ossification is limited, giving a different configuration from the mature bone.

The normal angle in infants is between 30 and 50°[9] and there is a progressive decrease in

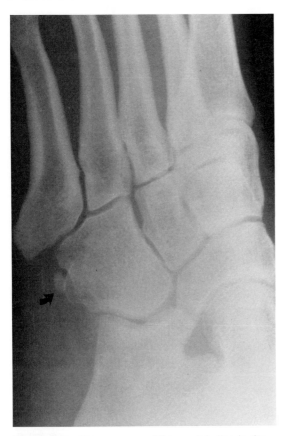

Figure 4.7 Os peroneum. This ossicle lies in the tendon of peroneus longus and is seen on the oblique view of the foot (arrow).

the angle until the age of five when it is between 15 and 30°

In the lateral projection, the midtalar–midcalcaneal angle does not change with age and ranges between 25 and 50° and is usually between 37 and 45°.[10]

The normal relationship of the talus and calcaneus may also be assessed by relating it to the metatarsals on the AP view. The midtarsal line passes through or just medial to the first metatarsal and the midcalcaneal line passes through the fourth or fifth metatarsal. Such relationships are not significantly affected by inversion or adduction.

On the lateral view, the extension of the midaxial line of the talus aligns closely with the first metatarsal. In certain normal children under five with a relative degree of hindfoot valgus the talar axis may pass medial to and below the first metatarsal on the two respective

views.[9] The relationship between the hindfoot could be better made with the midfoot rather than the metatarsals but in infants and small children there is insufficient ossification on the bones. However, the relationship of the navicular to the talus may be a valuable indication of malalignment in older children. In normal circumstances it lies immediately anteriorly to the talus in both AP and lateral views.

The forefoot is quite flexible and the appearances may therefore change with weightbearing and non-weightbearing films. However, on the AP films there is generally convergence and slight overlaps of the base of the metatarsals, while considerable superimposition is the norm for the lateral, where the first metatarsal is superior and the fifth inferiorly positioned.

Due to the limited ossification of bones and the abundant plantar fat, the arch of the foot is difficult to assess in the infant. However, when pressure is applied the angle between the calcaneus and fifth metatarsal is usually obtuse on the lateral. In the older child on standing films an angle of 150–175° is usually seen.

Abnormal alignment

Pure hindfoot malalignment at the subtalar joint results in altered relationship between the talus and the metatarsals but the relationship of the midfoot and forefoot to the calcaneus is maintained. The ankle mortise limits movement of the talus relative to the tibia and therefore the calcaneus moves relative to the talus.

Hindfoot valgus

The calcaneus is displaced laterally in the axial plane and on the AP view there is an increase in the talocalcaneal angle, with abduction of the calcaneus (Fig. 4.9A,B). The midfoot and forefoot moves laterally and as the talus is inhibited in axial movement by the ankle mortise, the longitudinal axis of the talus lies medial to the first metatarsal. If the navicular is ossified it will lie lateral to the anterior surface of the talus. On the lateral weightbearing view there is increased talar plantar flexion as the lateral movement of the calcaneus reduces

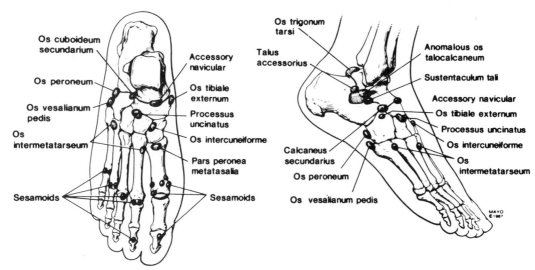

Figure 4.8 The accessory ossicles in the foot are demonstrated. Reproduced from Berquist *et al.*[17]

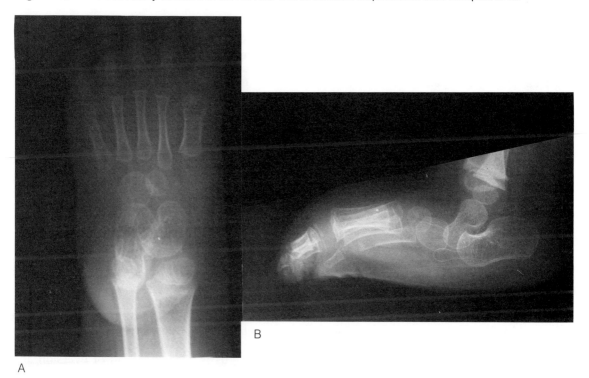

A

B

Figure 4.9 Congenital vertical talus. A. On the AP view the calcaneus is displaced laterally to the talus, although in this case the degree of hindfoot valgus is limited. B, The lateral view shows the vertical talus. The navicular is not yet ossified.

support for the anterior talus. In severe cases an almost vertical talus may be produced. In these circumstances, the normal longitudinal arch is lost. The navicular may descend with the talus or will dislocate dorsally and relate to the dorsum of the talus (Fig. 4.9B). Hindfoot valgus occurs in planovalgus, congenital vertical talus and neuromuscular abnormalities.

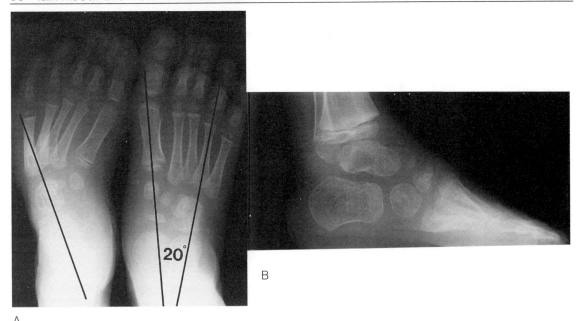

Figure 4.10   A, Talipes equinovarus of the left foot. The talus and calcaneus are superimposed and the longitudinal axis of the talus is lateral to the first metatarsal. There is inversion and adduction of the forefoot. In comparison, the right foot is normal, with an angle between the talus and calcaneus and the longitudinal axis of each bone passing along the first and fourth metatarsals respectively. B, The lateral view demonstrates the talus and calcaneus to be parallel to each other.

Congenital vertical talus may be associated with chromosomal abnormalities, arthrogryposis or myelomeningoceles. It is more common in males and muscle imbalance is a prominent aetiological factor.

Hindfoot varus

The calcaneus, midfoot and forefoot are displaced medially relative to the talus, with the additional inversion of the calcaneus. The longitudinal axis of the talus is lateral to the first metatarsal and the talocalcaneal angle is decreased (Fig. 4.10A,B). The navicular projects medially to its normal position. The adduction of the calcaneus leads to dorsal angulation of the talus on the lateral view, with the longitudinal axes of talus and calcaneus becoming parallel and more horizontal than normal (Fig. 4.9B). Hindfoot varus is commonly seen in congenital equinovarus and certain neuromuscular disorders.

Midfoot equinus is seen when the angle between the calcaneus and the tibia is greater than 90° and occurs in congenital equinovarus and vertical talus.

Forefoot abnormalities

Inversion and adduction of the forefoot combined is referred to as forefoot varus. Inversion is recognised on the lateral as a stepladder effect of the metatarsals and an increase in overlap on the AP views (Fig. 4.10A and B). Medial deviation of the forefoot alone is seen in metatarsus adductus (Fig. 4.11), and inversion is added in congenital equinovarus. Forefoot valgus is a combination of eversion and forefoot adduction with the radiographic signs being opposite and may be seen in congenital vertical talus and neuromuscular disorders.

Congenital equinovarus is a combination of forefoot adduction, hindfoot varus and hindfoot equinus. Medial subluxation of the navicular on the talus and a marked degree of inversion is generally present. On an AP radiograph, the talocalcaneal angle is decreased and

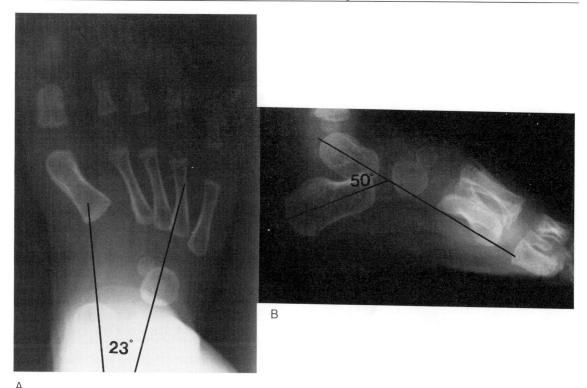

Figure 4.11   Metatarsus adductus. The relationship between the talus and calcaneus is normal, both in the AP (A) and the lateral (B) view. There is medial deviation of the forefoot.

the midtalar line lies lateral to the base of the first metatarsal. On the lateral view the calcaneus is plantarflexed and the talus and calcaneus nearly parallel. Medial deviation of the forefoot is present on the AP view with a greater overlap of the metatarsal bases (Fig. 4.10).

Pes Planus

When the calcaneus does not maintain its normal dorsiflexion, the longitudinal arch is decreased and the angle between the inferior surface of the calcaneus and the axis of the fifth metatarsal is increased. Pes planus is present in planovalgus foot, tarsal coalition, spastic flatfoot and congenital calcaneovalgus foot. Flexible flatfoot is the most common form of hindfoot valgus. The midtalar line projects medial to the first metatarsal. However, there is normal dorsi- and plantarflexion of the foot.

Pes Cavus

Increased dorsiflexion of the calcaneus and an associated increased plantarflexion of the metatarsals produce an abnormally prominent longitudinal arch. Cavus arch may be associated with hindfoot valgus or varus and is a prominent feature of some neuromuscular abnormalities, particularly Charcot–Marie–Tooth disease.

Fractures

The appearance of ankle and foot fractures in children depends upon the growth plate development, the relationship of the ligaments to the epiphyses and the mechanism of injury. Distal diaphyseal or metaphyseal fractures of the ankle may be of the greenstick type, with buckling of the anterior tibia and a cortical break posteriorly. However, fractures of the distal tibia and fibula frequently involve the growth plate[11] which may result in growth or articular deformity when the diagnosis and proper treatment are not made. In children the growth plates are weaker than the ligaments, so fractures of the physis occur more frequently than ligament injuries. Fractures of the growth plate are also more common in the first year and during rapid growth phases in the early teens. Such fractures are usually secondary to shearing or crushing forces and are described by the Salter and Harris classification (see Chapter 10). Type I are uncommon[11] and tend to occur more commonly in children under five years of age (Fig. 4.12). Type II are

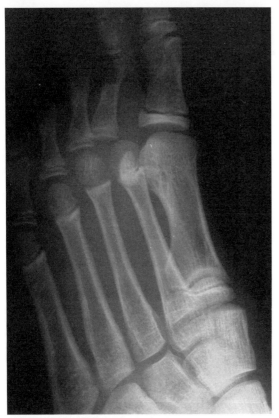

Figure 4.12 Type I fracture. The head of the third metatarsal is rotated following a fracture across the epiphyseal plate. The metaphysis is intact.

the most common and are often found in the over 10 year old. Type III spares the metaphysis and is usually caused by an intra-articular shearing force (Fig. 4.13A,B). Type IV requires

complete reduction to prevent growth disturbances[12] and makes up about 10% of physeal injuries (Fig. 4.14A,B). Finally Type V are the result of compression injuries and may involve other bones and joints and are the most uncommon.

Most epiphyseal injuries of the ankle may be clearly defined using the routine AP, lateral and mortise view. Fractures of the fibular physis are the most common and may be subtle. More complex physical injuries are sometimes best evaluated by CT, which clearly demonstrates the epiphyseal fragmentation and the distal tibiofibular relationship. It is important to define the degree of articular involvement and the degree of separation as displacement of more than 2 mm has significant treatment implications.[13]

The most common complication of growth plate fracture is premature or asymmetrical fusion. Type III and IV tibial fractures with greater than 2 mm displacement, comminuted fractures and Type V fractures have the highest risk, occurring in 32% of one series.[14] Growth plate deformity, due to arrest, will become evident from six months to a year after injury and may lead to leg length discrepancy or angulation deformity (Fig. 4.14B). Standing AP and lateral films of the ankle will suffice for follow-up but AP and lateral tomograms possibly supplemented by CT will be required in order to identify the extent of the tether when surgical treatment is contemplated. Leg length discrepancy is best measured by scannograms, which may either be performed with a special grid system or by CT.

Injuries to the tarsal bones

Fractures or fracture dislocation of the talus are rare in children.[15] The talus serves to support the body weight and to distribute the forces to the foot. It ossifies from a primary centre in its neck with maturation completing between 16 and 20 years. Articular cartilage covers a substantial amount of the surface and there are no direct muscle or tendon attachments. This limits the blood supply which is mainly provided by a branch of the posterior tibial artery, which supplies the inferior neck and most of the body. Branches of the dorsalis pedis artery enter the superior aspect of the

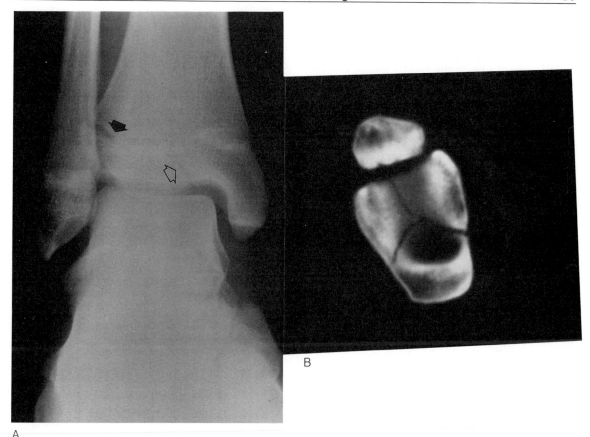

A

B

Figure 4.13   Type III fracture. A, There is a vertical fracture through the epiphysis (arrow) and along the epiphyseal plate, causing slight displacement (arrow). B, The value of CT is clearly demonstrated in evaluating the extent of the fracture.

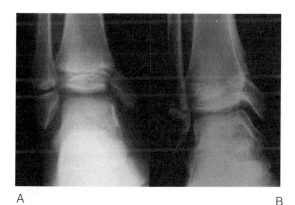

A   B

Figure 4.14   Type IV fracture. A, the vertical fracture of the medial aspect of the epiphysis extends through to the metaphysis. B, Subsequent epiphyseal tethering is leading to further distortion of the joint as growth progresses.

talar neck and supply the dorsal portion of the neck and the head of the talus. Finally, part of the lateral wall is supplied by the peroneal artery.

Fractures of the talar neck are rare in children[16] and are usually caused by abrupt dorsiflexion of the foot. Direct trauma to the dorsum of the foot may also be responsible. Talar neck fractures may be subtle and may be overlooked, especially as up to 20% may have medial malleolar fractures, which are often more obvious.

Fractures of the talar body are caused by axial compression between the tibia and the calcaneus and are often due to a significant fall. Routine AP and lateral views of the ankle and AP, lateral and oblique views of the foot are obtained and will usually show the fracture. However, either linear or computed tomography may be required in order to show an undisplaced fracture and when no injury is seen in these films the presence or absence of a bone injury can be confirmed by means of Tc99 MDP bone scans.

Complications are particularly common following displaced talar neck fractures but may occur with all types of talar injuries. Avascular necrosis is difficult to diagnose on a radiography in the early stages but Tc99 MDP bone scanning has provided a means of early identification, showing an area of low activity due to absent perfusion. However, magnetic resonance is the most specific and sensitive method of diagnosis, with loss of the normal high marrow signal on T1 weighted images. The presence of disuse osteoporosis leading to subchondral lucency in the talar dome in the early non-weightbearing period is an indication of an intact blood supply. Avascular necrosis becomes evident in the radiographs around eight weeks with areas of increased density within the bones due to the laying down of new bone on dead trabeculae and the collapse of bone trabeculae, which may lead to fragmentation of the articular surface.

Delayed or non-union is not uncommon after talar neck fractures partially due to their intra-articular nature, lack of periosteum and decreased blood supply. Serial radiographs or CT may demonstrate widening sclerosis and irregularity of the fracture line in non-union. However, MRI will demonstrate a high signal in the fracture line on the T2 weighted sequence due to the presentation of fluid when non-union is present and low signal when fibrous union has occurred.[17] CT may be valuable in demonstrating articular deformities, particularly in the subtalar joints, resulting from malunion.

Osteochondral fractures of the talar dome are uncommon in children under 16 years of age. Lateral fractures are due to inversion or inversion–dorsiflexion injuries and produce a narrow flake-like fragment.[18] Medial lesions are deeper and when associated with trauma are due to lateral rotation of the plantarflexed ankle.

Talar dome fractures are most easily detected on mortise views or occasionally the AP view. The lesion will not be easily seen on the lateral view but any effusion in the joint will be best evaluated on this view by the dis-placement of the anterior and posterior capsular fat line. Occasionally linear tomograms or CT coronal cuts may be required in order to visualise dome fractures as over 20% of cases may otherwise be missed[19] but CT in the axial plane may miss small dome lesions. Technetium bone scanning is valuable for identifying unexpected lesions in some cases. Double contrast arthrography may be used to assess the continuity of the articular cartilage and recently magnetic resonance imaging has been used to show the cartilage defect and the underlying marrow changes (Fig. 4.15A,B).

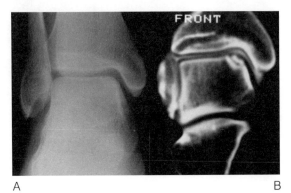

A   B

Figure 4.15 Osteochondral fracture. A, The defect on the medial margin of the talar dome is difficult to visualise on the AP view. B, Ankle arthrography with CT coronal cuts shows the defect clearly and demonstrates the intact cartilage outline.

Regardless of treatment methods osteoarthritis may eventually occur and has been reported in up to 50% of adults.[18]

Subtalar joint

The majority of eversion and inversion motion occurs at the subtalar joint. Inversion is limited by the interosseous ligaments, peroneal tendons and the lateral ankle ligaments, while eversion is restricted by the deltoid ligament, posterior tibial tendon and anterior tibial tendon. The talus and calcaneus are connected by joint capsules, lateral, medial, interosseous and cervical ligaments. Subtalar dislocation is rare in children but may be bilateral in cases of Ehlers–Danlos syndrome. When dislocation occurs, articular fractures are common, particularly in lateral dislocations. Routine views of the foot are usually sufficient in order to diagnose subtalar dislocations but CT is particularly valuable for demonstrating small fractures.

Calcaneal fractures in children are much less common than in adults; they are usually less extensive and compression is less likely to occur. Sixty-three per cent of calcaneal fractures in children are extra-articular, rising to 92% in patients less than seven years of age. Axial loading from falls or from motor vehicle accidents are the most common cause. Different classification systems have been proposed in order to define calcaneal injuries but the radiographic evaluation is similar for all types. Routine lateral oblique and axial views will demonstrate most fractures and measurement of the angle of the superior surface of the talocalcaneus (Bohler's angle) may be helpful. Any reduction below 22–48° will indicate a compression fracture. Conventional and computed tomography are the most valuable additional techniques to demonstrate more complex fractures and also the avulsion injuries of the margins of the calcaneus. CT enables joint alignment to be assessed, detects intra-articular fragments and the integrity of the sustentacular portion of the calcaneus. The talocalcaneal joints are best seen on the coronal (frontal) scans and the talonavicular and calcaneocuboid articulations are more clearly demonstrated on the axial scans. When tendon and ligament injuries are suspected, magnetic resonance may be helpful. Three-dimensional reformatting may be of value in planning treatment of complex fractures.

Midfoot and forefoot injuries

There is minimal motion in the articulations of the navicular, cuboid and cuneiform and stability is greater laterally than medially. Classification of injuries is based upon the deforming forces and resultant displacement but medial and longitudinal injuries form the majority. Isolated fractures of the tarsal bones, without associated joint involvement, are very unusual in children. Avulsion fractures caused by twisting or eversion forces occur in the navicular due to the pull of the talonavicular's capsule or anterior fibres of the deltoid ligament. Most body fractures are associated with frac-

ture dislocation of the midfoot. Subtle subluxations, avulsion fractures or undisplaced fractures may be difficult to identify due to overlap of bones with the result that AP, oblique and lateral views are required. Soft tissue swelling may provide a clue to the site of fracture. The line of the articular surfaces which should all be parallel must be carefully scrutinised. Fluoroscopically positive spot views and CT may be required to show subtle fractures.

Tarsometatarsal injuries

The lower lateral metatarsals are connected at their bases by transverse metatarsal ligaments. The first and second metatarsals are not connected in this way, with the second metatarsal attached medially to the medial (first) cuneiform. The plantar ligaments and tendons provide more support than the dorsal soft tissues and thus most dislocations occur dorsally.[20] Typically the injury occurs with forced plantar flexion of the forefoot with or without associated rotation but it may also occur with falls with the forefoot fixed or compression of the heads when the toes are on the ground. In most cases the displacement is lateral and variations occur depending upon whether the first metatarsal is involved or the extent of any fracture.

Routine views of the foot are usually sufficient to diagnose obvious fracture dislocation but subtle ligament injuries require greater precision. Loss of alignment of the medial margin of the second metatarsal and second cuneiform is a useful sign on the AP view but the os intermetatarsus should not be misdiagnosed as an avulsion fracture. The lateral border of the first metatarsal and first cuneiform should also align as should the medial base of the fourth metatarsal and the medial margin of the cuboid. The preservation of parallelism of articular surfaces is the way in which to diagnose. Subtle fractures of the base of the first metatarsal, which are associated with ligamentous disruption, should not be overlooked. CT evaluation of the arch of the foot in the axial plane may help to demonstrate the separation of the components.

Metatarsal and phalangeal injuries are common in children and usually result from direct trauma. The common site is the neck of

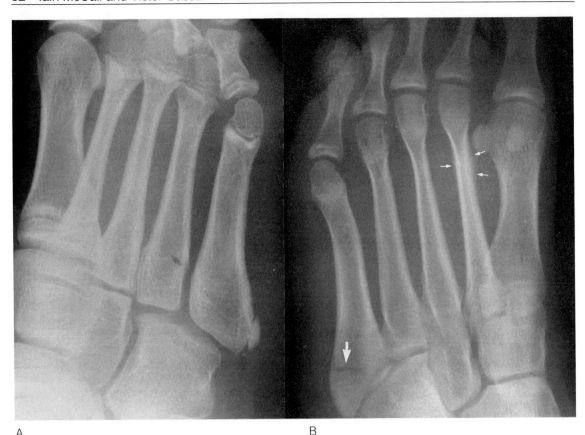

A   B

Figure 4.16   A, Normal epiphysis of the base of the fifth metatarsal. B, The fracture of the base of the fifth metatarsal is perpendicular to the cortex (bold arrow). There is also periosteal reaction around the distal shaft of the second metatarsal, due to a stress fracture.

the metatarsal due to its relative weakness compared with the shaft. Fractures may be incomplete, with greenstick type lesions. The base of the fifth metatarsal is a particularly common site and may be either an avulsion fracture of the epiphysis or a transverse fracture. The growth plate runs parallel with the shaft whereas the fractures are perpendicular to the shaft (Fig. 4.16A,B).

Fractures of the phalanges are usually due to the toe striking a firm object and such fractures may be spiral or with involvement of the articular surface (Fig. 4.17). Dislocation may be associated. AP and oblique views are usually sufficient to delineate all fractures.

Stress fractures are caused by muscle tension on normal bone[21] and are usually associated with some activity which may be recently initiated or may have been undertaken excessively. Pain is the presenting feature and ten-

derness is usually present. Paediatric stress fractures are most commonly found in the upper tibia but lower fibula and metatarsals may also occur, albeit less frequently. The majority of metatarsal stress fractures involve the second and third metatarsals. Calcaneal, navicular and sesamoid stress fractures are uncommon.

Radio-isotope studies with Tc99 MDP are the most sensitive method of identifying stress fractures in the early stages when radiographs may be normal.[21] The activity will be increased on both the early blood pool and later bone phase, due to the increased vascularity at the fracture site. Periosteal new bone will become evident along the shaft of a long bone and will be reasonably localised to the site of the fracture (Fig. 4.16). When the lesion is primarily cancellous, a linear increase in sclerosis within the cancellous bone may be all that is seen.

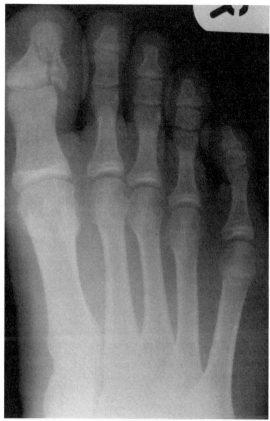

Figure 4.17 Crush fracture of the distal phalanx of the great toe.

Navicular stress fractures may present with a lucent line or sclerosis involving the medial third of the bone.

Tarsal coalition

This is a congenital condition in which varying degrees of union occur between two or more tarsal bones. In the younger child varying degrees of restriction of motion between involved tarsal bones may become apparent but the condition is not likely to become obvious until pain develops and this usually occurs between 8 and 12 years of age for calcaneonavicular coalition and during adolescence with talocalcaneal coalition. The increase in body weight and strenuous sporting activities may be responsible for the onset or the increase in pain in the subtalar or midtarsal region. Shortening of the peroneal muscles

gradually occurs over the course of time resulting in restricted subtalar motion, hindfoot valgus deformity, abduction of the forefoot and tautness of the peroneal tendon, the so-called peroneal 'spastic' flatfoot.

The overall incidence is probably less than 1% and the most common form is the medial talocalcaneal bridge (62%) with the calcaneonavicular (29%) and posterior talocalcaneal bridge (4%) much less frequent.[22] Isolated fusions between other tarsal bones occur in a few cases. There is evidence to suggest that it is an inherited autosomal dominant disorder, with almost full penetration.

The radiological demonstration of tarsal coalition is dependent upon the site and upon whether the bridge is fibrocartilage or bone. Plain radiographs are of little value in the younger child, where much of the cartilage skeleton is unossified. However, in adolescence most lesions may be demonstrated on routine radiographic studies.

Calcaneonavicular coalition is best demonstrated on the 45° oblique views of the foot as there is tarsal bone overlap on the AP and lateral views. When the bridge is ossified it completely obliterates the gap between the calcaneus and the navicular but when it is fibrous or cartilaginous, the anterior medial ends of the calcaneus may only be in close proximity to the navicular. In this situation, the contiguous surfaces are flattened and may be sclerotic and irregular, similar to a pseudoarthrosis (Fig. 4.18). Occasionally, the anterior process of the

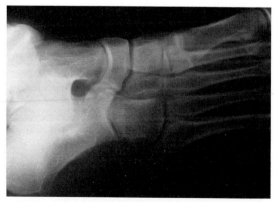

Figure 4.18 Calcaneonavicular coalition. There is a widening sclerosis and irregularity of the adjacent bone ends, with loss of the normal space between the calcaneus and navicular on the 45° oblique view.

calcaneus may appear as a slender prolongation, due to the presence of a cartilage bar.

Talocalcaneal coalition is more difficult to diagnose but medial coalition may be suspected from the lateral view when the sustentaculum tali is elongated and prominent due to bony thickening. However, confirmation of bony bridging may be demonstrated on the axial view of the calcaneus taken with good bone penetration (Fig. 4.19A,B). The angle of the axial view may vary between 30° and 45°, depending upon the plane of the sustentaculum *tali*. When the coalition is fibrous or cartilaginous, a radiolucent line is present along the joint but the margins are irregular and lack cortication. In addition, the plane may be inclined medially and downwards, in contrast to the horizontal position of the normal joint. When there is doubt about the status of the joint, a CT scan in the coronal and axial plane of the ankle and hindfoot will demonstrate the joint clearly (Fig. 4.19C,D).[23] The normal appearance is of well corticated smooth subarticular bony margins, clearly separated by the normal articular cartilage. Complete bony bridging is well demonstrated and may be sclerotic. Fibrous or cartilage union may be more difficult to diagnose as there is a narrow space between the long surfaces. However, these surfaces will usually be irregular and less sclerotic.

Coalition of the posterior and anterior subtalar joints is uncommon. The former may be demonstrated on medial and lateral oblique axial projections. When doubt occurs CT in the coronal plane to the ankle will demonstrate the joint clearly. The anterior joint is demonstrated on the oblique lateral dorsiplantar projection of the normal tarsus. In this view the medial border of the foot is placed on the film with the sole tilted at 45° to the cassette. The tube is centred just below and anterior to the lateral malleolus.[24]

The restriction of movement between the talus, calcaneus, navicular or cuboid may result in other changes on the plain films and such changes may be best shown on the standing lateral. There may be beaking on the dorsal and lateral aspect of the head of the talus adjacent to an otherwise normal talocalcaneal joint (Fig. 4.19A), which may be due to impingement of the dorsal part of the navicular on the films during dorsiflexion. Narrowing of the posterior talocalcaneal joint space and broadening of the lateral process of the talus may also be seen as calcaneonavicular coalition. This may be associated with flattening of the undersurface of the neck of the talus.

When a fibrous coalition is suspected but doubt remains, arthrography of the subtalar joints either with air or contrast may be helpful. This is best combined with the plain films and CT. The contrast is injected into the talonavicular joint on its dorsal aspect and should outline the talocalcaneonavicular joint space. On the lateral view or on the coronal CT, contrast should be seen extending above the sustentaculum *tali*, which will not be seen in cases of coalition. The posterior and anterior compartments do not communicate but arthrographic demonstration of the former may be achieved through direct puncture from a medial approach although clinically this is rarely warranted.

The use of magnetic resonance in this condition has not been fully evaluated but the fibrous coalition, which is dark on T1 and T2 weighted images, can be differentiated from a narrow joint or osseous coalition.

Inflammation

The most important inflammatory process to affect children is juvenile rheumatoid arthritis. It is a generalised disease and there are a number of variants, depending upon the extent of involvement and also the presence or absence of systemic manifestations (see Chapter 6). The feet and ankles are commonly involved in juvenile chronic arthritis. The plain radiographs will initially demonstrate increased density of periarticular soft tissues and displacement of the anterior fat lines, the ankle and the periarticular fat lines around the metatarsophalangeal joints, due to the presence of joint effusions and synovitis. Osteoporosis in the juxta-articular bone is another important early feature. Joint space narrowing and periarticular erosions are a late feature as the articular and epiphyseal cartilage of children is thick. Periosteal new bone is common in this condition and involves the small tubular bones of the feet. It is often thick and is seen early in the disease. Bone growth, maturation and epiphyseal fusion is acceler-

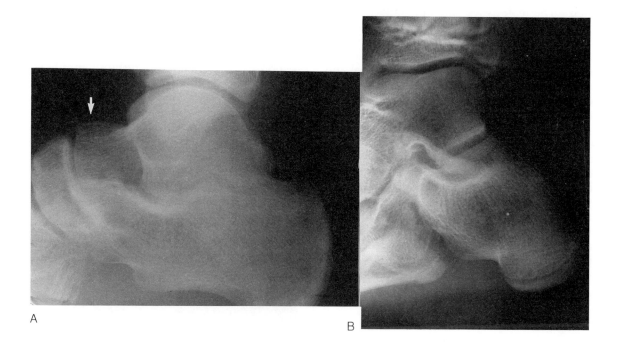

A

B

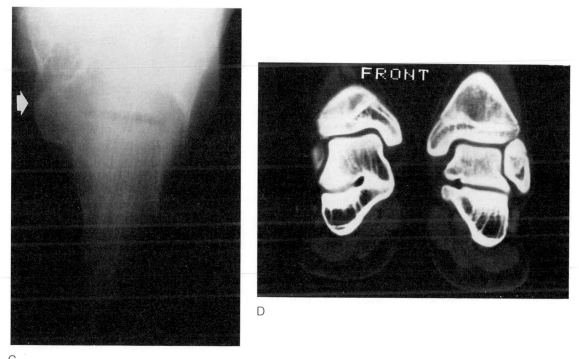

C

D

Figure 4.19   Talocalcaneal bar. The lateral (A) and lateral oblique (B) views show poor differentiation of the middle subtalar joints. Mild beaking is demonstrated in the anterosuperior aspect (arrow). C, The axial view of the calcaneus shows bony bridging of the middle subtalar joint (arrow). D, The coalition is confirmed by the CT scan. The normal side demonstrates a clear middle subtalar joint space.

ated. The epiphyses may be enlarged but longitudinal bone growth may be retarded due to the premature epiphyseal fusion. The most commonly affected joints are the ankle, proximal interphalangeal, metatarsophalangeal and intertarsal joints. Frequently joint ankylosis occurs late in the disease and may be asymmetrical.

Ankylosing spondylitis may affect patients in their teens and although involvement is predominantly in the spine and sacroiliac joints, calcaneal changes are not uncommon. Fluffy erosive changes in association with osseous proliferation occur at the insertion of the Achilles tendon and plantar fascia on the calcaneus and radiographic changes may be seen around the metatarsal and interphalangeal joints.

Infection

Most frequently pyogenic osteomyelitis occurs in infants and children and is three times more common in males than in females. It may be of haematogenous origin or may be caused by external inoculation during puncture wounds. Haematogenous osteomyelitis most commonly affects the calcaneus with other tarsal bones less frequently involved. Clinically there is pain and limp with soft tissue swelling and tenderness. In infants, vessels in the long bones extend through the growth plate into the epiphysis, whereas in children the vessels terminate in sinusoidal lakes in the metaphysis. This accounts for the higher incidence of epiphyseal and joint space involvement in infants with osteomyelitis and the higher susceptibility of the metaphysis in children. Early diagnosis is best achieved using Tc99 MDP bone imaging, which will demonstrate a marked increase in uptake of isotope on both the early blood pool and late bone phase. Comparison with the asymptomatic joints is essential as increased uptake is seen in normal epiphyseal plates. The earliest radiographic change is swelling of the deep soft tissues, which displace the adjacent fat planes, and this is best seen on radiographs accomplished by reducing the kilovoltage across the X-ray tube. Radiographic changes in bone occur later with lytic areas, loss and distortion of trabecu-

lar pattern and periosteal new bone formation. The periosteum is more loosely attached in infants and infection therefore elevates and penetrates it more frequently. The degree of response also depends upon the type of bone affected. When adequate treatment regimens are instituted, such changes will resolve leaving a normal bone. When chronic infection develops, there will be areas of sclerosis and lucency in the bone and sclerosis and distortion of the cortical surface. Areas of necrotic or dead bone (sequestra formation) may be demonstrated, which are more dense than the surrounding osteoporotic or hyperaemic bone (Fig. 4.20).

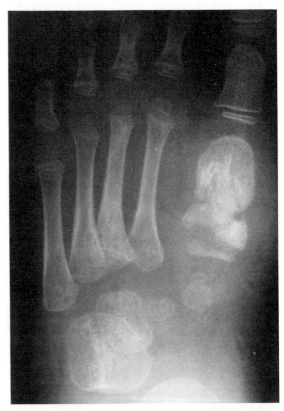

Figure 4.20 Chronic infection. There is considerable soft tissue swelling around the first metatarsal, which is sclerotic with areas of necrosis.

Localised bone abscesses (Brodie's abscess) may occur, which are usually metaphyseal lucencies, with well margined dense surrounding sclerosis. Central sequestra may be present and cortical involvement may produce considerable sclerotic reaction, not unlike an osteoid osteoma. CT will demonstrate the lucency and the central sequestra very effectively. Osteomyelitis, due to salmonella infection, often affects the diaphysis and may be associated with bone infection, particularly in a patient who has underlying haemopoetic disorders such as sickle cell anaemia.

Tuberculous osteomyelitis may involve children of all ages although bone and joint involvement only occur in 3–5% of patients with tuberculosis. When present it is usually due to haematogenous spread to the metaphyseal region of the long bones in children. The shafts of the metatarsals may show obvious layered periostitis, with multiple metatarsals being involved. Soft tissue swelling of the foot is also a prominent feature. Congenital syphilis may produce similar bone changes but without the soft tissue swelling.[25] Circumscribed cystic lesions may also be demonstrated but these are rare in the foot.

Rubella and cytomegalic inclusion disease in neonates may present mild periosteal changes with mixed lucent and sclerotic changes in the metaphysis.

Infection of bone following fracture may be particularly difficult to appreciate due to the disuse osteoporosis and periosteal callus formation as part of the healing process. Serial radiographs will be necessary in order to identify a failure of the normal healing process and also isotope studies are frequently helpful.

CT is useful in order to demonstrate localised destruction of the tarsal bones and is also the most effective method of demonstrating sequestra in chronic osteomyelitis. Magnetic resonance demonstrates infection as a dark area on T1 weighted images, while on T2 would be due to oedema, contrasting with the bright signal of normal marrow and fat on T1 weighted images. Therefore it demonstrates infection earlier than routine radiographs and identifies the extent of soft tissue involvement.

Differential diagnosis of infection includes Ewing's sarcoma. Differentiation may be difficult as this tumour produces a mixed lytic and sclerotic pattern especially in the calcaneus and tarsal bones. Cystic lesions with eosinophilic granuloma may be seen and reaction to a foreign body and stress fracture may also cause confusion.

Septic arthritis

Contamination of the joint may occur from the haematogenous route either by direct spread from soft tissue and adjacent bone or following trauma. Direct spread from adjacent osteomyelitis is more common in infants due to the vascular supply across the growth plate.

Monoarticular involvement is common and initially the radiograph demonstrates periarticular swelling which is identified as a slight increase in density and by displacement of the pericapsular fat line and muscle planes. Some juxta-articular osteoporosis may be present in the early stages. As the infection progresses, destruction of cartilage occurs, leading to joint space narrowing and finally bone destruction on either side of the joint. As with osteomyelitis, two phase technetium bone scans will identify joint infection early. CT scanning is unlikely to add any specific information apart from demonstrating joint destruction in the tarsal bones in the later stages. However, magnetic resonance will clearly identify the joint effusion as a bright signal within the joint on the T2 weighted images. Cartilage destruction may also be directly visualised. Aspiration of the joint and culture of the fluid is an urgent requirement for the treatment of septic arthritis.

Osteochondrosis

Osteochondrosis or osteochondritis are terms which have been used for ischaemic disorders of the epiphyses in children. Some of the conditions previously ascribed to this group are normal variations of ossification. This is the case for the changes in the calcaneal apophysis which has been called Sever's disease. The apophysis is often sclerotic and fragmented, especially towards the end of the first decade of life and is of no significance as the apophysis develops normally.

Osteochondrosis involving the navicular, known as Kohler's disease, is more likely to be due to ischaemia, although the aetiology remains controversial. It is observed between the ages of three and seven years and the appearances are of irregular ossifications and flattening of the bone although the space of the

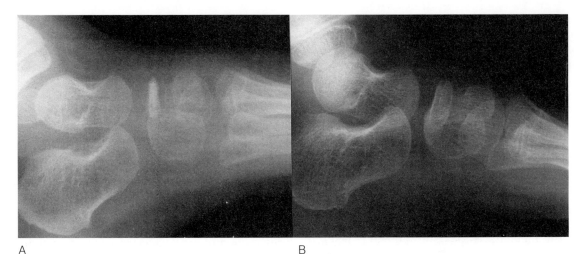

A   B

Figure 4.21   Kohler's disease. A, the navicular is flattened and sclerotic and the apparent joint space is increased. B, Fifteen months later the bone growth has returned with the outline of the sclerotic bone still visible inside the new ossification. A small calcaneal spur is seen which is a normal developmental variant.

cartilage model is intact (Fig. 4.21A,B). It is difficult to differentiate from normal irregular ossification in the absence of symptoms of local pain, swelling and a decrease in movement, although the frequently unilateral nature of the disorder allows comparison with the normal foot. Tc99 MDP bone scans are often equivocal as activity may vary from a low level to a significant increase over normal epiphyseal activity. The natural history is of bony reconstruction and a normal end result.

Collapse of the metatarsal heads associated with sclerosis is a further form of this condition. Originally described by Freiberg (1914) it is thought to be due to ischaemic necrosis secondary to repetitive trauma. The second metatarsal is most commonly involved, probably due to its greater length, but the changes in the third and fourth metatarsals are also seen. Symptoms occur most commonly in adolescence. Radiographically there is flattening and irregularity of the articular surface of the epiphysis of the metatarsal heads and frequently there is a rim of sclerosis on the endosteal margins of the defect. Healing occurs with reconstitution of the sharp subchondral line but flattening of the head persists.

Osteochondrosis of the sesamoids of the first metatarsal may also occur and once more repeated trauma is probably an important aetiological factor. Adult females are more commonly affected and sclerosis and irregular-ity of the sesamoid is seen radiographically. The isotope bone scan may show increased uptake.

Dysplasias

A large number of dysplasias have been described and many will have involvement of the foot. It is inappropriate in this text to give a detailed account of all these conditions. However, there are a few important points that should be stressed.

Deformity and irregularity of a number of epiphyseal centres are most likely to be due to a dysplasia, with multiple epiphyseal dysplasia being the most likely condition, although similar epiphyseal changes may be seen in some of the mucopolysaccharidoses. Multiple epiphyseal dysplasia produces shortened long bones in the feet with irregular frayed metaphyses, small irregular epiphyses and widened epiphyseal plates (Fig. 4.22). The tarsal centres are small and irregular. After fusion, the metatarsals are short and the heads are widened and flattened. In spondyloepiphyseal dysplasia the peripheral joints are less involved but talipes equinovarus or midfoot valgus may occur. In achondroplasia the long bones of the foot are short and broad and in Moquio–Brailsford syndrome, the shortening of the metatarsals and phalanges is due to

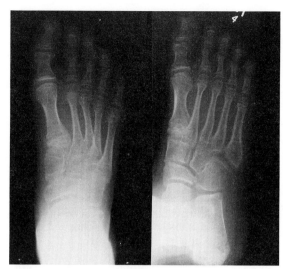

Figure 4.22   The epiphyses are widened, flattened and irregular and the metaphyses are splayed. The outline of the tarsal bone is more irregular than normal.

premature epiphyseal fusion but with normal modelling. Rockerbottom deformity with vertical talus may be seen.

Ossification from multiple centres may be due to dysplastic epiphysealis punctatae but hypothyroidism should also be considered, especially with delayed maturation.

In osteopetrosis, the metaphyses of the metatarsals are expanded and osteosclerotic, without distinction between cortical and cancellous bone. A bone within a bone appearance may be present in the small bones of the feet and healing stress fracture may occur.

Osteopoikilosis also results in increased sclerosis but the sclerosis has a multiple spotted appearance in the bone ends. It is of no clinical significance and is very rare.

Overgrowth of the foot may be associated with vascular anomalies such as arteriovenous (AV) malformations and haemangiomas and also with neurofibromatosis. Hemihypertrophy has been reported in association with Wilms' tumours.

In Marfan's syndrome the feet are unusually long, with joint laxity which may produce pes planus. Talipes equinovarus has also been found.

Acromegaly produces overgrowth of bones and this is both in the length and width of the long bones. Cartilage thickness is also increased, leading to joint space widening, and increased skin thickness of the toes and heel pads is common.

Hypoplasia may be associated with central neurological defects or as a focal peripheral underdevelopment involving one or more sclerotomas. The thalidomide embryopathy is a well known effect on the extremities.

Microdactyly of the first toe is an associated feature of myositis ossificans progressiva.

Osteogenesis imperfecta is characterised by thin osteoporotic bones with multiple fractures and shortening of bones due to healing fractures.

Abnormalities of bone modelling may be due to diaphyseal aclasia which affects the ankle but rarely the foot. Multiple small exostoses of the distal tibia and fibula may deform the lower ends and may lead to poor formation of the ankle mortise.

Ollier's disease produces irregular translucent areas in the metaphyses, with streaks of cartilage alternating with areas of increased density. The diaphysis is not usually extensively involved.

Fibrous displasia produces a lack of bone modelling with sclerosis. Bone maturation may be advanced.

In cleidocranial dysostosis the main feature is short terminal phalanges with cone-shaped epiphysis and pseudoepiphyses.

Neoplasm

Skeletal tumours of the foot are unusual and constitute only about 3% of primary bone tumours.[26] It is even more unusual for children's feet to be involved. However, all the recognised tumour types that affect children have been reported in feet. All imaging modalities have some value in the diagnosis and evaluation of bone tumours but the plain radiograph is usually the source of initial diagnosis. However, it is important to define the exact site and extent of any lesion and CT and MRI are particularly valuable in this regard. Distant extension and involvement are best assessed with bone seeking isotopes.

Benign tumours

Osteochondroma is the most common benign tumour but despite this it is still unusual in the foot. It usually manifests in the second decade and may be associated with lesions elsewhere as multiple hereditary exostoses. The radiographic features are those of a peripheral bony projection with flaring or undertubulation of the affected bone. The trabecular and cortical bone of the lesion is continuous with that of the bone of origin. The periphery of the lesion may be irregular in outline and some cartilaginous calcification may be present. Subungual exostoses are radiologically similar to osteochondroma and arise from the distal phalanx beneath the nail bed and have a predilection for the great toe. This probably represents reactive growth to trauma or pressure.

Osteoid osteoma is a highly cellular tumour of bone containing fibrovascular tissue, immature bone and osteoid, which may generate a vigorous osteoblastic host response. In the diaphysis of long bones, it produces a prominent periosteal reaction but in the bones of the foot it is more often intra-articular and the perifocal sclerotic reaction is not prominent. In these circumstances there may be osteoporosis or osteosclerosis and the lesion may be more lucent. Epiphyseal enlargement may also occur. The lesions produce increased activity on both the early and late phases of Tcm bone scan and may be identified visually with CT.[27]

Aneurysmal bone cyst is rare in the foot but has been found in the tarsals, metatarsals and phalanges. It is composed of cavernous blood-filled spaces with thin fibrous walls. The radiological appearances are of expansion of the bone by the lucent lesion, which has a well defined endosteal margin and thin shell of bone on the outer margin. Enlargement may lead to a break in the outer shell, with soft tissue extension.

Simple bone cyst occurs in the first two decades and in the foot the most common site is the calcaneus near the junction of the anterior and middle third. There is a well defined, purely lytic lesion, with mild expansion of the cortex and fine trabeculation (Fig. 4.23). The cyst contains straw coloured fluid.

Enchondroma is a benign hypocellular neoplasm of cartilage, which is most commonly found in the phalanges when affecting the

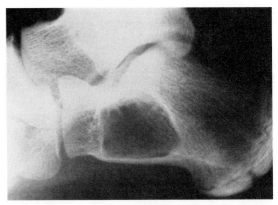

Figure 4.23 Simple bone cyst. A well defined lucency is seen in the junction of anterior and mid-third of the calcaneus.

foot. They are intramedullary, expand the cortex and have well defined margins. Punctate calcification may be seen within the lesion.

Chondroblastoma is a tumour of cartilage which invariably involves an epiphysis or apophysis. Thus they occur in children but are rare in the foot. The bones affected are usually the talus and the calcaneus and the appearances are of a sharply marginated lucent expansile mass.

Malignant tumours

Osteosarcoma although rare is still the most common malignant tumour to affect the ankle and foot in childhood. It may be either osteolytic, osteosclerotic or a combination of the two. Destruction of the cortex with an ill-defined endosteal margin is present. In the long bones, periosteal reaction is present and this may be partly destroyed by tumour extruding into the adjacent soft tissue.

Ewing's sarcoma is a highly malignant round cell tumour, which affects children and may affect the foot and ankle, with all bones being potential sites. The tumour produces a moth eaten effect in bone, involving the diaphyses. Periosteal reaction may be a prominent feature but this is variable and a soft tissue mass is common.

Soft tissue tumours are often difficult to demonstrate on routine radiographs but soft tissues can be seen on CT and to greater advantage on MRI. Intravenous contrast enhancement may assist the demonstration of lesions in muscle in

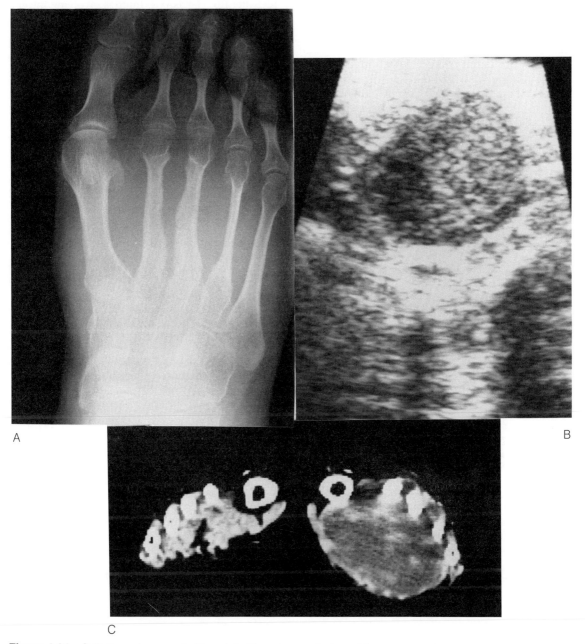

Figure 4.24   Soft tissue tumour. A, The plain films shows playing of the metatarsals, with bony deformity due to a soft tissue mass. B, The ultrasound demonstrates the round mass, which is shown to be solid by the multiple bright echoes within it. C, The normal and abnormal feet are compared, showing the large, substantially homogeneous, soft tissue mass, which was proven to be a fibroma.

CT. Benign lesions tend to have sharp margins with a homogenous CT density and MR signal. Malignant lesions often have an ill-defined margin and a variable texture, due to internal necrosis or haemorrhage. Local invasion or adjacent bone destruction is a feature of malignancy. Tumours which occur in children include lipoma, fibroma and haemangioma (Fig. 4.24).

References

1 Solomon MA, Gilala LA, Oloff LM, Oloff J, Compton T. CT scanning of the foot and ankle 2. Clinical applications and a review of the literature *AJR* 1986; 146: 1204–14.

2 Fornage BD. Achilles tendon ultrasound examination. *Radiology* 1986; 159: 759–64.

3 Olson RW. Ankle Arthrography. *Radiol Clin North Am* 1981; 19: 255–68.

4 Freiberger RH, Kaye J. *Arthrography*. New York, Appleton-Century-Crofts; 1979.

5 Hoerr NL, Pyle SJ, Francis CC. *Radiographic Atlas of Skeletal Development of Foot and Ankle*. Springfield, Thomas, 1962.

6 Keats TE. *An Atlas of Normal Roentgen Variants*, 3rd edn. Chicago, Year Book Medical Publishers, 1984.

7 Harrison RB, Keats TE. The cleft epiphysis. *Skeletal Radiol J*. 1980; 23.

8 Caffey J. *Paediatric X-ray Diagnosis Year Book*. Chicago, Medical Publishers Inc., 1978.

9 Templeton AW, McAlister WH, Zim ID. Standardisation of terminology and evaluation of osseous relationships in congenitally abnormal feet. *Am J Roentgenol*; 1965; 92: 374–81.

10 Vanderwilde R. Staheli LT, Chew DE, Malagon V. Measurements on radiographs of the foot in normal infants and children. *J Bone Joint Surg* 1988; 70A: 407–15.

11 Rogers LF. Radiology of epiphyseal injuries. *Radiology* 1970; 96: 289–99.

12 Salter RB, Harris WR. Injuries involving the epiphyseal plate. *J Bone Joint Surg* 1963; 45A: 587–622.

13 King TF, Bright RW, Hensinger RN. Distal tibial physis fractures in children that may require open reduction. *J Bone Joint Surg* 1984; 66A: 647–57.

14 Spiegel PG, Cooperman DR, Laros GS. Epiphyseal fractures of the distal ends of the tibia and fibula. *J Bone Joint Surg* 1978; 60A: 1046–50.

15 Canale ST, Kelly FB. Fractures of the neck of the talus. *J Bone Joint Surg* 1978; 60A: 143–56.

16 Letts RM, Gibeault D. Fractures of the neck of the talus in children. *Foot Ankle* 1980; 1: 74–7.

17 Berquist TH, Ehman RL, Richardson ML. *Magnetic Resonance of the Musculo Skeletal System*. New York, Raven Press, 1987.

18 Canale ST, Belding RH. Osteochondral lesions of the talus. *J Bone Joint Surg* 1980; 62A: 97–102.

19 Morrey, BF, Cass IR, Johnson KA, Berquist TH. *Foot and Ankle. Imaging of Orthopaedic Trauma and Surgery* (Ed. TH Berquist). Philadelphia, WB Saunders, 1986, pp. 407–98.

20 Anderson LD. Injuries of the forefoot. *Clin Orthopaed* 1977; 122: 18–127.

21 Daffner RH. Stress fractures. *Skeletal Radiol* 1987; 2: 221–9.

22 Harris RI. Retrospect–Peroneal spastic flat foot (rigid valgus foot). *J Bone Joint Surg* 1965; 47A: 1657.

23 Deutsch AL, Resnick D, Campbell. Computed tomography and bone scintigraphy in the evaluation of tarsal coalition. *Radiology* 1982; 144: 137–40.

24 Isherwood I. A radiological approach to the subtalar joint. *J Bone Joint Surg* 1961; 43B: 566.

25 Resnick D, Niwayama G. *Diagnosis of Bone and Joint Disorders*. Philadelphia, WB Saunders Co, 1981.

26 Dahlin DC, Unni KK. *Bone Tumours; General Aspects and Data on 8,542 Cases*. Springfield, Thomas, 1986.

27 Cassar-Pullicino VN, McCall IW, Wan S. Intra-articular osteoid osteoma. *Clin Radiol* 1992; 43: 153–60.

5 Cutaneous Diseases in Childhood

John Thomson

Embryology

The epidermis starts to form at about the fourth week of life as a single cell layer which then soon divides into an outer periderm and an inner germinative layer. Starting with the basal cells, the layers of the epidermis develop sequentially, slowly at first, then speeding up until all are complete at about six months (Fig. 5.1). At this stage the periderm is shed and this helps to form the fetal greasy coating which is called the vernix caseosa.

By eight weeks the dermis is a thin layer which over the next three months gradually resolves and separates from the subcutis. The development of the dermis compared to that of the epidermis is always delayed especially in respect of bulk. This explains the somewhat 'wasted' appearance of some newborn, especially the premature, where the vascular networks can be seen with the naked eye.

The nail fold and matrix start to show at approximately the third month with the development of a nail plate shortly thereafter.

Towards the third month some of the basal germinative cell layers start to crowd together. This is the primitive hair germ and hair shaft which start to develop around the fourth month. In association with the hair, sebaceous glands start to form. These glands are functional at around the 16th week and they also contribute to the vernix caseosa. The eccrine

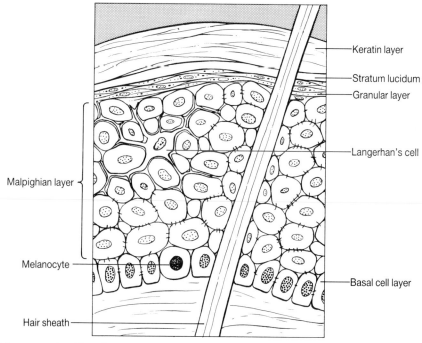

Figure 5.1 The normal epidermis.

glands form first on the palms and soles beginning at the third month, with those on other areas developing more slowly.

Reaching a diagnosis

In common with most clinical subjects the dermatological diagnosis is reached by a logical progression through the history, the examination, to the special investigations (Appendix I). Attempts to make a diagnosis without a history should be avoided. Occasionally the diagnosis may be correct but inevitably vital information such as the patient's drug history will be missed. Similarly any special investigations should be an adjunct to the history and examination and not the principal means of diagnosis.

In the child the history may need to be taken from or augmented by an adult as certain vital questions require to be answered. For example, what was the duration of the condition and where was its initial site? What was the initial type of lesion and what was the subsequent pattern of spread? Is the rash symptomless, itchy or painful? Are there fluctuations in severity? Is there a past history of previous skin problems, as some are recurrent? In addition certain skin affections tend to be familial; thus it is essential to enquire about the family history. An awareness of a general medical problem may be invaluable in diagnosing its cutaneous manifestations. At this stage it is pertinent to ask what drugs the patient is being prescribed. Specific enquiry may need to be made regarding, e.g. aspirin, tonics, cough bottles, as these are all preparations which the patient or his family may not regard as drugs.

Previous treatment may modify the condition and render the diagnosis more difficult. However, when treatment seems to have been adequate and appropriate to the clinician's initial diagnosis but unsuccessful, an alternative diagnosis should be considered. Hobbies and sports all need to be ascertained as they may well have a vital bearing on the diagnosis.

In dermatological diagnosis a thorough examination is necessary. The pattern or distribution of the rash may be the hallmark which gives the vital clue. It is appreciated that it may not be possible for the podiatrist to examine completely all the skin of the patient but readily available areas should be looked at and a careful history used as a substitute for inaccessible areas.

Individual lesions should be carefully assessed. When possible a primary lesion should be examined and its type classified, e.g. macule, papule, pustule or vesicle.

Secondary skin lesions may evolve from primary lesions by scratching or infection, e.g. excoriation, crusting and ulcers, and these are very much less useful diagnostically.

Finger and toe nails should also be examined; for example, rows of sharp pits may indicate psoriasis in an otherwise obscure red scaly rash.

When possible the mucous membranes should be viewed. In the case of the podiatrist this will be restricted to the patient's oral mucosa. However, appropriate changes there may suggest the presence of lichen planus.

Ichthyosis

Ichthyosis (literally a 'fishy condition') is a term applied generally to the group of conditions in which the skin is dry and scaly and which is usually without any redness. This group includes a large heterogeneous number of conditions and the two commonest forms are ichthyosis vulgaris and sex linked ichthyosis.

Ichthyosis vulgaris

As the vulgaris part of the name would suggest this is a fairly common condition occurring in approximtely 1 : 300 persons in the United Kingdom. It is inherited as an autosomal dominant condition with a high penetrance.

There may be a lipid metabolism abnormality but the basic cause is unknown.

Clinically ichthyosis vulgaris is not apparent at birth but some evidence appears any time after three months. The severity of the condition varies from the very minor to the more obvious forms. However, the scales tend to be small and white and it is usually not too much of a problem to the patient. Most areas of skin are involved but it is classically worse on the extensor aspects of the limbs with sparing of the antecubital and popliteal fossae. The face may be affected and hyperlinear palms and soles are common. Hyperkeratoses around hair follicles (keratoses pilaris), especially on thighs and arms, is often associated with this condition. The patient complains of 'roughness' of the skin and chafing and eczema may complicate the problem, especially in cold damp weather. Irritant and contact dermatitis are more likely due to the inferior barrier function of the involved skin. The condition is lifelong.

Most would accept the association of this type of ichthyosis with atopic eczema (see section on atopic eczema later in this chapter).

The histology of ichthyosis vulgaris shows a degree of hyperkeratosis coupled with parakeratosis. The main feature, however, is the total absence, or very marked reduction, of the granular layer.

Treatment options vary in proportion to the severity. Patients with minor degrees of the condition may choose to ignore it. More severe forms are usually controlled by emollients which may be simple greases, e.g. emulsifying ointment; some may contain urea which can act as a hydrating agent. Propylene glycol 60% in aqueous cream may act in a similar fashion. Combining keratolytic agents with the emollient may alleviate the symptoms, e.g. salicylic acid ointment in equal parts with glycerin of starch. In only very severe forms would alteration of keratinisation by systemic retinoids be considered since these drugs may well produce severe side effects.

Sex-linked ichthyosis (X-linked ichthyosis)

Sex-linked ichthyosis is due to a gene carried on the X chromosome and males only are affected. It is inherited as a recessive characteristic with a prevalance of approximately 1 : 6000.

In persons with this condition there has been found to be a deficiency in the enzyme steroid sulphatase. It is postulated that this leads to an increase in cholesterol sulphate which may adversely affect skin shedding.

Clinically the condition usually occurs within the first year. Males only are affected

and the clinical picture may mimic autosomal dominant ichthyosis vulgaris. However, the scales are usually larger, darker and more adherent. The patient is often accused of not washing himself properly. The sides of the neck, the extensor aspects of the limbs and flexural involvement are commonly affected areas. Pre-auricular scaling is thought to favour sex-linked ichthyosis as a diagnosis since it is much less common in ichthyosis vulgaris.[1]

The pathological appearances are of hyperkeratoses and parakeratoses. However, the main feature distinguishing it from ichthyosis vulgaris is the presence of a granular layer which may be increased in thickness.

Treatment is similar to that for ichthyosis vulgaris but usually requires to be more aggressive. There is some controversy as to whether systemic retinoids will help. In severely affected families genetic counselling may be appropriate.

The other forms of ichthyosis are rare.

Palmoplantar keratoderma

The palms and soles may be affected in some of the ichthyoses with considerable thickening of these areas. Some other conditions selectively affect the palms and soles and are grouped as the palmoplantar keratodermas (keratoderma palmaris et plantaris). The term tylosis (literally heavy callus) is sometimes used to denote keratoderma.

Many conditions causing scaly patches elsewhere, e.g. psoriasis or eczema, may affect the palms and soles alone or in conjunction with other areas. Hyperkeratosis from any cause may lead to loss of flexibility and the development of painful bleeding hacks.

When treatment is to be purely symptomatic, emollients are often effective, e.g. aqueous cream, urea-containing preparations. Occasionally the effect of emollients may be enhanced by occluding the lesions with polythene for short times.

The hyperkeratosis should be reduced either physically or chemically, e.g. salicylic acid 10% which acts as a keratolytic. Propylene glycol 60% in water or aqueous cream may also be of help.[2]

Epidermolysis bullosa

Epidermolysis bullosa describes a group of conditions and is not a single disease as the term suggests. The main feature is the formation of a blister in the skin which develops after very minor trauma.

In general terms the deeper the level of the epidermal separation the more likely is the condition to be inherited recessively and the more liable it is to cause scarring.

The podiatrist is more commonly asked to help in the less severe forms of the condition where there is a superficial blister which will heal without scarring. Some forms are present at birth but some do not become manifest until after puberty or early adult life and are perhaps related to the wearing of heavy footwear.

Frictional forces, especially in warm weather, cause the most problems with the feet being more affected than the hands.

Management of epidermolysis bullosa requires a team approach. In the more severe forms, genetic counselling and prenatal diagnosis with the offer of termination may be appropriate. In more minor cases on the feet, good hygiene, mild antiseptic washes and meticulous attention to the fitting of footwear are necessary. Avoidance of friction is helped by appropriate appliances in shoes. Shoes should ventilate and avoid overheating the feet. Mild solutions of, e.g. 2% formaldehyde, may harden the skin. Established blisters may be decompressed and any secondary infection will require treatment. Oral phenytoin may help some forms of dystrophic epidermolysis bullosa.

Ehlers–Danlos syndrome

The Ehlers–Danlos syndrome can now be shown to be not a single entity but a group of about 11. The common link is abnormal connective tissue which leads to the clinical features. There are differing modes of inheritance, biochemical abnormalities and clinical patterns. Most types exhibit joint hyperextensibility leading ultimately to joint damage. The skin is hyperextensile and may be pulled out into grotesque patterns. The abnormal connective tissue in the blood vessels may lead to bruising or cardiac and valve abnormalities.

Marfan's syndrome

Marfan's syndrome is an inherited disorder of connective tissue which occurs in approximately 1.5 births per 100 000. It is inherited as an autosomal dominant but sporadic cases occur. There may be a relationship to increased parental age.

Patients with the syndrome are usually much taller than the average with a depressed sternum. The increased height owes much to disproportionately long lower limbs but the upper limbs are also similarly affected. All limbs are thin and become especially abnormally long distally, producing very long 'spider' digits.

Many of the clinical problems relate to the abnormal hyperelastic connective tissue. The skin may exhibit striae distensae especially over the thighs and shoulders.

Skeletal abnormalities in conjunction with the lax joint capsules lead to many foot problems. Pes planus may be aggravated by diminished subcutaneous fat and abnormal joint positions including hyperextensibility of the knees and an associated kyphoscoliosis. Abnormal foot function may lead to the appearance of callosities on areas subject to trauma and may be an early manifestation.

No treatment other than symptomatic is possible.

Hereditary haemorrhagic telangiectasia (Osler–Rendu–Weber disease)

This is an autosomal dominant disease affecting most of the small blood vessels, which start to dilate around puberty. There is a predilection for mucous membranes and the condition often presents as epistaxis or gastrointestinal bleeding. These may possibly lead to anaemia which may be severe at times. In the skin, the face and lips are the commonest areas to be affected; also the hands and less commonly the feet. Treatment is usually symptomatic.

Neurofibromatosis (Von Recklinghausen's disease)

This condition is due to an abnormal gene which is inherited as an autosomal dominant. Various types are recognised.

Clinically hyperpigmented areas and tumours start to appear in later childhood. The pigmented areas vary in size from about 2 mm upwards and exhibit different shades of colour, e.g. some have the appearance of milky coffee and are designated as café au lait spots. Freckle-like lesions aggregate in the axillae and these are considered pathognomonic. The cutaneous lesions vary from raised domes, soft pedunculated lesions to large plexiform swellings. On firm pressure the soft cutaneous lesions appear to herniate through the deep fascia and this is a useful test. Some tumours may occur in internal organs causing problems by pressure. In the skin and elsewhere they may become sarcomatous. In some organs endocrine abnormalities may be provoked. The eye may be involved with iris haematomas (Lisch nodules). The foot may be directly involved or secondarily by the effects of kyphoscoliosis.

Microscopically, elements of nerve tissue are usually found with associated cells.

The management may consist of genetic counselling and surgical excision of appropriate lesions.

Arthropod bites and stings

Insects[3] may be divided into two main groups (1) those who sting, usually in defence, and (2) those who bite, often in order to ingest blood. The damage may be direct trauma (e.g. horsefly or cleg), by tissue damage from a noxious chemical (e.g. bee sting) or an antigen–antibody reaction in a previously sensitised person. Secondary events such as superficial infection are introduced and disease may ensue.

The clinical symptoms vary considerably and there are also many differences to be found on examination. Exposed areas are vulnerable although some arthropods like humid sweaty areas, e.g. under clothing bands. The foot and ankle are especially vulnerable and lesions may be solitary, grouped or linear.

The clinical appearance depends on the mechanism of damage involved: (1) there may be a central puncture mark: (2) an urticarial weal may occur within a few moments progressing to a papule in the next day or so, resolving slowly over the next few days; (3) more severe reactions may occur, e.g. blisters or tissue necrosis. Lymphangitis, lymphadenopathy, cellulitis, malaise or fever are all possible sequelae. Very occasionally collapse due to an anaphylactic shock may occur in hypersensitive patients. A current problem, especially in the USA, is Lyme disease, which results from a bite from a tick (*Ixodes ricinus* – the common deer tick), producing an annular reaction in the skin. Joint, cardiac and neurological complications have been described.

Arthropods may induce skin disease of many types, e.g. a common one relevant to podiatrists is scabies.

Scabies

Scabies (Plate 1) is due to infestation with the human scabies mite, classified as one of the suborders of Acarina and referred to as *Sarcoptes scabiei* var. *hominis* (Fig. 5.2). The mite

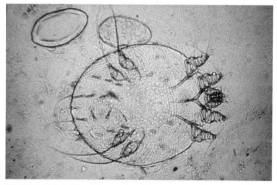

Figure 5.2   Scabies mite (*Sarcoptes scabiei* var. hominis).

cannot exist for more than a few days without a host and thus transmission is usually by close personal contact with an affected person.

The history usually reveals some involvement of other household members or of persons with whom the sufferer is closely involved. The predominant symptom is itching especially at night or when the patient is warm. This may relate to increased activity of the mite. Itching is also thought to be associated with the development of an allergic reaction to the *Sarcoptes* or to degeneration products. This would explain the variable latent period after infestation before pruritus commences. On subsequent occasions itching begins earlier.

During the early stages the condition is usually symptomless but in four to six weeks a hypersensitivity reaction occurs giving rise to a rash and itching with the classic sites of involvement being the interdigital webs, anterior wrists, axillary fold, ankles and feet.

The typical lesion is the burrow which is usually seen as a small greyish line. Scratching often converts these burrows into excoriated papular and/or secondarily infected areas.

Usually the diagnosis is easily made after a good history and examination but it may be missed on occasions. The finding of a mite confirms the diagnosis.

The treatment of scabies is a good example of the importance of the management. It is essential to explain the condition to the sufferer. Scabies engenders shame and misconceptions about dirt and poor hygiene; thus a sympathetic approach is needed. It is absolutely mandatory that the entire household (and any other involved households) be treated simultaneously. Failure to treat will almost inevitably lead to re-involvement of others and constant recurrences.

A modern treatment is gamma benzene hexachloride which is effective with one adequate application.

The itching of scabies may take approximately three weeks to settle after effective treatment. In a few patients purplish nodules, usually in axillae, peri-umbilical areas, buttocks or genitalia, remain as persistent nodular scabies.[4] The itching of these may be alleviated by topical steroids or by oral antihistamines and the nodules will slowly regress.

Bacterial infections

Normal skin is not sterile after the immediate postnatal period and resident and transient bacteria and yeasts are present. These organisms are not spread evenly and they tend to aggregate; e.g. moist areas such as the toe-clefts may harbour above average numbers.

Intermittently pathogens may invade, e.g. staphylococci and streptococci. Entry is made through breaks in the skin integrity and by diminished immunological defences, e.g. the scaling of psoriasis, weeping areas of dermatitis and open ulcers.

The immediate aim is to treat the infection but at the same time attention should be directed to the inner and outer defences with appropriate treatment when possible; e.g. the urine should be tested for sugar lest there might be hitherto undiagnosed diabetes mellitus.

Impetigo contagiosa

This is a superficial skin infection due to *Staphylococci* or *Streptococci* and sporadic cases occur but the condition may spread rapidly in closed vulnerable communities. The organism gains access probably via a minor abrasion or through macerated skin. For this reason children with running noses are often affected on the face. Impetigo may complicate other skin conditions especially where the skin integrity is breached and therefore some conditions, e.g. eczema or scabies, may be secondarily impetiginised.

The common history is of a facial lesion rapidly crusting. The child remains well and non-toxic but other lesions may soon appear at adjacent or distant sites. Other contacts, especially in the household, may be affected. The primary lesion is a blister. As it is so superficial its walls are delicate and rupture so that the clinician usually sees only secondary crusting which is traditionally described as 'honey coloured'. In some patients blisters remain, e.g. in areas where the keratin layer is thick such as the palms and soles. Isolated acute blisters in such areas may pose a diagnostic problem.

Topical or systemic antibiotics may be used in treatment, e.g. oral flucloxacillin for a staphylococcal infection and phenoxypenicillin for a streptococcal infection. When using topical antibiotics, crusting must be removed. Usually this is done using warm olive oil, or hydrogen peroxide, and very occasionally a starch poultice may be required. Common topical antibiotics are chlortetracycline, fusidic acid and mupirocin.

Underlying skin diseases such as eczema or scabies should be treated. The disease and its treatment must be explained to both the patient and parents and they must all be reassured that scarring will not ensue. Towels and other fomites should be individual. Physical contact between children should be avoided if possible.

Erysipelas

Erysipelas is an infection of the skin with *Streptococcus* usually of the Group A type with the organism gaining entry through a minor and perhaps unnoticed breach in the skin. Nowadays this condition is much less common.

There is usually a fairly abrupt onset with malaise and some fever. The affected area is swollen resembling the skin of an orange but is red in colour. The plaque is raised and has an easily palpable and spreading edge. These appearances are characteristic and usually lead to the diagnosis. The face is a common site but the condition is reported on the limbs. In the foot a pre-existing fungal infection in the toe webs can allow the *Streptococcus* to gain access.

Treatment should be started promptly. This is especially important when the face is involved as the infection may pass to the cavernous sinus and thence to the brain. Penicillin usually rapidly settles erysipelas but it should be given for at least a week's course. Erysipelas can be recurrent and may lead to lymphoedema and here long-term antibiotic therapy may be justified.

Cellulitis

Cellulitis is a deeper infection than erysipelas. The commonest causative organism is *Streptococcus pyogenes* followed closely by *Staphylococcus*, but others are possible. Access to the tissues usually occurs by a breach in the skin, e.g. a wound or ulcer or a macerated toe web. The characteristic signs of inflammation occur with redness, swelling, heat and pain and these are often associated with lymphangitis, lymphadenopathy, fever and extreme malaise.

The body's defences respond with an increase in polymorphonuclear leucocytes.

Antibiotic therapy is usually with flucloxacillin or cloxacillin which are penicillinase resistant antibiotics. Treatment usually has to be commenced prior to bacteriological examination but if a proven streptococcal infection is found Penicillin V or Phenethicillin may be given orally. When the infection is more serious parenteral penicillin is necessary.

Viral infections

Viruses are infective agents which are smaller than bacteria and which cannot multiply on their own. They may damage or destroy the host cell in a variety of ways.

Once they have replicated their increased numbers cascade into the blood stream where they may be trapped in capillaries near the skin. However, they may be unable to replicate further in local cells as the body's various defence mechanisms come into play. This may explain the skin rash (exanthem) of many systemic viral diseases.

Viral infections may affect the skin as (1) a transient exanthem of another systemic viral disease, or (2) direct infection.

Rubella (German measles)

A short spell of malaise is followed by enlarged lymph nodes of the head and neck and then a rash which is characteristically of pink macules commencing on the face, 'running down' the trunk and limbs and then coalescing especially centrally. The rash is evanescent and many atypical types are seen adding to the diagnostic difficulties.

Measles

Measles has an incubation period of approximately 14 days which is asymptomatic and this is followed by a prodromal phase of fever and malaise. After three to four days there is an apparent severe cold with cough, suffused eyes and running nose. The eruption begins in the mouth with small white spots (Koplik's spots) which resemble grains of salt on a red background. The skin rash begins as a slightly purplish blotchy eruption behind the ears and spreads to the trunk and limbs with involvement of hands and feet. Marked desquamation of the hands and feet may ensue.

Herpes – Varicella/zoster (chickenpox/shingles)

The herpes virus group consists of a number of DNA viruses. Some of the human ones have a predilection for cells of the nerve tissue and skin. One of the commonest is the varicella/zoster virus which causes chickenpox and shingles. Chickenpox is the result of initial exposure in a susceptible person. A symptomless incubation period of up to three weeks is followed by the macular rash which is soon replaced by tense unilocular blisters which become pustular and crusted. Different stages are seen together which was useful in the days when it had to be differentiated from smallpox.

The eruption is most marked on the trunk and is thus described as centripetal but there are often palmoplantar lesions. It is usually very itchy. Fever and constitutional symptoms tend to run concurrently with the rash. Scars may be left as the condition resolves.

Warts (verrucae)

Deoxyribonucleic acid (DNA) containing papillomaviruses (PV), a subgroup of the Papova virus family, are the responsible agents for viral warts.[5]

The PV is species specific and the human agent is designated as human papillomavirus (HPV). Within this group there are a number of subtypes – currently over 50 and ever increasing. The subtypes may cause wart infections of specific types or sites. As far as warts of the hands and feet are concerned, subtypes 1, 2 and 4 are the norm. HPV can exist in a dormant but infectious form outside the body for a very long time. The virus probably requires a portal of entry via an injury to the epidermis. Children have a finer skin than adults and are therefore more liable to minor trauma. Persons with abnormal skin barriers as in eczema have an increased incidence. Communal bathing, shower areas and swimming baths with abrasive non-slip moist sur-

rounds are examples of high risk areas for contracting plantar warts. Once inoculated the incubation period appears to be infinitely variable.

After the clinical lesions develop there is also a variable time before regression; 20–30% will clear spontaneously in six months. Humoral antibodies (IgM and IgE) have been identified and are involved. Cell mediated immunity is very important and warts can spread rapidly in the immunosuppressed patient.

It is thought that the virus stimulates the basal epidermal cells to divide but viral DNA and other products are found only to the depth of the granular layer. It is postulated that one or two seeds are in the basal cells and that they are only able to start multiplying at a certain stage of cell development which occurs around the level of the granular layer.

The common wart is usually easily diagnosed. The area presents with projecting columns of hyperkeratosis interspersed with black dots which represent thrombosed capillaries. The skin markings often seem to be 'pushed aside'. The lesions may vary in number from solitary to many hundreds and they may remain single or coalesce into masses. Bleeding may occur from trauma or self-treatment.

A similar picture is seen with plantar warts. On the weightbearing areas warts rarely project to the same extent. They can produce a prominent capsule of hyperkeratosis which obscures the wart and which may delude the observer into thinking that the lesion is a corn (Plate 2). There may be single or multiple lesions and sometimes small warts spread locally forming plaques of lesions. Warts may spread around nail folds and thus give rise to nail plate distortion.

The patient's main complaint is the appearance. However, pain may be a problem in areas of pressure. This is especially apposite to plantar warts. The sufferer may be unable to walk or he may have a distorted gait. The pain may be tolerable except just after rising or after direct pressure from standing on a pebble.

The diagnosis is usually straightforward but difficulties may occur with plantar warts; e.g. the single lesion under a pressure point where there is much overlying hyperkeratosis – partial reduction of the area may reveal petechial points. When reducing a corn shiny sheets of keratin, a central core, and skin markings continuing over the lesion would be expected.

Histologically most types of warts show hyperplasia of all epidermal layers especially the keratin, granular and prickle cell layers. The basal cell layer is intact. The dermal papillae seem to claw into the centre under the wart and blood vessels reach high up into the substance of the lesion. There may be large keratinocytes with an eccentric nucleus surrounded by a halo called koilocytes or 'bird's eye' cells. These represent balloon degeneration damage to prickle cells caused by the virus.

There is no specific antiviral drug effective against HPV and therefore any treatment is destructive to the infected area and tends to be painful.

Destructive measures may be carried out by the use of chemical or physical modalities, e.g. chemically: keratolytic agents such as salicylic acid in different formulations may be used; tissue denaturing agents such as formalin, glutaraldehyde, mono and trichloroacetic acid all have a place; podophyllum may be used but should be avoided if there is the remotest possibility of pregnancy as complications have been described. All the chemicals react more favourably when they gain access to the wart tissue and any hyperkeratosis should first be reduced. With podophyllum a violent reaction can ensue. At times intense pain is due to the formation of a walled off area of tissue necrosis and much relief can be obtained by draining this.

Methods of tissue destruction relying on cold are described as cryotherapy. Less scarring ensues than with, for example, cautery. Cryotherapy is commonly used in the treatment of warts. Cooled carbon dioxide (dry ice) used as a hard stick or as a slush when mixed with acetone is more difficult to use and only achieves $-78\,°C$ as a maximum and in consequence has largely fallen from favour. Liquid nitrogen is the most commonly used and in theory at least reduces the tissue temperature to $-198\,°C$. It can be applied by a cotton bud or by a spray system such as CRY-AC. The HPV virus may be able to survive liquid nitrogen and the dip method has theoretical possibilities of virus dissemination. Both the dip and spray methods are mainly used on areas other than the palms and soles. In these areas a cold probe may be used; those which are

fuelled by nitrous oxide are slow and tedious. Liquid nitrogen probes are much quicker but in order to overcome technical difficulties, expensive equipment is required. The appropriate tip is applied to the area and contact enhanced by a lubricating jelly (e.g. KY jelly). All methods should freeze the appropriate area and a 1 mm surround. Individual practitioners vary the time that freezing is maintained, but it should not exceed 30 seconds. A greater cell kill is achieved with two or more freeze/thaw cycles. The patient should be warned regarding the possibility of subsequent blisters.

Cautery for warts is less commonly used and great care is needed not to provoke scarring. Diathermy, using the Birtcher Hyfrecator type of machine or similar, has the same potential problems. Apart from very small filiform lesions a local anaesthetic is required. The injection site must *not* be cleansed with alcoholic solutions such as a Mediswab because these are highly inflammable.

Surgical curettage may be useful in solitary warts on the dorsa of the feet or when the diagnosis is in doubt and histology is required. When curetting is carried out the plantar wart should be cored out from its hyperkeratotic capsule. Great care and skill is required to strike a balance between ineffective curettage and post curetting scars. Having obtained anaesthesia there is a tendency to err towards the latter.

Hand, foot and mouth disease

Hand, foot and mouth disease is an uncommon condition which has been reported world wide. The causative virus is usually Coxsackie A16 but others have been implicated.

The condition affects young children and presents with general malaise for about 24 hours. This malaise is followed by a sore mouth caused by small blisters which rapidly progress to shallow ulcers. Variable numbers of vesicles then appear on the hands and feet and usually on the dorsa with a predilection for the periungual area. These vesicles are oval and resemble grains of rice. They may affect the flexures or the crease areas of the feet and hands. Clearing usually occurs within the week. Contacts may be affected.

Histologically there is an intra-epidermal blister. No specific treatment is necessary.

Molluscum contagiosum

Molluscum contagiosum is a common viral disease, especially in children, and is due to a pox virus which is frequently contracted near swimming pools.

After a variable incubation period of possibly two to seven weeks, the lesions develop. They are usually multiple and are commonly although not exclusively found in or around axillae or groins. Vast numbers may occur in the atopic, immunosuppressed patient or in those who have been inappropriately treated with topical steroids. The individual lesion (1–5 mm) is a flesh-coloured, dome-shaped papule with a characteristic central depression. From this umbilicated area, white caseous material may be expressed. The appearances may be modified by secondary infection with inflammation and pus. Solitary lesions may occur which may become very large and may be difficult to diagnose mimicking, for example, basal cell carcinoma.

When there is clinical doubt, the diagnosis may be confirmed by smearing the expressed material on a slide and examining a potassium hydroxide microscope preparation. Large balloon cells which resemble frog spawn are easily seen.

The natural history of molluscum contagiosum is towards spontaneous resolution in a number of months. Destruction of the lesions by liquid nitrogen, by hyfrecation or simply by expressing them, speeds the clearance.

Fungal diseases

Fungi differ from bacteria although some bacteria may mimic fungi. As a group fungi are very successful and their subgroups reach six figures ranging from small organisms to large mushrooms.

Fungi can multiply asexually when small fragments replicate into whole new organisms. All their characteristics remain the same but this is not good for adaptation. Some can replicate by sexual means and here nuclei fuse and divide.

Because of these variations classification of fungi is difficult and it often changes. Under the microscope most fungi have an appearance of a tangled skein of threads. Classifications are made on microscopic examination as to the degree of branching, whether they are compartmented (by septa), their type of replication and the formation of buds or spores.

Fungal disease in humans is referred to as mycotic disease and it falls into two main headings: (i) the superficial mycoses which purely affect the skin, nails and/or hair, and (ii) the deep or systemic mycoses which affect deeper structures alone or with secondary skin changes. With immunosuppression, e.g. HIV disease, more fungal infections of all types are being encountered.

The superficial mycoses are usually subdivided into two groups:

1. Dermatophytes
2. *Candida* and allied groups.

This is an artificial subdivision in so far as the dermatophytes tend to produce the classic annular eruption known as ringworm on the open skin. However, the term ringworm may also be applied to nail and hair infections. In addition dermatophyte infections may be designated as tinea (t). The part of the body affected is added as a latinised genitive, e.g. tinea pedis, t. capitis, t. corporis or t. unguium.

The dermatophyte group can be further subdivided into three main groups: *Microsporum*, *Trichophyton* and *Epidermophyton*. These in turn may all be split, giving rise to names such as *Trichophyton mentagrophytes* var. *interdigitale*. Some dermatophytes may cause one specific disease while other conditions may be due to one of several fungi.

The dermatophytes invade keratin but may be prevented from deeper penetration by a serum inhibitory factor. In the epidermis they affect the keratin layer and in the nail the entire plate may be affected as far as the growing matrix. In the hair they grow down within or outside the hair shaft beneath the skin surface and therefore shaving cannot eradicate the infection.

Histologically the offending agent may be seen in keratin in sections stained by haematoxylin and eosin. The ease of demonstration is much enhanced by the use of PAS (periodic acid–Schiff) stain.

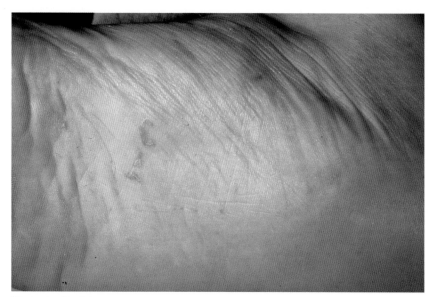

Plate 1 Scabies

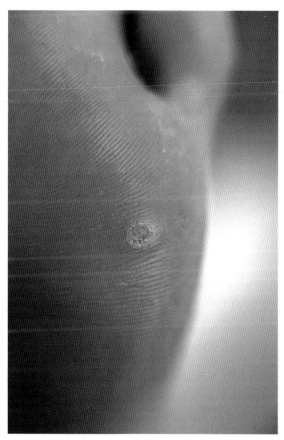

Plate 2 Verruca Plantaris

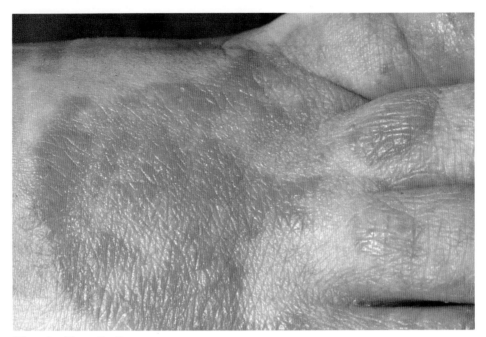

Plate 3 Tinea Pedis

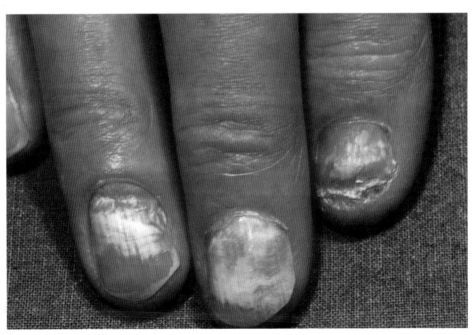

Plate 4 Fungal Leuconychia

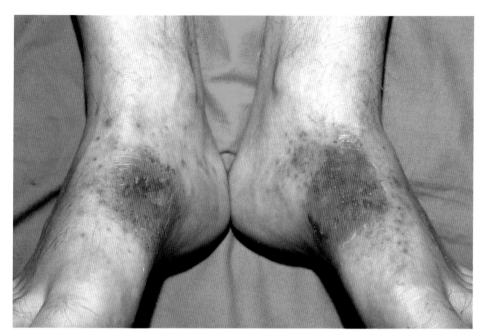

Plate 5 Shoe Contact Dermatitis

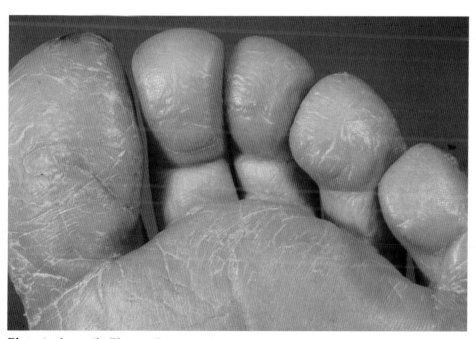

Plate 6 Juvenile Plantar Dermatosis

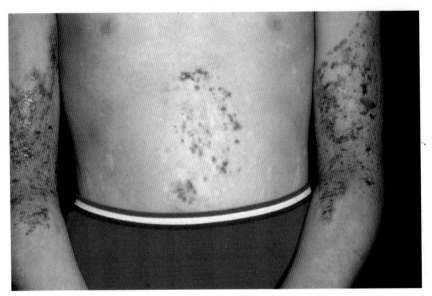

Plate 7 Atopic Eczema

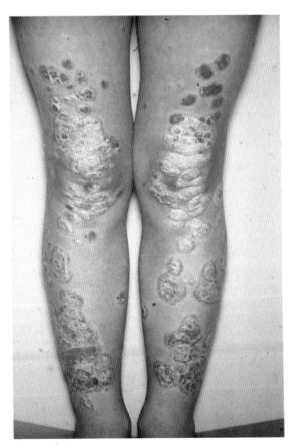

Plate 8 Plaque Psoriasis

The *Candida* (C) group may also be split up into different members. *C. albicans* is the most common and *C. parapsilosis*, *C. tropicalis* and others may be pathogenic. The different types make little difference to therapy for cutaneous lesions. *Candida* may be a normal commensal on the body, although not all persons carry it, and it is usually found near orifices such as the mouth, anus or vagina. The total colony present is kept in balance by the rest of the skin flora. However, *Candida* is a great opportunist and waits to invade when this balance is upset.

Histologically signs of acute inflammation with microscopic pustule formation are observed. PAS staining is helpful in enhancing the visualisation of small numbers of fungus.

Tinea infections

Tinea infections may be due to one of a number of dermatophytes obtained either directly from an infected person or animal or indirectly from soil or fomites. The initial lesion may be seen as a small reddish area which soon spreads to form the typical ring with a clearing centre akin to the 'fairy ring' which may be seen in some field mushrooms. The border appears more active and indeed contains more fungi. The scaly edge tends to overhang centrally with less or no scaling to the outside.

With all forms of dermatophyte infection a secondary eruption may occur at distant sites. Other skin conditions may give rise to a similar phenomenon which is described as an 'id' or 'ide' reaction and this word may be used alone or more correctly as a suffix such as dermatophytide of trichophytide when the aetiological agent is known.

Tinea pedis (athlete's foot; foot ringworm)

Tinea pedis is the commonest dermatophyte infection and 10% of the general population (larger in closed communities) may be affected. The condition is very prevalent in the civilised world – civilisation here being defined as the wearing of shoes, especially occlusive ones. Moisture macerates the skin thereby weakening its defences and thus allowing entry of the fungus. A particular weak spot is the interdigital web between the fourth and fifth toes. The causative fungi lurk around wet areas of showers and swimming pools. Anti-slip surfaces surrounding such areas further abrade the skin and facilitate infections.

Three varieties of dermatophyte predominate, viz. *Trichophyton rubrum*, *T. mentagrophytes* var. *interdigitale* and *Epidermophyton floccosum*. Some variations in the clinical picture are seen with the different types.

The commonest clinical picture (Plate 3) is of scaling and maceration between the toes with the fourth and fifth interdigital webs almost invariably affected either alone or in conjunction with some others. In many such patients this is asymptomatic and they may be unaware that they suffer from the disease.

Any of the causative organisms may be isolated from this type along with other infectious agents such as bacteria.

A dry red scaling may affect the plantar surfaces and this scaling is usually due to *T. rubrum*. Fine scaling covers this and is accentuated by scraping the surface lightly. This occurs spontaneously at skin markings and a network of criss-crossing white lines is seen.

Less commonly small blisters form, usually due to *T. mentagrophytes* var. *interdigitale*, and they tend to appear in hot weather. Occasionally a violent very acute infection coupled with an associated dermatitis reaction may be crippling and devastating.

The proximity of the toe nails renders them liable to be infected (see tinea unguium). Recurrent tinea pedis may be due to a reservoir of fungus in the nails. Palmar ringworm (tinea manuum) may be consequent upon foot infection particularly with *T. rubrum*. All forms of tinea pedis may lead to one of the ide eruptions previously described. They are rare in minor infections but are more common in severe ones.

When possible the clinical diagnosis should be confirmed by direct examination with potassium hydroxide or a culture (see special investigations, Appendix I). However, it should be remembered that the fungus may be difficult to visualise and may be unpredictable in culture.

Treatment may have limited success but:

1. Cleanliness and hosing down around communal bathing areas may reduce the incidence.

2. Meticulous attention to drying of the feet, especially interdigitally, will reduce physical maceration and so reduce the likelihood of penetration by fungus.
3. Hyperhidrosis is common and should be treated concomitantly.
4. The wearing of more occlusive types of footwear should be discouraged.
5. Patients with severe infections should be banned from public swimming pools.
6. The wearing of plastic socks for swimming may help (but this may not be popular with children and also it is almost impossible to avoid the foot coming into contact with the wet surface at some time).

Topical treatment involves application of one of the imidazoles, e.g. miconazole nitrate cream. These drugs damage the wall of the fungi and lead to inhibition of growth and ultimately cell death. There are many variations on the imidazole theme but no one preparation would appear to have any significant advantages over the others. The use of antifungal dusting powders for shoes and/or hosiery is difficult to evaluate.

Tinea unguium (onychomycosis; nail ringworm)

Most of the predisposing factors for tinea pedis, which can coexist, are pertinent to toe nail ringworm. The trio of *T. rubrum*, *T. mentagrophytes* var. *interdigitale* and *E. floccosum* are again implicated with the emphasis on the first two.

Clinically infection first manifests itself at the distal end of the nail plate. There may be some subungual alteration and the nail plate may change colour. On viewing the nail plate end on, a honeycomb of crumbly nail underlying the smoother upper surface may be seen and this is sometimes called distal subungual onychomycosis. Leuconychia (Plate 4) (white superficial onychomycosis) may develop due to *T. mentagrophytes* var. *interdigitale*. When severe infections of both types are present the fungus may ultimately break through rendering the upper surface of the nail plate rough and scaly. Onycholysis may be a prominent feature. Onychomycosis, which occurs much more commonly in toe nails, involves one or two nails initially but gradually others may be affected.

The differential diagnosis includes psoriasis, trauma and other nail dystrophies. Traumatic changes usually affect only one or two nails and also the patient may relate the particular incident. Changes due to eczema and other skin diseases are usually identifiable after history taking and general examination. Pure nail dystrophies may be more difficult.

In the management of tinea unguium concomitant tinea pedis (or manuum) should be treated. Current topical therapies may not necessarily cure the affected nail. However, they may be used around all the nails and digits in an effort to prevent further spread. Tioconazole paint has still not yet been fully evaluated and it is expensive.

Systemic griseofulvin has been used but its success rate, especially in toe nail infection, is poor. Itraconazole, a systemic imidazole, has been introduced. Oral terbinafine shows great promise but cannot yet be used in children.

Tinea incognito

This term refers to the modification and masking of a fungal infection by the inappropriate usage of strong topical steroids.

Initially the eruption seems to improve with lessening of symptoms and paling of the area. However, the symptoms never completely clear and when the steroid is withdrawn the condition may flare up. The characteristic scaling edge and clearing centre may be lost or diminished rendering accurate diagnosis more difficult. The area is slightly reddish and frequently nodules are present.

Once diagnosed the topical steroid application should be stopped and appropriate antifungal treatment given.

Candidiasis

Candidiasis (also referred to as candidosis) is due to infection with one of the yeast-like fungi of *Candida* of which *Candida albicans* is the main offender. When it is present on mucous membranes it may be described as thrush, e.g. oral or vaginal thrush. It may be a normal com-

mensual in small numbers but it is an opportunist.

Supercolonisation may occur when the
balance of power is upset by broad spectrum
antibiotics, diabetes mellitus, systemic steroids, immunosuppression or drug addiction.
When the skin defence is reduced by another
rash *Candida* may colonise such an area. It is
more common in the obese, especially those
patients with diabetes mellitus.

On mucous membranes, candidiasis causes
pain or discomfort. Whitish patches on a red
background may be rubbed off with a swab
and a raw bleeding area remains.

Moist skin folds are the target of *Candida*.
The interdigital webs of toes are potential sites
for invasion. Nail folds may be colonised leading to paronychia with a swollen 'bolstered'
area which causes cuticle destruction and nail
dystrophy.

On the skin, a salmon pink patch extends
into the depth of the crevice. Frequently there
is a fine scaly fringed edge with small pustules
which rapidly burst and crust. Small outlying
satellite lesions with redness and crusting outside this plaque are common.

The diagnosis is made by examination of
appropriate scrapings. It is important to bear
in mind that the finding of a few *Candida* on a
swab may be within normal limits.

When treating transient improvement may
be obtained by the use of drugs alone but the
underlying cause for the candidal infection
must be sought and remedied where possible.
Correction of diabetes mellitus, stopping the
use of broad spectrum antibiotics or inappropriate steroids play a major part. When the
moist areas can be dried, *Candida* will die out
or will be loath to recolonise.

Nail folds should be kept dry. Hygroscopic,
mildly antiseptic agents may help, e.g. thymol
4% in chloroform. Shoes and socks should be
less occlusive thereby reducing sweating.
Several different preparations of nystatin are
available but it is not absorbed from the gut
and requires to be applied topically. Nystatin
is ineffective against dermatophytes.

The imidazoles are active against dermatophytes and *Candida* and are useful when the
practitioner does not have access to laboratory
diagnostic facilities or when he is unsure of the
offending organism. Topical drugs are usually
used in an appropriate vehicle.

Eczema/dermatitis

Eczema and dermatitis refer to inflammatory
conditions of the skin and these terms should
be considered as interchangeable. The classical
features of inflammation will be seen and the
relative degree of each of these will vary from
patient to patient. Eczema or dermatitis is not
the final diagnosis and the cause must still be
sought.

The aetiology falls into two main groups:

1. Exogenous, e.g. contact dermatitis.
2. Endogenous e.g. atopic eczema, seborrhoeic eczema, pompholyx, lichen simplex.

As far as the skin is concerned the end result
may be very similar but they must be separated by careful history taking and by their pattern, rather than by individual lesions.

The diagnosis of eczema is one of the differential diagnosis of red scaly rashes. The degree
of redness and swelling present is proportional
to the intensity and the edge of the lesion is
not clearly demarcated. Blisters, usually visible
to the naked eye, may be seen ranging from
tiny vesicles to large bullae. The area may
weep profusely from these or be dry, hard and
fissured. Moist raw areas are liable to secondary infection and may be covered with loosely
adherent yellowish crusts. Associated lymphadenopathy may ensue but no scarring will
result from uncomplicated dermatitis.

The symptoms of dermatitis are those of
inflammation. The patient may complain of
pain, heat or intense itching. Swelling, especially on the face and at the extremities, may
be very troublesome. On the foot swelling may
render walking impossible and on the hand,
loss of joint mobility is extremely incapacitat-
ing. Complicating superadded infection leads
to an offensive malodour.

Oedema develops in the epidermis and
upper dermis. The epidermal cells appear to be
pushed apart and cling on to their intercellular
attachments (spongiosis). The oedema may
collect as epidermal vesicles of variable sizes.
The epidermis thickens (acanthosis) and disruption of the normal maturation of the epidermal cells means that nucleated cells are
seen within the keratin layer (parakeratosis).
Reddening of the area results from dilatation

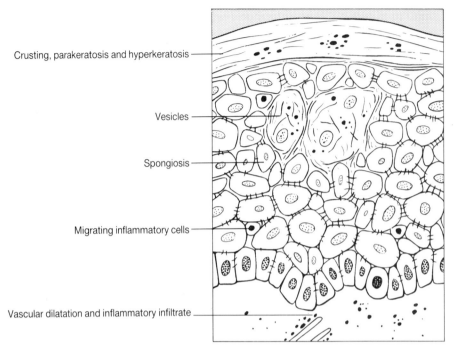

Crusting, parakeratosis and hyperkeratosis

Vesicles

Spongiosis

Migrating inflammatory cells

Vascular dilatation and inflammatory infiltrate

Figure 5.3   Histology of acute eczema.

of the dermal blood vessels and this dilatation allows the cells of inflammation to rush in (Fig. 5.3).

In the management of eczema where possible the cause should be identified and treated. In the endogenous eczemas no remedial cause may be identifiable and in these cases, and in others, treatment of the dermatitis may be undertaken to give symptomatic relief.

Rest of the area is advisable. Elevation of swollen areas gives great relief, especially in the foot, from throbbing discomfort. Firm bandaging may help but should be non-occlusive. Protection from irritants either by complete avoidance or by suitable protective wear is essential.

As a general rule the more moist the skin lesion is the more moist the base should be. Thus an acute weeping eruption would suggest the use of a lotion, perhaps as a soak or as a compress. As the area becomes drier a cream (water miscible), or an ointment (water insoluble), or a paste may be applied. Pastes may be difficult to apply directly on to the skin and may require to be spread first on to calico or old linen with a flexible knife.

Many topical steroid preparations are avail-

able and the first consideration is the strength of the steroid. Topical corticosteroids are classified into different groups ranging from mildly potent to very potent. Certain patients are shown to be developing an acute contact dermatitis to the steroid molecule itself. Strong topical steroids should be used on a time limited basis and very great care should be taken in their use on thin skinned areas since long continued use will lead to atrophy of the skin, marked skin striae and rebound of the condition for which they are used.

Secondary infection may occur and may well supervene and therefore the incorporation of an antimicrobial agent into a therapeutic preparation is advantageous. Antiseptic agents are usually based on iodine and many of these are iodinated quinolines, e.g. vioform hydrocortisone.

Antibiotics may usefully be incorporated though some prefer to give them orally. Allergic contact dermatitis may be caused by the antibiotics themselves. This is occasionally masked by the strong steroid with a delayed flare thereafter and it is difficult for patient and practitioner to recognise the iatrogenic nature. Neomycin is an example of such an antibiotic.

Contact dermatitis

Contact dermatitis is a vitally important condition and it is essential to understand it and to be very certain before a diagnosis is made.

There are two main types:

1. Irritant contact dermatitis.
2. Allergic contact dermatitis.

Irritant contact dermatitis (Plate 5)

Normal skin is a highly efficient protective envelope and is capable of withstanding quite remarkable onslaughts but certain substances may overwhelm it, e.g. strong acids and alkalis. Contact with these will provoke an instant caustic burn which may be described as an acute irritant dermatitis. This will occur in everyone and is related to direct cell injury with immunological mechanisms taking no part, at least initially. When these agents are weakened there will eventually be a stage when the skin can resist them and no reaction occurs. This point will be individual to the particular patient and may be termed as his threshold. Most patients with irritant dermatitis have been in contact with subtler substances than caustics, e.g. detergents. Usually the initial contact does not cause a reaction but through time the skin's protective barriers diminish until the individual's threshold is reached and the disease is manifest. This may be termed cumulative insult and the time taken to reach the threshold is infinitely variable.

As a result, patients are often confused and do not realise the time scale involved. They tend to blame the eruption on a new substance in their environment and discount the irritants since they have been in contact with them for 'a long time'.

The pattern of the dermatitis depends on the area of contact, e.g. perspiration and occlusive footwear such as wellingtons, may localise the condition to the feet.

The areas of dermatitis are themselves indistinguishable from those due to any other cause as is the histology.

Irritant dermatitis is an important diagnosis to make because it should be possible to clear it within a reasonably short time. When suitable avoidance can be undertaken the prognosis in that patient should be good. Treatment should be prompt in order to prevent chronic forms of eczema developing. Also the breached integument can permit access to allergens and this is a common initial happening before the development of allergic contact dermatitis.

The dermatitis should be treated as previously described.

The specific treatment is avoidance and of protection from potential irritants. Barrier creams can never be anywhere near absolute and when used should be employed with this in mind as they only complement avoidance and physical protection. However, regreasing the skin is advantageous and simple non-perfumed creams should be used, e.g. Simple cream.

Washing should be continued but the use of hot water, abrasive degreasing, heavily perfumed soaps or solvents must be avoided.

Allergic contact dermatitis

The allergens involved in allergic contact dermatitis are usually substances of low molecular weight and in the skin of the vulnerable individual these allergens combine with normal tissue proteins forming antigens. Langerhans' cells convey this complex to the regional lymph node where a specific antibody is produced. The ability to produce this antibody is dependent upon T cells recognising the antigen. These cells then circulate and give an innate potential against the specific antigen or original substance (Fig. 5.4). Any ensuing reaction produces the allergic contact dermatitis clinical pattern. The entire process takes time – usually 14–21 days – and is thus called delayed hypersensitivity. Cells, rather than humoral factors, are involved and thus it is an example of cell mediated immunity.

When the reaction is over, a small reserve of memory cells remain and if the original complex, or one similar enough, returns these remaining T cells can multiply very rapidly without all the fabrication process in the lymphatic tissue and a more rapid clinical response ensues. Therefore once sensitised the individual remains so essentially for life. Desensitisation is impossible. Allergic contact dermatitis becomes commoner with advancing age but children too may well have allergic contact dermatitis.

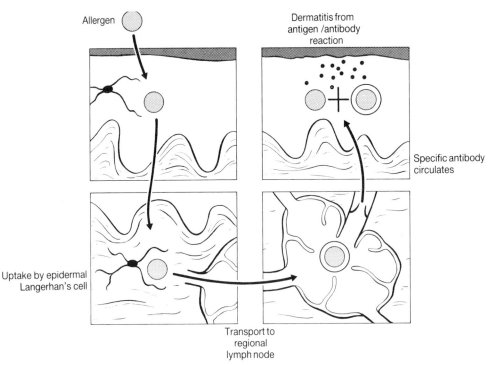

Allergen

Dermatitis from antigen /antibody reaction

Specific antibody circulates

Uptake by epidermal Langerhan's cell

Transport to regional lymph node

Figure 5.4 The skin and associated lymphocyte (T) system (the SALT system).

Many factors lead to unmasking the innate sensitivity. The more prolonged the contact with the antigen, the more likely it is to develop. When the normal skin barrier is damaged, e.g. by irritant dermatitis, this predisposes to allergic contact dermatitis. It is vitally important to know the area of first involvement and what might have been in contact with the skin. Time must be spent to understand the patient's pastimes and hobbies, clothing and jewellery. Perfumes, toiletries and local applications prescribed or bought over the counter must be identified.

Usually contact dermatitis will occur initially at the area of contact. However, this may be much more than at first thought and is termed 'wandering contact'.

Many substances may cause allergic contact dermatitis and it is good practice to try to identify the offender clinically, thereafter progressing to specific patch testing.

Once allergic contact dermatitis is confirmed, the management commences. Written instructions as to where a substance may be encountered and where suitable substitutes may be found are essential. Avoiding contact

with certain agents is easy but virtually impossible with others, e.g. nickel. However, unless contact is prevented by avoidance or by the insertion of a suitable barrier, the problem will not be solved.

The dermatitis reaction is treated as previously described. Any aggravating features such as concomitant irritant contact dermatitis or hyperhidrosis of the feet should also be treated.

Juvenile plantar dermatosis (Plate 6) (atopic winter feet; glazed feet; forefoot eczema)

This condition is confined to children and its aetiology is unknown. However, the appearance and increased incidence suggest that modern, more occlusive footwear which is less able to absorb perspiration may be implicated. As a general rule patch tests have been negative for contact factors. There may be an increased incidence of atopy.

The clinical picture is usually very characteristic. A child of up to 14 years presents with a rash on the weightbearing area of the forefoot while the instep, interdigital webs and toe arches are not affected. However, the heel or entire sole may be. There is a pink shiny glazed appearance and scaling may be present. The flexibility of the skin may be lost and this results in fissures which may bleed and may be exquisitely tender thus rendering walking impossible.

There may be a seasonal variation with the condition worsening in winter but this is inconstant. Spontaneous clearing usually occurs in the early to mid teens.

Histological changes are unhelpful although there may be sweat gland occlusion.

Many cases are misdiagnosed as tinea pedis (Fig. 5.5) but it should be possible to separate

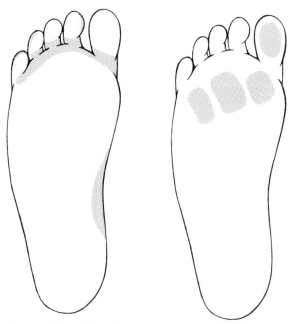

Figure 5.5 Differential diagnosis of athlete's foot and juvenile plantar dermatosis. Left, typical pattern for athlete's foot; right, typical pattern for juvenile plantar dermatosis.

these clinically and appropriate specimens should be taken when in doubt. Care should be taken not to overlook the possibility of occasional genuine allergic contact dermatitis.

Treatment is unsatisfactory, but less occlusive footwear, thin cotton socks and cork insoles are all helpful. Emollients when used liberally may make the skin more supple but topical steroids have little place.

Pompholyx

Pompholyx refers to eczema of the palms (cheiropompholyx) or soles (podopompholyx). Blisters are a feature of this condition and hence the term pompholyx ('a bubble').

The exact cause is undefined but it may represent an eczematous reaction which is precipitated by a number of different noxious stimuli. Vesicles tend to be prominent due to the normal hyperkeratosis and there is a fairly good link between distant fungal infections in certain cases. The suggested association with irritant contact dermatitis, allergic contact dermatitis, atopy or stress is less obvious. All cases seem to worsen in hot weather.

Histology shows the picture of an eczema with vesicles surmounted by a thick keratin layer.

Clinically a burning sensation is frequently followed by intensely itchy blisters which are usually small but which may occasionally coalesce to form large bullae.

Pompholyx is characteristically bilateral and localised to the hyperkeratotic areas of the palms and soles or along the sides of the digits. The vesicles may be deep and difficult to see but may be felt by firm rubbing and they are likened to 'sago grains'. They progress to the surface, burst, crust and desquamate in approximately a fortnight. Secondary infection or spread to other areas may occur and recurrent episodes of pompholyx are not uncommon.

In the management of the condition, any convincing precipitating factors should be treated. Dermatitis is dealt with in the conventional manner. Potassium permanganate foot baths may prevent secondary infection.

Severe cheiro/podopompholyx is a grave disability as manual dexterity and mobility is lost. Under these circumstances hospital admission may be required. The distressing pain of oedematous hands and feet is alleviated by elevation of the appropriate limb.

Atopic eczema (Plate 7)

Atopy refers to a complex of conditions of which the skin manifestations are only one aspect although often the most prominent. Many other problems may occur in the atopic, e.g. asthma, hayfever or allergic conjunctivitis.

Atopic eczema, whose aetiology is unknown, is a common disease perhaps reaching about 3% of the general population and there is a positive family history in approximately 70% of patients.

Immunological abnormalities may be demonstrated in atopic eczema. An elevated level of immunoglobulin E (IgE) is a common finding but it is thought that the rise in IgE is a non-specific intermittent feature. Cell mediated immunity in the atopic is diminished and clinical examples of this are seen in the lessened capacity of the patient to cope with many viral skin infections. Encounters with herpes simplex, wart, molluscum contagiosum and other viruses may result in surprisingly extensive and severe disease. The atopic may have similar problems with some fungal and bacterial infections. T cell lymphocytes are the agents of the cell mediated immune reaction and many variations in their number can be found in atopic eczema.

There is the possibility of food allergy being causative or provoking exacerbations as there is no doubt that certain foods seem to exacerbate certain patients and this is particularly so in children.

The small blood vessels in the atopic patient show a tendency to constrict and this may be secondary to the plethora of vasoactive substances whose proportions are upset in the condition. Firm stroking of the normal skin should provoke a red raised line or weal but in the atopic this line is white and is described as white dermographism. However, some non-atopics, e.g. those with seborrhoeic eczema or acute contact dermatitis, may exhibit the sign.

The increased tendency to vasoconstrict may account for the facial pallor seen in many atopics. Numerous other elevations or decreases have been described in the chemical substances related to inflammation and there may be problems at receptor sites for some of these.

Atopic eczema may begin at any age but is common between 2 and 6 months. At this stage it may be designated infantile eczema but there are other causes for dermatitis in infancy. Usually the first sign is a weeping eczematous facial eruption but many variations are possible. The relative sparing of the napkin area may be helpful in differentiating it from these other eczemas.

As a toddler approaches childhood the distribution pattern tends to change, exhibiting a pronounced flexural predilection involving wrists, elbows, knees, ankles and the sides of the neck.

Approximately half of patients with atopic eczema have ichthyosis similar to the autosomal dominant type. The atopic has the worst of both worlds in that the ichthyosis often affects all areas except the flexures – the very areas singled out by the eczema (Plate 7). This associated ichthyosis, which may be itchy and uncomfortable, has a very important bearing on many aspects of atopic eczema. Ichthyosis plays a considerable part in the temperature intolerance of many atopics as sweating in hot humid weather is a problem.

In conjunction with the ichthyosis the atopic palm is often dry and hyperlinear and in later life this may contribute to dermatitis localising there. Under the eyes there may be an extra skin crease (Morgan–Dennie fold) due to skin oedema.

Many patients with atopic eczema note that the condition gradually settles in late childhood to go through a spell of increased activity in the teens. Most, although certainly not all, will settle in the late teens or early twenties with much less trouble thereafter. This can never be guaranteed and there are some in whom the first presentation is at this age.

The changes in atopic eczema may resemble those of any other eczema and the diagnosis relies on the history and the pattern. However, some differences exist; e.g. the pruritus of atopic eczema is usually much more intense than in other forms of dermatitis. Cutaneous markings are more easily seen and are supposed to resemble the bark of a tree, i.e. lichenification. This is highly characteristic of, although not unique to, atopic eczema.

The eczema, the ichthyosis and the pruritus with associated scratching together render the skin liable to secondary infection. Certain people are of the opinion that infection triggers the eczema and vice versa but probably both occur.

Stress plays a considerable part in atopic eczema but does not cause the condition although many exacerbations are related to periods of stress.

Non-skin manifestations of atopy include asthma and the condition is occasionally called the eczema–asthma complex. Hayfever and conjunctivitis are other 'allergic manifestations'.

Lichenification and lichen simplex

Thickening of the skin develops in response to rubbing or scratching. It may be secondary to any, usually itchy, skin condition of which atopy is a prime example. When these changes occur with no apparent initial skin disease the condition is called lichen simplex. Neurodermatitis is the term used by some to refer to both.

Clinically both conditions are rare in childhood. They are intensely itchy and the skin markings stand out like tree bark. Treatment consists of removing any cause. Usually the standard measures for the therapy of dermatitis are ineffective but occlusion by bandages, or by thick pastes may break the itch/scratch cycle.

Psoriasis

Psoriasis is common and affects approximately 2% of the world's population with ethnic variations around this figure. The aetiology is unknown but there is a greatly increased epidermal cell turnover. The normal epidermal basal cell requires about 28 days to progress to the flexible cohesive acellular keratin layer. This period of time is reduced in the active psoriatic patch to three or four days. The keratin layer is cellular and non-cohesive resulting in scaling or flaking.

These changes may be triggered or modified by heredity, ultraviolet light, drugs and stress. Many alterations in cells' immunity and mediator systems have been noted but in most instances it is unclear which is cause and which is effect.

An appreciation of the histology helps to understand the clinical features of the disease (Fig. 5.6). The epidermis becomes thicker (acanthosis), although paradoxically there is thinning over the rete ridges which contain a dilated capillary, hence giving the patch its red colour. Polymorphonuclear leucocytes migrate into the epidermis, and aggregate in small collections known as Munro's microabscesses. The keratin layer is cellular and scaly (parakeratosis).

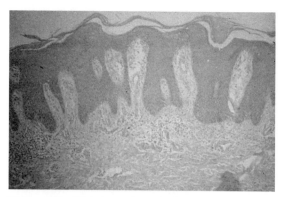

Figure 5.6 Histology of psoriasis.

The onset of psoriasis may be at any age from early infancy to advanced years with the peak incidence occurring in the late teens or early twenties. The first episode of psoriasis may occur with no obvious precipitating factors.

Psoriasis may occur with no family history but in the majority of patients another family member is affected. The inheritance pattern is autosomal dominant with incomplete penetrance.

Some drugs may induce or aggravate pre-existing psoriasis or may produce a psoriasiform eruption. These drugs include lithium, beta blockers and gold. In the past many varieties of psoriasis were described on the basis of the configuration of the lesions but this descriptive classification has now been abandoned. However, it is important to recognise different types.

Acute guttate psoriasis

This is the commonest form in the young. There is rapid development of a widespread rash with no particular distribution and this is frequently subsequent to a minor infection, e.g. a streptococcal sore throat. The spots are small, red, drop-like (hence guttate) and scaly and are symptomless. They reach a peak in numbers and subside in approximately six weeks, either by clearing completely or by progressing to plaque psoriasis.

Plaque psoriasis (Plate 8)

This is the commonest form of psoriasis. It consists of patches of red, scaly skin and has a predilection for the scalp, knees, elbows and sacral region, although any area may be affected. The condition is roughly symmetrical and occurs mainly on the extensor surfaces but less frequently it may affect the flexures. The latter may impinge on the podiatrist because of the involvement of nail folds or interdigital web maceration.

The individual patches are round or oval, red and scaly. The scaling is silver coloured and dry. The prime diagnostic feature is the clear demarcation of the plaque (c.f. eczema). Light scraping accentuates the silvery colour which is due to an increase of air under the scale. This then acts as a reflector and the line is supposed to sparkle like mica. Around the patches there may be a white halo known as the ring of Woronoff.

Small bleeding points are seen when the scales are torn off. This is due to damage to the thinner areas of skin overlying the dilated capillaries in the rete ridges and is known as Auspitz's sign.

Injury to the lower epidermis and upper dermis leads to the isomorphic or Koebner phenomenon in patients with active psoriasis and psoriasis will appear in that area within two weeks. This test may be useful diagnostically. However, the Koebner phenomenon occurs in certain other skin diseases and is therefore not unique to psoriasis.

A variant form of psoriasis which is more common in children, is a stocking or glove pattern which may be difficult to differentiate from eczema.

The mucous membranes and nails of all patients with red scaly eruptions must always be examined. In psoriasis the mucous membranes are very rarely affected. Nail changes are common and are to be observed in about 50% of patients who present with psoriasis. There may be sharp pits, which are frequently in a linear pattern in one or more nails. This presentation is referred to as pepper-pot pitting or thimble nails and is pathognomonic of psoriasis.

Onycholysis may be due to psoriasis. A common, although not invariable picture, is a triangular pattern at the distal lateral parts of the nail plate. Subungual hyperkeratoses, discoloration or thickened crumbly nails are encountered. None of these changes are unique to psoriasis and therefore other conditions must be excluded.

Pustular psoriasis

Pustular psoriasis occurs when the Munro microabscesses become large enough to be seen by the naked eye. There are localised and generalised forms. The localised form tends to occur on the palms and soles. Crops of deep seated pustules form on a reddish backdrop gradually 'ripening' to a golden brown colour and then progressing to desquamation. It is a very recalcitrant disease and is rare in children.

Fortunately generalised pustular psoriasis is also very rare in children.

Erythrodermatous/exfoliative psoriasis

This also results in a gravely sick patient who presents with problems of central core temperature and of maintaining fluid and electrolyte balance. Exfoliative erythroderma can result from other causes. Because the individual plaques become confluent and lose their characteristics, the diagnosis must be made from the history or nail changes when these are present.

Psoriatic arthritis (arthropathic psoriasis)

Various types of arthritis may occur in a minority of psoriatics (2%). Sometimes severe mutilating forms occur but these are observed infrequently in children. Psoriatic nail changes in affected digits may be diagnostically helpful.

Psoriasis is a capricious disease which will clear and settle frequently for no known reason. There is a kaleidoscope of different clinical pictures which affect people of all ages and circumstances. Treatment must be tailored to the individual.[6]

The majority of sufferers are treated with topical therapy.

1. Emollients such as soft yellow paraffin or simple creams which are bland are mainly used in the treatment of less severe forms of psoriasis although they do assist in softening some of the thicker scales.
2. Tars are so messy that many patients find

the disease itself preferable. Coal tar 1–10% in yellow soft paraffin is used on the body and wood tars (e.g. oil of cade 6–12% in emulsion), on the scalp.

3. Salicylic acid, 5–20% in yellow or white soft paraffin, may utilise its keratolytic effect and thus help psoriasis.
4. Dithranol (anthralin in USA) has the disadvantage of producing considerable staining.
5. Ultraviolet light may be considered under topical therapy. Sunlight contains UV A + B, (i.e. 280–400 nm) and it helps most psoriatic patients. The effect of sunlight is enhanced with concomitant tar therapy while the application of an emollient, e.g. coconut oil, also helps by the reduction of reflection of light from the patches.
6. Topical steroids have a small part to play in the therapy of most psoriatic patients. They are effective initially but may produce side effects. The more potent of them produce more satisfactory results but they should be used with caution.
7. Very few psoriatic patients require treatment with systemic drugs and such patients tend to have more severe forms of the disease. Most of the drugs used are toxic to the cells as they divide and the basic aim is to slow down the epidermal cell turnover. Methotrexate is the commonest drug but etretinate, hydroxyurea and cyclosporin A have all been used. The aforementioned common improvement with ultraviolet light is harnessed by giving a photosensitiser (psoralen) plus UVA, called PUVA therapy. The psoralen makes the patient more reactive to UVA (320–420 nm) and this is then given intensely.

Nail psoriasis is a condition which may be encountered by the podiatrist and this is one of the most difficult areas to treat. Steroids must be applied either directly as ointments or as an impregnated tape.

Physically induced skin disease

The skin is a tough encasing envelope which may be damaged by certain physical agents, e.g. cold, heat or trauma.

Chilblains (perniosis)

The commonest problem due to cold is a chilblain (perniosis) in which abnormal vasoconstriction in response to cold occurs. Too rapid rewarming opens up the arterioles earlier than the venules and this leads to local oedema and the development of a red swelling in the affected area. Pain and intense itching occur and the lesion slowly subsides to a livid purplish colour within two or three weeks.

Children are more prone to chilblains than most adults in whom a search for underlying disease should be made, e.g. lupus erythematosus. Treatment is symptomatic but prevention may be aided by the use of warmer clothing. Rapid rewarming of cold areas, especially by direct heat, should be avoided.

Burns

Burns may be caused by dry or wet heat, chemicals, friction or electrically. The extent and depth of a burn varies tremendously. The scarring provoked by many burns requires lifelong medical attention. Prevention of burns is thus extremely important and the podiatrist should take great care with corrosive chemicals and with diathermy in the presence of inflammable materials, e.g. certain alcoholic skin cleansers.

Water is the best first aid measure in all but a very few instances and is used either to dilute the chemical or to reduce the temperature as rapidly as possible.

Only small superficial burns would be within the province of the podiatrist's treatment. Sterile covers or antibiotic creams which prevent secondary infection are useful.

Trauma

Sudden acute blows or crushes produce tissue damage to various depths with consequent bruising and oedema. The diagnosis is usually apparent from the history.

Corns (Clavi)

Corns result from long-term continued pressure combined with friction. Initially the response leads to hyperkeratosis or to a callosity which may be protective. When pressure is continued, the keratin is compacted in such a way that a central 'nail' develops which tend to point towards a bony prominence. Some corns develop in unique sites and may be related to hobbies or pastimes while the majority are associated with an abnormal architecture of the foot or with the wearing of unsuitable footwear.

The main aim of treatment is reduction of the lesion, the removal of pressure from the area which should then have suitable padding applied to it. A thorough biomechanical examination of the feet should be carried out and advice given about footwear.

Blisters

Sudden unaccustomed frictional forces, e.g. school sports days, may lead to the development of blisters rather than to callosities. Moist sweating skin and new or ill-fitting footwear are predisposing factors. Prior applications of weak solutions of formalin may 'harden' the skin and thus reduce sweating. It may be possible to alter the plane of friction by the judicious application of tape. Once blisters develop they may be drained but it is better to avoid debriding them when exercise is continuing since the collapsed roof forms a dressing. Secondary infection should be prevented.

Post-traumatic punctate skin haemorrhage (talon noir)

Post-traumatic punctate skin haemorrhage is the result of bleeding into the skin and occurs when sudden shearing forces rupture the rete peg capillaries. It is characteristic of sports in which there are sudden acceleration/deceleration moves and may be termed as badminton or as tennis heel. It may occur anywhere but the borders of the heel are common and a very black slightly speckled area develops. The intensity of the colour may be mistaken for a malignant melanoma, so therefore a careful history must be taken.

Child abuse (non-accidental injury)

Bizarre, repeated or unexplained trauma must always raise the possibility of child abuse. In common with other health professionals, the podiatrist must bear this in mind. Great care must be taken to be certain or at least that there is a reasonable chance of abuse before mention is made of such a possibility. To diagnose it wrongly or to miss the diagnosis are both disasters of equal magnitude.

Nails

The podiatrist spends much time examining, maintaining and treating nails and the anatomy of the nail is well known. The nail plate is recessed into the lateral and posterior nail folds, the latter being sealed by the cuticle. The nail plate is composed of three layers: the upper layer formed from the dorsal matrix at the proximal end of the nail; the middle layer from the intermediate matrix and is seen as the half moon or lunula; and the ventral layer from the nail bed matrix.

Nail growth is affected by many factors but the normal toe nail will take approximately nine months to grow 1 cm. Finger nails grow three times faster than toe nails and all rates of growth slow with age.

After a severe illness there may be an upset in the nail growth. Thereafter a transverse indentation (Beau's line) may be seen on several or all nails.

Bacteria, e.g. staphylococci, may invade the nail fold thus causing acute paronychia especially in finger nails. Antibiotics with or without surgical drainage is the treatment for such a condition. Elevation of the affected area alleviates pain. When paronchia becomes chronic, the invading organisms change and the predominant pathogen is *Candida* which is reinforced by bacteria. The cuticle is destroyed thus allowing infecting agents to enter. The skin overlying the fold becomes swollen and 'bolstered' and occasionally beads of pus may be expressed. Ultimately nail dystrophy, denoted by the nail plate exhibiting a wavy surface, develops.

Treatment is aimed at drying out the nail fold. Hygroscopic, mildly antiseptic preparations are useful, e.g. 15% sulphacetamide in 50% surgical spirit or 4% thymol in chloroform. These drugs are flammable and should be kept securely away from children. The use of antibiotic/fungal creams is not too successful.

Paronychia affects the lateral nail fold in toe nails. An abnormal nail plate, whether it be congenital, diseased or acquired, presses into the fold and thereby damages it. This damage provokes the formation of granulation tissue. Parts of the edge of the plate fragment and shards are driven into the area. During treatment these shards must be removed and the nail prevented from gouging further by reduction of its width by correction of its curvature. Granulation tissue may be chemically cauterised by copper sulphate (bluestone) or by silver nitrate, and any infection present must be treated.

Many types of trauma may damage the nail. Acute injury, which may lead to a subungual haematoma, may occur with no apparent history, especially when it is associated with acceleration or deceleration sports.

A concern in the differential diagnosis is that such presentations are rapid onset malignant melanomas. However, the diagnosis may be confirmed when altered blood can be demonstrated by puncturing the nail plate with a red hot paper clip or by drilling gently through it with a scalpel blade. Alternatively it may be possible to gain access from under the distal end of the plate. Observation and accurate measurement to ascertain if the discoloration is progressing distally may be justified but when there is doubt, it is necessary to remove the nail and then carry out a biopsy.

Nail biting, habit tics, manicure incompetence, ill-fitting footwear, certain hobbies and prolonged immersion in water variously lead to nail plate dystrophy, cuticle destruction and onycholysis. Long-standing periungual eczema may lead to problems especially near the posterior nail folds and these problems are frequently associated with cuticle loss. The nails may show pits which mimic psoriasis. Here a careful observation reveals that these pits are larger and that they do not show sharp edges. Another change is the thickening of the nail plate coupled with bands of increased colour. Some of these bands may be whitish in colour while others may appear muddied with particles.

Psoriasis commonly induces nail changes and has already been discussed. There are many other nail dystrophies some of which are associated with developmental abnormalities.

Connective tissue disease

The main characteristics of these diseases will be described elsewhere (Chapter 6) and this section will be restricted to a short description of the skin changes in the child.

Lupus erythematosus (LE)

Lupus erythematosus is broadly divided into two types: the purely cutaneous or discoid LE (DLE) and the systemic form (SLE). Both types may occur in childhood but are relatively rare.

In SLE the vast majority of patients present with a rash at some time. The commonest rash is a photosensitivity type which appears in exposed areas. A classical description is one of the 'butterfly' or 'batswing' red facial eruption with involvement of the cheeks and the bridge of the nose. Many other rashes have been described, e.g. palmar/plantar erythema, capillary nail fold dilatation. Mothers who have SLE may give birth to infants with neonatal SLE. Self-limiting annular rashes are seen and, more seriously, heart block may occur.

In DLE there are, by definition, always skin lesions. The face is the most common site but other areas including hands and feet may be affected with the concentration on light exposed sites. The lesions are variable with the commonest type being a round patch. This patch begins as a raised papular area and progresses to a roughened scaly patch. The scales exhibit a marked follicular pattern and are particularly pronounced on the scalp. These scales project down the destroyed hair follicle which when extracted are said to resemble a 'tin tack'. Scarring occurs with pigmentary abnormalities and hair loss.

Histologically, the main changes are centred around damage to the epidermal basal cell layer which shows liquefaction degeneration. Swelling, fibrinoid change and hyalinisation occur in the upper dermis. There is an upper dermal lympho-histiocytic infiltrate which tends to aggregate around skin appendages. Follicular keratin plugs may be observed. PAS staining shows thickening of the basement membrane and immunofluorescence shows a band of immunoglobulins at this site which usually consist of IgG with or without IgM or IgA. The pathologist may suggest SLE when the changes are more acute and with the presence of more immunoglobulins and less scarring, but depending on the site of the disease separation may be difficult.

The main treatment of LE is detailed elsewhere (Chapter 6). As far as the skin is concerned sun avoidance and sunscreens should be advised. Topical steroids may help to prevent scarring and very potent examples should be used, even on the face, when indicated.

Systemic sclerosis (SS)

Systemic sclerosis (SS) is rare in childhood. The main brunt of the skin changes is borne by the hands and face.

There is usually a history of Raynaud's phenomenon in the hands. The skin may be swollen at first and then becomes bound down and inelastic thus inhibiting finger movement. The distal finger ends may become whittled down resembling a pencil end and the nails may overhang to be described as 'parrot beaks'. Parts of the digits may be lost. Small, painful and difficult-to-heal ulcers may develop over bony prominences. Less frequently similar changes may occur on the feet.

Sclerotic skin changes on the face lead to a taut shiny forehead, beaking of the nose and microstomia with pursed radial fissuring. This latter feature makes dental hygiene difficult. In the child the tissue sclerosis and prominent parotids give the appearance of 'mumps'. Particularly, but not exclusively, telangiectasia develops in large 'mat-like' areas on the face.

All parts of the skin may exhibit an increase in pigmentation. Subcutaneous calcification which is painful and difficult to treat may be extruded through the skin especially in areas overlying bones.

A skin biopsy is not the way in which to diagnose systemic sclerosis. Initial changes may be minimal with gradual miniaturisation. The collagen may swell, become homogeneous and pale especially in the lower dermis. Immunofluorescence is not helpful.

A sympathetic rapport is essential when treating systemic sclerosis. Raynaud's phenomenon may be helped by the use of electrically heated gloves or socks. Care of skin and prompt treatment of infected areas is essential and prevention of trauma by competent podiatry is important.

Dermatomyositis

Although there are different causes, known and unknown, of dermatomyositis the cutaneous changes in each type, including the juvenile form, are broadly similar. The emphasis between the skin and muscle involvement is infinitely variable.

Photosensitivity, indistinguishable from LE, may be the presenting sign. The classic rash of dermatomyositis affects mainly face and hands. There is a lilac or heliotrope colour on the face with periorbital oedema particularly of the upper eyelids. Frequently periungual redness due to capillary dilatation and ragged nail cuticles may be observed on the hands. Erythema over knuckles gradually extends in a linear pattern over extensor tendons and bony prominences. Less commonly, similar changes occur on the feet. A vague erythematous area may be noticed on the 'shawl' area of the trunk. Extruding subcutaneous calcium deposits are a problem, especially in childhood dermatomyositis.

The skin histology is not usually helpful as it frequently just shows a mild lymphocytic infiltration. At times it may mimic LE.

There is no specific skin treatment although symptomatic therapy may be required.

Ainhum

Ainhum derives from a word meaning 'to saw' and may be due to an abnormal blood supply. The condition may commence in childhood with a painful hack which gradually encircles the digit, usually the fifth toe, and which then transforms to a tight band which finally amputates the digit. It is commoner in African blacks but very rare in other races. Certain conditions which mimic it are known as pseudoainhum.

Naevi

A naevus is an abnormality which may be composed of bizarre cells, by themselves nonmalignant, although some have an increased tendency to transform to cancer. The commonest naevi in the skin affect the vasculature and the pigment producing cells such as the melanocytes.

Vascular naevi

The medical classification of telangiectasia, capillary and cavernous haemangiomas are used differently by different authors and this results in confusion. Therefore it seems easier to employ the non-medical terminology.

1. Salmon patch relates to a small linear pink area. The occipital area is frequently affected, e.g. 'the stork mark', which tends to persist. Other involved areas, e.g. on the head and neck, tend to fade and contrary to popular thought such areas are not due to forcep marks or other pressure.

Histologically there is simply a dilation of blood vessels. Treatment is cosmetic.

2. Portwine naevus presents as a red area at birth which does not involute but which increases in size proportional to body size and which then darkens to the well known purplish or port wine colour. Nodules may develop but initially the skin texture is normal. Very occasionally there may be deeper angiomatous malformations, e.g. on the meninges, which lead to epilepsy. The histology shows capillary and cavernous vessels. The current best treatment is cosmetic in order to camouflage but modern lasers may be therapeutically helpful.

3. Strawberry birth marks are not usually visible at birth. At about two to five weeks they present and grow rapidly in size. Rarely do they exceed 5 cm in diameter but at times they may be larger. Subcutaneous vessels may also be involved. Their colour varies from red to deep purple and the surface from smooth to puckered. Spontaneous involution after some years is the norm and this may be hastened by superadded infection and ulceration. Histologically there are thin-walled dilated blood vessels which gradually obliterate with ageing and with a concomitant increase in connective tissue stroma. Treatment should be expectant with firm reassurance to the parents. Skin texture is expected to return to completely

normal but occasionally gigantic lesions break down blood cells and such lesions require the administration of steroids. Surgery has no place unless pressure symptoms lead to hazards, e.g. occlusion of the urethra.

Benign pigmented naevi (melanocytic naevi; moles)

At 12 weeks pigment producing cells from the primitive neural crest migrate as melanoblasts which reach the dermo-epidermal junction at 20 weeks. Certain of these melanoblasts appear to become 'stuck' at various points in this migration and in the deeper dermis these can lead to various pigmented naevi. Certain naevi may develop from epidermal cells 'dropping back' into the dermis or from other cells with a common neural crest origin. In any event the benign pigmented naevi (or moles) are very common and numerous different classifications have been suggested the easiest of which is to consider them as congenital or acquired.

1. Congenital pigmented naevi may not be present at birth but should be visible within the first few weeks. They may be subdivided by size into small, under 1.5 cm; medium, 1.5–20 cm; or large, 20 cm plus. Any site may be involved with the larger ones being predisposed to affect the lower trunk. Mottled pigmentation may be seen with an outer irregular edge, and coarse hair may grow through the naevus. Once developed congenital naevi persist. Generally the larger they are the more likely there is to be malignant change.

Histologically smaller naevi tend to show aggregations of naevus cells in nests while larger ones are more 'crowd-like'. The naevus cells have abundant cytoplasm and may contain melanin. Certain of them possess spindle-like cells and some epithelioid cells.

Surgical treatment is not practical for larger naevi. Small ones may be resectable depending upon the site but these are usually left until later childhood in view of the more remote chance of malignancy. However, these should be observed regularly and preferably with photographic records.

2. *Acquired benign pigmented naevi* develop in children with a peaking of development in teenage and in early adult life. Many such naevi disappear slowly with age. In the newly developed most of these naevus cells are found in 'pockets' or groups in the junction between the dermis and epidermis, hence the name 'junctional naevus'. When dermal naevus cells are also present the term 'compound naevus' is used and when they are purely located in the deeper dermis they are termed 'intradermal naevi'.

Junctional naevi may show a uniform scattering of pigmentary stippling which is more easily seen with some magnification and after coating with some mineral oil. Although any site may be involved the soles, the palms and the genitalia are common areas. Such lesions are flattish and do not age or fade to the same extent as in other sites. Compound and intradermal naevi should show fairly homogeneous pigmentation although the intensity of the colour fades in the older intradermal ones. The edge should not be ragged. The lesion of the compound and intradermal variety may be dome-shaped but the skin markings should not be interrupted. Hair may grow through these especially in the intradermal type. Histologically naevus cells of various types are seen in the appropriate site. In the junctional type pockets are observed in this zone. In the deeper varieties the nests tend to transfer to cords and the cells have less cytoplasm.

In most cases surgical removal is only required on account of constant trauma or clinical doubt regarding the benign nature of the lesion. When prevailed upon to remove them for cosmetic reasons the possibility of a less attractive scar ensuing should always be borne in mind and this should be discussed with the patient and parent.

Malignant melanoma

Of all the pigmented lesions seen very few are malignant and of these very few occur in childhood. However, there is an increase in such lesions and they may occur in children. The reasons for this increase are not clear but there is considerable evidence that sun exposure abuse should be avoided. One severe episode of sunburn may be more hazardous than longer term gradual ones.

Suspicious symptoms and signs would be complaints of itching, inflammation, bleeding and/or discharge unless there was a convincing history of recent trauma. Increase in size (especially to over 1 cm) would cause concern and an alteration in pigmentation with loss of homogeneity and an irregular edge would be ominous, as would abnormalities of the skin surface.

Malignant melanomas spread by horizontal or vertical paths with the latter having a much worse prognosis in respect of secondary metastases.

Histologically atypical melanocytes with bizarre nuclei and frequent mitoses are seen. The thickness is important in the prognosis and is classified by the pathologist who uses an absolute measurement (Breslow's thickness) or who relates it to the depth level of other structures (Clarke's levels).

Any pigmented lesion suspected of being a malignant melanoma should be assessed by an appropriate doctor as soon as possible.

References

1 Okano M, Kitano Y, Yoshikawa K, Nakamura T, Matsuzawa Y, Yusa T. X-linked ichthyosis and ichthyosis vulgaris: comparison of their clinical features based on biochemical analysis. *Br J Dermatol* 1988; 119: 777–83.

2 Baden HP, Alper JC. A keratolytic gel containing salicylic acid in propylene glycol. *J Invest Dermatol* 1973; 61: 330–3.

3 Alexander J O'D. *Arthropods and Human Skin*. Berlin, Springer-Verlag, 1984.

4 Thomson J, Cochrane T, Cochran R, McQueen A 1974. Histology simulating reticulosis and persistent nodular scabies. *Br J Dermatol* 1974; 90: 421–9.

5 Bunney MH. *Viral Warts: their Biology and Treatment*. Oxford University Press, 1982.

6 Zachariae H. Management of difficult psoriasis. In *Recent Advances in Dermatology* (Ed. RH Champion and RJ Pye), No. 8. Edinburgh, Churchill Livingstone, 1990.

6 Paediatric Rheumatology
Madeleine Rooney and Brian Ellis

Rheumatic diseases are a group of conditions whose underlying pathology is inflammation of the connective tissues. Although many organs may be involved, there is a predilection for joint inflammation, i.e. redness, swelling, heat and pain.

The study of rheumatic diseases in childhood is a relatively new specialty. Although George Frederic Still is usually considered to be the 'father of paediatric rheumatology', after his description of the condition in 1896, the specialty per se has really only been developed since the Second World War.

Juvenile chronic arthritis

For many the term juvenile chronic arthritis (JCA) is synonymous with adult rheumatoid arthritis. In both, arthritis is the predominant feature; however, there the similarity ends.

In children, large joints such as the hips, knees and ankles, as opposed to the small joints of the hands, are much more commonly affected. The number of affected joints is often lower in children, i.e. an oligoarthritis as opposed to a polyarthritis. Seropositivity for rheumatoid factor (see below) is very uncommon. The most important difference lies in the fact that children are growing. The impact of inflammation on a joint not only affects that joint but also the adjacent epiphysis, thus interfering with normal limb growth.

The management of children with chronic arthritis not only involves the treatment of the inflammation, but also the fostering of normal growth patterns.

Epidemiology

The incidence of juvenile chronic arthritis is in the order of 0.01% of children under the age of 15.

Pathology

In health the typical synovial joint consists of two bones with articulating surfaces coated in articular cartilage cuffed in a diaphanous membrane – the synovial membrane (SM). Externally the structure is supported by the joint capsule, ligaments, tendons and muscle (Fig. 6.1a). Articular cartilage is avascular and receives its nutrition from the small quantities of synovial fluid (SF) produced by the synovial membrane. The fluid, in coating the articular surfaces, dramatically reduces friction thus minimising structural wear. At arthroscopy the healthy joint does not contain collections of fluid but glistens. The SM is as fine as chiffon.

The synovial membrane

The SM has a one to two cell deep lining layer with an incomplete or fenestrated basement membrane lying beneath it. This lining layer is supported by a loose bed of connective tissue (which allows the membrane to be stretched and compressed during movement) containing the subsynovial capillaries (Fig. 6.1a). The membrane becomes more fibrous as it extends outwards to fuse with the joint capsule. The lining cells are made up of two functional cell types, A and B. B cells are secretory, producing hyaluronic acid and other components, which mix with an ultrafiltrate of plasma which passes through the walls of the synovial membrane capillaries and the basement membrane to produce synovial fluid. The A cells are phagocytic, engulfing joint debris and are the general housekeepers of the joint. It is probable that A and B cells are from the same stem cell, performing different functions at different time points.

The aetiological agents responsible for any of the forms of JCA remain unknown. However, the changes observed within the synovial membrane could be explained on the basis of a

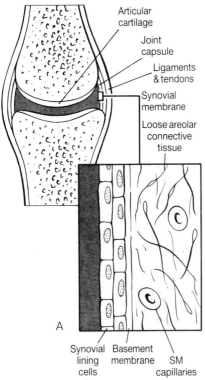

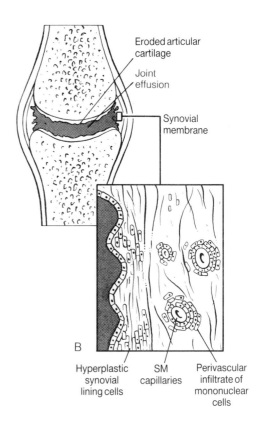

Figure 6.1   A, The healthy joint. B, The inflamed joint.

chronic cell mediated immune response; thus for clarity this is the model which will be used here.

A foreign or altered self protein (antigen) encounters the endothelial cells lining the small capillaries within the synovial membrane. These cells become activated and express molecules on their surfaces which are adhesive to circulating mononuclear cells. During activation, these endothelial cells swell and the vessel walls become 'leaky', allowing passage of 'primed' and selected mononuclear cells into the subsynovial matrix. Thus one of the earliest changes within the synovial membrane is a perivascular infiltrate of mononuclear cells (Fig. 6.1B). The synovial membrane contains macrophage like cells that are highly specialised in that they express molecules on to their surface (class II HLA/DR molecules) that are the linchpin of an immune response. These cells in vitro are able to process foreign proteins and antigens and express them on to their surface in conjunction with the HLA DR molecules which enables T cells with appropri-

ate receptors to 'recognise' this antigen and become activated (Fig. 6.2). Activated T cells produce large quantities of small proteins (peptides) which act as intercellular messengers, leading to recruitment and activation of the T cells with a resultant cascade effect, with large aggregates of T cells forming within the synovial membrane. In addition, by mechanisms which are not understood, the one to two cell deep lining layer becomes markedly increased. This leads to a several thousand fold increase in the surface area of the synovial membrane within a joint (Fig. 6.1b). The combination of a large surface area and increased transudation of fluid from leaking synovial vessels leads to the collection of large volumes of fluid within the joint, i.e. joint effusion. Many of the substances produced by activated cells within the joint are known in vitro to be able to destroy cartilage and may explain the changes such as the erosion of cartilage which may be seen on X-ray and in pathological specimens.

Many of the early histological changes are

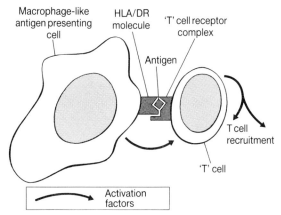

Figure 6.2   Diagram of T cell mediated immune response.

similar to those seen in any 'healthy' immunological response, for example chronic infection. However, in health, once the foreign antigen has been cleared or destroyed, the immune response is switched off and the infiltrates disappear. For some reason, in JCA the immune response remains 'switched on', possibly because the offending foreign material is not adequately removed or more likely, that in a genetically defined group of individuals, there is a defect in the normal inhibitory mechanism employed in downregulation of the immune response.

Current concepts in the pathogenesis of JCA

Despite a significant body of scientific research, no cause for JCA has been found to date. For many years, an infectious aetiology has been sought and although there have been sporadic reports of bacteria having been isolated from the synovial membrane, these findings have not been corroborated. Viruses appear a much more likely candidate especially since some, such as the parvo and Coxsackie viruses, can cause a transient arthritis (see below) very similar to JCA. Nevertheless exhaustive research has failed to prove any consistent viral link. In recent years, however, our knowledge of virus 'behaviour' and the host response to them has increased dramatically. A whole new group of viruses has been defined such as the human T cell leukaemia virus (HTLVI). Many of these viruses can infect cells without, at least initially, causing any detectable changes in the immune system of the host. Thus, many of the methods used for their detection in the past would have been inadequate. The possibility of a viral aetiology remains speculative. However, a search for possible viral agents using more sophisticated techniques must still be continued.

Profound immunological disturbance can be found in JCA. Whether these are causative or merely the result of the underlying cause (epiphenomenon) remains unknown. That genetics have a part to play is undisputed. Other autoimmune diseases occur more frequently in the first degree relatives of these children than can be explained by chance. Further, certain histocompatibility antigens, which define 'self' occur more frequently in the disease population than in the control. However, the genetic contribution is far from 100%. For example, there is less than a 50% likelihood of an identical twin developing any form of JCA when the other twin is affected.

Therefore, both genetic and environmental factors must be involved in the pathogenesis of these diseases.

Classification

Juvenile chronic arthritis divides into three broad groups, each with several subgroups. This classification has been defined by the Juvenile Rheumatoid Arthritis criteria subcommittee of the American Rheumatism Association[1] (JRA ARA) which was subsequently revised in 1977.

The three subgroups are:

1. Pauci-articular JCA.
2. Polyarticular JCA.
3. Systemic JCA.

The salient features of each are listed in Table 6.1.

Pauci-articular JCA

Pauci-articular JCA accounts for 40% of affected children and refers to an arthritis where, during the first six months of the disease, four or fewer joints are affected. The arthritis is often asymmetrical with the knees, ankles and wrists most often involved. It occurs most commonly in preschool girls with a sex ratio

Table 6.1 Clinical and epidemiological features of JCA subsets

	Systemic JCA	Pauci-articular JCA	Polyarticular JCA
% Patients at onset*	Approx. 25	Approx. 50	Approx. 25
Age at onset	Usually before 5th year	1–4 years	Throughout childhood
Sex ratio	F = M	F >> M	F > M
HLA type	No clear link ? DR4	DRw5 associated with eye disease F >> M B27 associated with spondyloarthropathy later onset M > F	DR4 associated with RF
ANA antibodies % ±		50+	25%
RF (Rheumatoid Factor) ±		–	10% with disease onset in adolescence

* Within first six months.
% are averages of multiple series.

F : M of 9 : 1 (when children with a B27 related spondyloarthropathy are excluded). Systemic disease is absent. However, there is a curious association with a chronic inflammation of the anterior chamber of the eye, chronic anterior uveitis, which when left undiagnosed or untreated can lead to blindness. The chronic anterior uveitis occurs in about 20% of children with pauci-articular JCA and is associated with antinuclear antibodies (see below) in the serum of these children in 75% of cases. The condition is asymptomatic; thus when these children are not recognised and the possibility of uveitis investigated, the only serious and most treatable complication of pauci-articular JCA can have devastating effects.

The diagnosis of pauci-articular JCA is primarily clinical, based on the involvement of four or fewer joints (often knees and ankles) after the exclusion of other causes of arthritis, e.g. viral or septic. Antinuclear antibodies are found in 50–90% of these children when children with the HLA antigen B27 (usually older boys) are excluded.

Antinuclear antibodies (ANAs). As the name implies these are circulating antibodies directed against nuclear antigens. Since nuclear material is not normally exposed to immunocompetent cells, it is not clear how these antibodies develop. The frequency of detection of such antibodies depends upon the cell types used as substrate, e.g. rat or mouse liver. In more recent studies using the HEp–2 cell line (derived from human laryngeal epithelial cells) as a substrate for ANA assays, 60–70% of chil-

dren with pauci-articular JCA are positive. This increase in sensitivity leads to some decrease in specificity with 5% of healthy children giving a low positive result. Although ANAs are found in all subgroups of JCA they occur with greatest frequency in the pauci-articular subgroup when the risk of eye disease increases by 50%.

Since only a few joints are affected, the arthritis can be treated locally. Topical non-steroidal anti-inflammatory preparations can reduce swelling and stiffness in moderately inflamed joints, whereas intra-articular administration of crystalline steroid preparations such as triamcinolone hexacetonide can provide long-lasting relief. Non-steroidal anti-inflammatory drugs (NSAIDs) can be very beneficial for pain and stiffness when several joints are involved to a similar degree. When inflammation is persistent within a joint, rapid growth at the adjacent epiphyseal plate may result in initial overgrowth of the limb and then, with subsequent early epiphyseal fusion, in shortening (Fig. 6.3).

Inflammation in any joint results in the adoption of a flexed posture. This occurs partly because flexor muscles are stronger than joint extensors and because the flexed posture lowers intra-articular pressure within the joint. Thus flexion is the most comfortable position for the limb. When this attitude is allowed to persist, capsular and muscle contraction will result in the development of a fixed flexion deformity. Indeed, in children, soft tissue contractures rather than bony abnormalities are the main cause of disability in JCA.

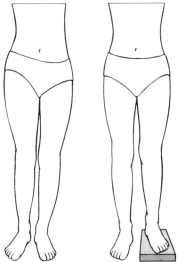

Figure 6.3 Shortening of the left leg due to long-standing disease of the left knee. The leg was initially larger but, following early epiphyseal fusion, the limb was ultimately shorter. Note the pelvic tilt until leg length was corrected with an appropriate raise.

The greatest effort must therefore be made to maintain the joint, while inflamed, in its extended position at the same time encouraging a full range of movement. The joints which cause the greatest problem in this respect are hips, knees, wrists and ankles.

Hips. The inflamed hip rapidly develops a flexed internally rotated and adducted deformity. When not treated early, correction may only be possible by surgical intervention, which requires hospitalisation with stressful separation from family and the disruption of schooling. Children do not tolerate prolonged periods of immobilisation. The aim is to enable such children to lead as normal a life as possible. Thus an effort should be made for physical therapists to fit into the normal daily routine of a child with the minimum of disruption. School and play are essential and children should not be discouraged or prevented from involving themselves in physical activities. Children are their own best monitors. Thus a child with a very painful hip will not play football or climb a tree. When walking is painful, cycling should be encouraged thus keeping the child mobile and in contact with his peers. Where flexion deformities are developing, reg-

ular periods of physiotherapy should be undertaken before and after school. Following an initial course performed by the physiotherapist, many parents are able to learn the techniques and to provide the treatment themselves.

During sleep, hip flexion is frequently the posture adopted by the child. However, this is the ideal time to immobilise the joint in its neutral position. Where minimal flexion deformities are present or where such deformities are to be prevented, the child should be encouraged to sleep in the prone position. Where significant flexion is present, light traction may be applied to the limb during the sleeping times. Children rapidly tolerate this form of therapy provided it is not unduly painful. Pleasurable activities such as watching TV can be adapted; e.g. the child may be encouraged to watch TV lying prone on the floor with a cushion wedged under his chest for periods of 30 minutes or so.

Swimming is by far the most important form of exercise. It is beneficial to all joints, exercising all muscle groups without placing a load on inflamed joints; but perhaps most importantly it encourages socialising.

Knees. As with the hip, knee joints rapidly develop fixed flexion deformities when inflamed. When untreated, tendon or capsular contractures occur. Following local therapy, intensive physiotherapy should be commenced to regain a full range of movement, with night splinting in the form of back slabs in order to maintain extension. Modification of play, such as raising the seat of a tricycle to ensure full extension of the knee while pedalling, can be very effective.

Feet and ankles. Inflammation at the ankle or within the small joints of the foot leads to complex foot abnormalities due to the integral relationships of these joints. Inflammation at any of the foot articulations may lead to weakness of the intrinsic muscles of the foot with resulting varus and valgus deformity (Fig. 6.4). Stiffness in an affected joint such as the subtalar will lead to abnormal biomechanical function of the foot, abnormal loading and gait patterns. Loss of ankle movement again leads to abnormal loading during the gait cycle. Obviously abnormalities at the hip and knee will also affect normal functioning of the foot.

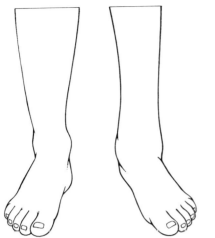

Figure 6.4 Valgus deformity of left ankle. Note the swelling around the ankle joint and the wasting of peroneal and calf muscles.

Management of ankle and foot problems in children is very problematic and includes maintenance of a neutral posture by the use of supportive shoes or trainers with ankle supports, heel cups and moulded orthoses. Exercises to improve intrinsic musculature are essential. However, the effectiveness of any of these measures has not been fully evaluated and much work and research remains to be done.

HLA B27 associated spondyloarthropathies. A subgroup of children with a pauci-articular onset of arthritis possess the histocompatibility antigen HLA B27. This antigen is found in approximately 90% of adults with ankylosing spondylitis. Such children have been arbitrarily grouped together. However, their disease 'complex' does follow a pattern: males are more commonly affected than females, with an onset in mid to late childhood with primarily a lower limb asymmetrical oligo- or monoarthritis. They are prone to enthesopathies, i.e. inflammation at the site of tendon insertion into bone such as plantar fasciitis or Achilles tendinitis. Unlike adult B27 associated ankylosing spondylitis, only a small proportion (approximately 10%) of these children develop clinically significant spinal disease. As a group these children are more at risk for developing any of the spondyloarthropathies such as Reiter's syndrome, psoriatic arthritis or the arthritis associated with inflammatory bowel disease. Painful anterior uveitis of the eye is the main extra-articular manifestation, and rarely cardiac involvement is noted.

Management is as for other forms of oligoarthritis.

Polyarticular JCA

In approximately 20% of children the mode of onset of JCA is polyarticular, i.e. five or more joints involved during the first six months of the disease. These may be divided into two groups: (a) those who are seropositive for rheumatoid factor and (b) those who are seronegative.

1. Seropositive polyarticular JCA. Rheumatoid factor is an autoantibody, usually an immunoglobulin of the IgM subclass, but also of IgG and IgA directed against self IgG immunoglobulin. The presence of IgM rheumatoid factor may be detected by a variety of methods, using either red cells (the sheep red cell agglutination test, SCAT) or latex particles (RA latex test) coated with IgG. When these are mixed with patient serum containing IgM rheumatoid factor, visible agglutination can be seen. Serum IgM rheumatoid factor is the hallmark of adult rheumatoid arthritis, although its pathogenic role is unclear. Five to ten per cent of children with polyarticular JCA are seropositive for rheumatoid factor. Girls are more frequently affected than boys and the disease usually commences in late childhood or during adolescence. It runs a polyarticular course involving the small joints of the hands and feet as well as cervical spine and large joints. The clinical and radiological features are the same as those seen in adult rheumatoid arthritis, with bony erosions. However, the disease is often more aggressive and destructive than that seen in adults, with a poor prognosis.

2. Seronegative polyarticular JCA. In a further group with a pauci-articular onset, the disease evolves to become polyarticular (extended pauci) over the months or years. This type occurs throughout childhood, again with a female predominance and with the pattern of joint involvement similar to that seen in the rheumatoid factor positive group. However, the disease is not as erosive or as destructive as the seropositive group, and the long-term prognosis is better.

Antinuclear antibodies are found in approximately 25% of these children and anterior uveitis does occur. Thus these children also require regular slit lamp examination of the eyes.

Other laboratory abnormalities include an anaemia and a raised ESR and thrombocytosis (see below) during active disease. The magnitude of the latter correlate fairly well with the number of involved joints and thus are useful in determining an index of disease activity and response to treatment.

As with other forms of JCA, the mainstay of treatment of polyarticular disease is physical therapy. Joint pain and early morning stiffness lasting several hours are the major symptoms. Non-steroidal anti-inflammatory drugs (NSAIDs) are particularly beneficial leading to increased patient mobility, independence and compliance with physiotherapy and are the first line of treatment. NSAIDs, however, do not alter the course of the treatment as they are not disease modifying drugs. When symptoms persist in spite of maximum NSAID therapy, i.e. the child still presents with multiple swollen, tender joints and a significant, persistent haematological upset with a raised ESR, thrombocytosis and anaemia, disease modifying anti-rheumatic drugs (DMARDs) are indicated. Hydroxychloroquine, Salazopyrin, gold and D-penicillamine have all been used with moderate success. Recent studies using methotrexate in polyarticular disease have been very promising. These drugs act by suppressing the immune system and thus have potentially toxic side effects including bone marrow suppression and renal damage. Therefore the decision to commence such agents is not taken lightly. DMARDs require regular monitoring and the long-term effects of some of these agents on children are not absolutely clear, but to date no significant disturbances in fertility, teratogenicity or neoplasia have been noted.

Corticosteroids. In a number of children the above measures are inadequate to control the disease and the symptoms and signs of joint inflammation are severe enough to require steroid therapy. As with the systemic form of JCA the benefits of therapy need to be balanced against the side effects of osteoporosis, growth stunting, obesity and skin changes. Steroid requirement is often much less than that required for systemic JCA. Alternate day therapy reduces growth retardation as do the new steroid analogues. Weight gain in children is particularly troublesome. When parents are aware of the increase in appetite and when carbohydrate intake is kept to a minimum, obesity may be avoided.

Systemic JCA

Systemic JCA refers to that subset of children in whom systemic extra-articular features are a prominent feature of their disease. The clinical features include:

Pyrexia
Skin rash
Lymphadenopathy
Hepatosplenomegaly
Pleurisy/pericarditis
Arthritis

Approximately 20% of children with JCA have the systemic form. Although it may occur at any age during childhood it is most common before the age of five years. Unlike other forms of JCA the sexes are affected equally. Although there is still some debate there are no definite genetic markers associated with this subtype. However, the influence of genes is manifested by the higher concordance with monozygotic as opposed to dizygotic twins.

Initial presentation is often with a daily high spiking fever to ~40°C returning to normal during a 24 hour period (Fig. 6.5) and accompanied by an evanescent salmon coloured rash. At the outset this fever will usually be attributed to an infection but it is unresponsive to antibiotics. Fevers and rashes are very common in childhood, thus a diagnosis of systemic JCA should not be entertained until all other causes of fever and rash have been excluded and the fever and rash are persistent, albeit intermittently, for at least six weeks. Generalised lymphadenopathy and abdominal pain are common features as is hepatosplenomegaly. The arthritis may be present at onset but frequently postdates the rash and fever by weeks or months. Children may be broadly divided into two groups: (i) those in whom the arthritis is an absent or a minimal feature

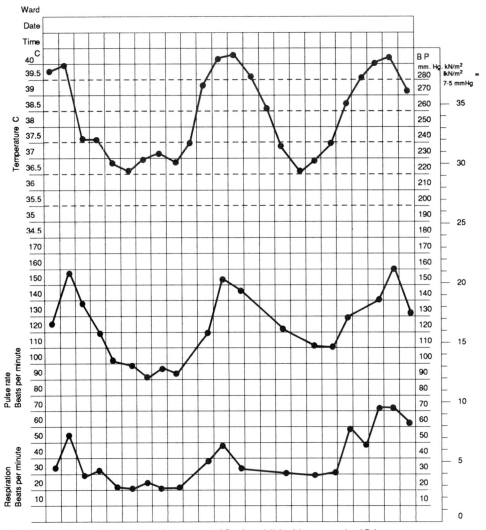

Figure 6.5   Classical daily high spiking fever to 40 °C of a child with systemic JCA.

where the prognosis is excellent, and (ii) those where the arthritis is prominent and often unremitting when the prognosis is rather poor.

Uveitis is extremely uncommon in these children.

Growth and development. Because of the systemic nature of this disease, chronic anaemia and growth retardation are not infrequent. Small stature in adulthood (below the 3rd centile) is a feature of early onset disease, disease uncontrolled throughout childhood and chronic steroid therapy (see above).

Pericarditis occurs in approximately 50% of children with systemic JCA during the initial episode. This is usually asymptomatic apart from mild chest pain and tachycardia and will respond well to steroid therapy. Rarely, however, cardiac tamponade due to a restrictive pericardial effusion or a severe myocarditis can lead to cardiac failure.

The most serious complication of systemic JCA is renal amyloidosis. Here a protein, serum amyloid A which is elevated in a variety of chronic inflammatory diseases, is deposited in body tissues, most importantly in the kidneys thus leading to renal impairment and in certain cases even failure. Renal amyloidosis accounts for approximately 50% of deaths from JCA.

The diagnosis of systemic JCA is one of exclusion, i.e. by excluding underlying infective or neoplastic conditions. There are no laboratory tests which diagnose this condition; thus good clinical acumen, the exclusion of other childhood febrile conditions and a follow-up of at least six weeks are necessary before a definite diagnosis can be made.

Investigations

Although there are no diagnostic laboratory investigations for systemic JCA there are a number which are almost always abnormal. These help to monitor disease activity and response to treatment. So common are these abnormalities that persistently normal results in the presence of clinically active disease should make the diagnosis questionable. These haematological abnormalities include:

1. *Anaemia*: where the haemoglobin content of the blood (in g/dl) is below that expected for the age. There are many types of anaemia. The commonest found in JCA is the normocytic (normal sized cells), normochromic (normal haemoglobinised cells), anaemia where fewer red cells are produced by the bone marrow.
2. *Leucocytosis*: an increase in the number of circulating white cells.
3. *Thrombocytosis*: an increase in the number of circulating platelets.
4. *Raised ESR*: the erythrocyte sedimentation rate is the rate at which red cells separate out of a thin column of whole blood into a red cell sediment and plasma. The commonest method used is that of Westengren when the distance the red cells have travelled in one hour is measured and expressed in millimetres. The normal for children is <10 mm.
5. *High levels of acute phase proteins* (produced by the liver in many inflammatory diseases): such as C-reactive protein.
6. *Hypergammaglobulinaemia*: an increase in the level of circulating immunoglobulins IgG, IgA and IgM, above that expected for age.

In the majority of children the fever, rash and arthritis may be controlled with adequate doses of aspirin or other NSAID approved for use in children such as naproxen, indomethacin or ibuprofen. When these features are inadequately controlled on maximum doses, or where there is evidence of major organ involvement such as cardiac, steroids will be required often initially in large doses. Children tolerate both NSAIDs and steroids much better than adults. Steroid induced osteoporosis and growth retardation may be minimised by using synthetic steroid analogues such as Deflazacort and alternate day therapy. The latter avoids suppression of the adrenal glands which are the body's natural source of steroid hormones.

In spite of the above therapies there are a small group of children in whom the polyarthritis runs an unremitting and destructive course. To date none of the disease modifying anti-rheumatic drugs such as gold, penicillamine or Salazopyrin, useful in other forms of arthritis, have been shown to be particularly effective. Currently there are a variety of new drug regimens under study such as intravenous immunoglobulins and methotrexate therapy. The outcomes of these studies are awaited.

A detailed description and the pharmacology of the drugs used in JCA are outside the scope of this book. However, an excellent review is listed in Further Reading at the end of the chapter.

General points of management

During active disease these children are often anorectic and therefore attention must be paid to calorie protein intake. Children will not over exert themselves when the disease is active and only in extreme circumstances should a child be confined to bed. Once the cause of the rash and fever is confirmed the child should be encouraged to go to school even when the disease is active. When joint disease is prominent they should be kept active and bed rest should be kept to a minimum; regular non-weight-bearing exercises and non-weightbearing play such as cycling and swimming should be encouraged.

The natural instinct of parents is to overprotect a systemically ill child. The detrimental physical and psychological impact of this on a child with a chronic disease can be immense. Therefore it is important to allow such children to indulge in normal childhood activities and this cannot be overstressed. With the exception of perhaps contact sports all normal activities should be encouraged even during active disease. Children are their own best monitors and will not play when in pain. Thus the risk of a child damaging himself by over-aggressive physical activity is far outweighed by the psychosocial damage of cosseting. Children are sensitive to parental anxiety and will rapidly adopt illness behaviours when it is to their advantage, i.e. complaints of fever or joint pain, if this will exempt them from attending school. The best weapon in the face of this potentially physically disabling disease is to enable these children to develop into well balanced and mature adults.

Septic arthritis

Septic arthritis occurs in all age groups of children. It is most frequently observed in those under two years of age and males are more often affected than females. Septic arthritis almost always involves one joint – a monoarthritis – the hip, knee or elbow being the most frequently involved. Septic arthritis can be a devastating condition. In cases where virulent organisms are involved such as *Staphylococcus aureus*, the joint may be destroyed in a matter of days. Thus there should be a high index of suspicion for a bacterial cause in a child with a monoarthritis and this should be excluded before any other diagnosis is considered. When diagnosed early and then treated with appropriate antibiotic therapy, prognosis is good. However, when diagnosis is delayed, the chances of the joint developing normally are very limited.

Unlike other forms of childhood arthritis, septic arthritis can be exquisitely painful and throbbing, night pain being a helpful indicator. However, in small children and babies, pain may be very difficult to assess. Fever is usually present. Thus in a febrile child who refuses to weightbear or to move the affected limb, joint aspiration should be performed for culture of the synovial fluid. Different organisms are encountered more frequently at different stages of development:

Neonate *Staphylococcus aureus*/Gram negative bacilli

1–24 months *Haemophilus influenzae*
Childhood/adolescent *Staphylococcus aureus*/streptococci/*Haemophilus influenzae*

Certain organisms are of low virulence such as *Mycobacterium tuberculosis*. Here the septic arthritis may be indolent and chronic and fever absent. Tuberculous arthritis is increasing, with a high prevalence rate among the Asian population and those children in contact with tuberculosis.

Viral arthritis

Arthritis frequently accompanies a number of viral illnesses in children. The natural history of viral related arthritides is for resolution in weeks or months. The importance of making this diagnosis is to separate such children from those with a similar clinical presentation where no viral aetiology is found and in whom the arthritis may well run a chronic course, e.g. JCA. Epidemiological studies have defined a number of viruses where rheumatic complaints are not uncommon.

1. Approximately 5% of children develop a transient symmetrical small joint polyarthralgia or arthritis following rubella vaccination.
2. Parvo-virus causes a childhood xanthoma, erythema infectiosum, with a characteristic 'slapped cheek' facial rash and a mild systemic upset with fever. Approximately 5% of children develop an arthritis similar to that seen following rubella vaccination. However, the arthritis may last for weeks and even months.
3. Enteroviral infection, e.g. Coxsackie B, leads to small or large joint arthritis in approximately 1 : 1000 cases. Resolution is usually complete within two weeks.
4. Case reports of arthritis due to adenovirus infection have been documented. Resolution appears to occur within one month.

Once the diagnosis has been made, both the child and parents can be reassured of the benign nature of the condition. A short course of NSAIDs is all that is required. Thus any child who presents with the sudden onset of an arthritis, especially when it is associated with a xanthoma or other febrile illness, should be screened for a possible viral cause.

Systemic lupus erythematosus

Systemic lupus erythematosus (SLE) is a multi-system immunologically mediated disease where the primary damage occurs in small arteries. The commonest tissues to be involved are those of the skin and joints, although any organ may be involved including the lungs, heart and kidneys with the latter being the greatest cause of morbidity and mortality. SLE is uncommon in children and rarely occurs before the age of five. Frequently first degree relatives are also affected. Classically children present with a photosensitive facial rash, arthralgia or frank arthritis. Other organ involvement is common, in particular, kidneys in the form of a glomerulonephritis which when left untreated will lead to renal failure. As well as the above signs, these children have evidence of systemic upset including mild fever and profound tiredness and lethargy. The disease mirrors that of adult SLE but is often more severe.

Ninety-five per cent of these children have IgG or IgM antibodies to a variety of nuclear antigens. Thus the presence of antinuclear antibodies (ANAs) is crucial to the diagnosis of SLE. However, since ANAs are present in a variety of other childhood arthritides, a positive test alone does *not* make the diagnosis. The presence of antibodies directed against double stranded DNA is diagnostic of the disease, but they are only present in approximately 30% of cases and although highly specific it is not a sensitive test. Other haematological and immunological disturbances include anaemia, lymphopenia, thrombocytopenia and hypocomplementaemia (low levels of circulatory complement components), the latter three of which are not found in other forms of childhood arthritis.

The arthritis is non-erosive and non-destructive and the pain and stiffness respond well to NSAIDs, although joint contractures do occur. The photosensitive skin rash may usually be controlled with sun blocks. In the presence of significant systemic upset or major organ involvement, steroids are the mainstay of treatment and are often life saving.

The anti-malarials hydroxychloroquine and chloroquine can be useful in controlling the skin rash and arthritic symptoms. However, both may very rarely cause retinal (macular) pigmentation leading to visual disturbance. These children therefore require six monthly or yearly fundoscopy (examination of the retina of the eye).

Dermatomyositis

Dermatomyositis is an uncommon disease of childhood and the primary tissues involved are the skin and muscles. Girls are slightly more frequently affected than boys and onset before the age of two years is rare.

In the skin the primary lesion is one of a perivascular infiltrate with vessel dilatation. In the muscle similar infiltrates occur leading to vessel necrosis with infarcted areas of muscle and consequent muscle fibre atrophy.

Two modes of onset are recognised. In the first the onset is acute and fulminant with fever and prostration and thought by some to be post infectious. In the second group the onset is insidious and the clinical features subtle. Thus the diagnosis is often delayed.

The skin of the face becomes oedematous and erythematous, with pronounced telangiectasia and a violacious discoloration around the eyes, and erythematous plaques across the knuckles of the hands (Grottron's plaques). Muscle inflammation is manifest by muscle weakness, usually of the proximal muscles – a proximal myopathy. Muscle pain is usually mild, but occasionally muscle pain and tenderness may be severe, depending upon the rapidity of onset.

Twenty-five per cent of children have an associated arthritis and a variety of other organs may be involved including lung and kidneys. Calcium deposition (calcinosis) in skin and subcutaneous tissue is a major complication. Large lumpy chalk-like deposits can form in pressure areas such as the buttocks or elbows, which are painful, unsightly and may ulcerate. Alternatively diffuse sheets of calcification may occur in fascial planes (which are only detectable by X-ray) which may impede muscle functioning.

Initial foot problems are often acute general pain followed by signs of peripheral oedema, an erythematous scaly rash extending distally from the knees, telangiectasia around the nail fold edge, muscle pain, walking difficulties due to muscle weakness and vasculitis resulting in skin ulceration. In addition there may be synovitis, Raynaud's phenomenon and muscle weakness affecting the pelvic girdle.

Diagnosis is made in the presence of characteristic skin changes, proximal muscle weakness and elevation of muscle enzymes (such as creatine phosphokinase (CPK) which is released from damaged muscle cells) in the serum. Electromyographic changes of myositis, or muscle biopsy evidence of myositis, may be necessary investigations, depending upon the clinical picture and the other laboratory results.

In the majority of cases the disease remains active for a number of years, then resolves, leaving a variable degree of disability as a result of muscle loss, soft tissue and skin contractures and calcinosis, all of which may improve, to some degree, with time.

During the inflammatory phase, steroids are the drugs of choice. In those children in whom steroids are only partially effective or when excessive doses are required to suppress the inflammatory component, immunosuppressive agents such as azathioprine or cyclosporin can be useful.

Physiotherapy is vital to prevent joint and soft tissue contractures and to improve muscle power until the inflammatory component has settled. Aggressive muscle building exercises should not be pursued during active disease, as there is evidence that these aggravate the underlying condition. Skin care is also essential in order to retain moisture and its suppleness. Precautions should also be taken to avoid trauma which may encourage calcification.

Scleroderma

Systemic sclerosis (scleroderma) is a rare disease which usually affects girls and like the adult form is often associated with a poor prognosis. Raynaud's phenomenon is often the initial presenting feature and may precede other symptoms by months or even years. The cyclical colour changes and numbness of the fingers and toes are usually triggered by exposure to cold. Skin changes vary substantially from mild thickening and induration of the finger tips (acrosclerosis, sclerodactyly) to extensive involvement of the face, arms and trunk. The affected toes are characterised by: pulp atrophy, tissue ulceration, arteriolar sclerosis, telangiectasia and pigmentary changes, with their overall appearance being one of tapered toes (poikiloderma). In cases of morphoea and linear scleroderma (which affect skin in a similar manner but which do not affect internal organs) the skin lesions have a clear line of demarcation with the normal skin. Arthralgia or arthritis of the digital joints combined with tightening of the skin may result in deformity and loss of joint movement. Tenosynovitis is seen in and around the ankle joint. The sclerotic changes can make walking and standing extremely painful.

Juvenile psoriatic arthropathy

The pattern of joint involvement is quite variable; the onset may be acute but it is predominantly slow, insidious and chronic. Monoarticular and pauci-articular onset is frequently seen. A common presentation is an asymmetrical pattern affecting a few joints, e.g. involvement of a metatarsophalangeal and the proximal and distal interphalangeal joints. Joint movements are often restricted and crepitus may be noted on passive movement. Heat, mild localised rubor and stiffness are characteristic changes overlying the affected joint. When this pattern of joint involvement is combined with a flexor tenosynovitis the characteristic sausage-shaped appearance of the toe, often with 'pencil-in-cup' deformity, is demonstrated.

Frequently the associated nail on the affected toe will show the characteristic changes of psoriasis, i.e. pitting, subungual hyperkeratosis, onycholysis and ridging, while adjacent toes may be free from both nail and joint involvement. The terminal result is often one of osteolysis of the phalanges and metatarsals and is accompanied by joint subluxations. Tendon sheath involvement may be a major part of the disease and this may overshadow any joint involvement.

Apart from the digital tendons being affected, the tendons which pass around the ankle joint are frequently inflamed. Pain in the area of the medial plantar aspect of the heel has been observed and has been attributed to enthesopathy of the plantar fascia. Rarely a very aggressive form of the arthritis may exist which results in massive bone erosions with or without ankylosis. This severe type of psoriatic arthritis especially affects the toes and is referred to as 'arthritis mutilans'.

Arthritis with inflammatory bowel disease

Arthritis is seen in association with ulcerative colitis and Crohn's disease in about 10% of cases. The onset for children with inflammatory bowel disease is usually after the fourth year, with male and female being affected equally. The development of joint symptoms may occur at the same time or some months or years following the bowel symptoms. Episodes of acute inflammatory synovitis lasting typically a few weeks affect large joints in the lower limb. The arthritis then runs a course parallel with bowel symptoms and disappears during remissions. There are seldom any residual effects on joint function. Erythema nodosum is an extra-articular manifestation which might be seen in the lower limb.

Reiter's disease

This is much more prevalent in teenage boys where the common cause is infective diarrhoea. The arthritis, which mainly affects several joints in the lower limb asymmetrically, varies from mild arthritis to widespread severe arthritis. The knee, ankle and digital joints are frequently involved resulting in subluxated metatarsophalangeal joints, flat feet and claw toes. The initial attacks of arthritis usually subside over a period of weeks to months but recurrences are common. Tenosynovitis affecting the Achilles tendon is frequently seen. The sole of the foot is often the site for the macular/papular rash of keratoderma blenorrhagica which at the time may closely resemble exfoliative dermatitis.

Other causes of monoarticular disease

Tuberculosis

In economically well-developed countries tuberculosis is rare today. Possible effects on the foot are tuberculous dactylitis and tuberculosis arthritis. Dactylitis presents as infection of the metatarsals and phalanges affecting several digits, which become swollen. Pain and disability are often minimal and the terminal outcome is shortening and contracture of the affected digit. The arthritis is monoarticular and insidious in its onset. The affected joint is of normal temperature but is stiff and has a 'boggy' (spongy) feel to it and the associated muscles will show signs of atrophy.

Charcot joints

Insensitivity to pain may occur as the result of peripheral nerve injuries, diabetic neuropathy and chronic diseases affecting the spinal cord. This insensitivity to pain may result in the rapid degeneration of joints and in diabetics the tarsal and metatarsal joints are most frequently affected. The presenting features are swelling, instability and the absence of pain.

Gout

In children gout is usually secondary to other diseases. As in adults the initial site may be the first metatarsophalangeal joint but any joint may become involved. The symptoms are redness, swelling, heat and pain and are often acute. Following the initial attack the disease may move on to affect other joints or may return to the original joint. When control is poor secondary arthritis will develop in the joints and gouty tophi may develop on tendons or in bursae.

Other causes of polyarticular disease

Post-infective arthritis (e.g. rheumatic fever)

Unlike in the late 1940s, rheumatic fever is rare in Britain today. Rheumatic fever seldom occurs before the age of five. The lower limb features start with a large joint polyarthritis in which the joint is very hot and tender. The progressive joint involvement can be described as 'flitting' in character. Prognosis for the joint symptoms is generally good. Ten per cent of cases may also present with the characteristic rash of erythema marginatum or with nodules along the path of tendon sheaths.

Haemostatic disorders

Haemophilia

This disease presents with uncontrolled bleeding into the tissues of the skin, mucous membranes and joints. In the lower limb large weightbearing joints, e.g. the knee and the ankle, are frequently affected. With intra-articular bleeding the joints become warm, discoloured, swollen and painful. The final outcome may be fibrous ankylosis. Another complication of repeated bleeding is either epiphyseal stimulation or early epiphyseal closure resulting in limb asymmetry.

Leukaemia

Articular manifestations of leukaemia are well documented. The lower limbs are frequently affected and in particular the knee joint. The typical symptoms are pain, swelling and muscle tenderness. In some children the presentation may be polyarticular, similar to juvenile chronic arthritis.

Psychogenic arthralgia

Not all joint pains are the result of pathological changes occurring within joints. Psychological problems, e.g. anxiety, fear and depression, may produce monoarticular or polyarticular symptoms. Often the patient walks with a limp and the symptoms are out of proportion to the clinical findings.

The role of the podiatrist in the management of foot problems associated with adult rheumatic disorders is well established. This role is quite varied and includes the referral of patients with undiagnosed rheumatic disorders to rheumatologists, the management of patients with chronic diseases and more recently the preservation of joints by means of podiatric orthoses. In contrast the role of the podiatrist in managing foot problems associated with rheumatic disorders in childhood has not yet fully evolved.

General principles of podiatric care

1. *The diagnostic role.* Since podiatrists play an ever increasing role in the screening of children, it is important that it is clearly understood how rheumatic disorders may present in the lower limb and the importance of early referral to prevent or limit joint damage thus reducing the possibility of irreversible complications, e.g. eye disease.

2. *Joint preservation.* Through an interdisciplinary approach podiatry has an important role to play in the prevention of foot deformities, through the knowledge and skills specifically developed in podiatric biomechanics and with the provision of orthoses where indicated.

3. *Foot health education.* The podiatrist plays an important role in increasing the child's awareness about good posture, physical activities and the role that inadequate footwear may have on the development of foot deformities.

Lower limb examination and assessment

The approach to the clinical examination will depend upon both the child's age and level of cooperation. Most children of five years of age and over may be examined in a way similar to adults. The younger child (especially when anxious) may require a modified approach to the examination. This may necessitate examining the child while he is sitting on his parent's lap. Relaxed and reliable clinical examinations which cause the child the minimum of stress are always underpinned by:

1. Establishing a good rapport with the child prior to the examination.
2. Providing an ongoing explanation of the examination.

3. Leaving any potentially stressful aspects of the examination to the end (this might include the examination of the child in the prone/supine position).

The physical examination should not differ significantly from a normal paediatric biomechanical examination, which would include:

- examination of all lower limb joints,
- assessment of digital/metatarsal lengths,
- evaluation of the forefoot/hindfoot relationship (frontal and sagittal planes),
- assessment of ankle joint dorsiflexion,
- calculation of relaxed and neutral calcaneal stance position,
- assessment of limb length,
- frontal, sagittal and transverse plane examination of the hip, thigh and lower leg,
- assessment of general body posture,
- observation of gait.

Aspects of the examination which should be highlighted in a child with a suspected rheumatic disorder are described below.

Clinical history

Podiatry predominantly relies on the 'clinical method' in order to arrive at diagnostic conclusions. Therefore the clinical history is central to the diagnosis of rheumatic disorders. It is important to obtain an accurate history of:

1. The symptomatic foot problem which would include, onset pattern, precipitating factors, type of pain, visible signs of disease and any effect/s on foot function or mobility.
2. The child's general health including previous illnesses, previous musculoskeletal symptoms and any history of trauma.
3. The family's history of disease or ill-health, special attention being given to any history of rheumatic symptoms or disorders.

Finally it is always worth considering whether or not there may be a social or psychological dimension to the presenting problem.

Joint examination

1. The first part of the joint examination should be visual, e.g. (a) changes in skin colour – erythema; (b) signs of swelling; look for a loss of joint definition, such as a balloon shape to the metatarsophalangeal joints, loss of the natural concavities or convexities around the subtalar joint.
2. Physical joint examination should include both active and passive examination, noting the quality and range of joint motion and the amount of pain elicited by these examinations. Where joint motion is restricted, note whether this is due to bony changes, joint swellings or muscular spasms. In joints which are swollen, distinction should be made between active synovitis and chronic synovial thickening. When active synovitis is present it is often possible to detect an increase in skin temperature and such joints have a characteristic 'boggy feel' to them.

Signs of muscular weakness

While it is easy to detect sizeable discrepancies in muscle bulk on visual examination, the girth of the thigh and leg should always be measured in an attempt to detect early signs of wastage. Power should be assessed in all muscle groups, e.g. hip and knee joint flexors/extensors, ankle joint dorsiflexors/plantarflexors and subtalar and midtarsal joint invertors/evertors. While it is difficult to assess the function of intrinsic muscles, a history of progressive toe deformity may suggest such a weakness. In addition, the specific function of tibialis anterior and tibialis posterior should be assessed as these muscles play an important role in foot function.

Many children find it difficult to create the active movements of inversion and eversion. Therefore, when testing for muscle power it is easier to put the foot into the desired position and then allow the child to resist the podiatrist moving it out of that position. When assessing muscle power a common fault is failure to isolate movements created by other muscle groups and this may distort the results. Muscle power may be graded against the Medical Research Council scale of muscle power.

Muscle tone may also be increased in those muscles which support a painful joint. Tone is passively assessed by observing the limbs' response to gravity and is then actively assessed by the clinician moving the limbs through a range of movements. Assessment of tone is quite problematic in terms of reliability and therefore it is important that clinicians examine many patients in order to develop experience of what is 'normal'.

Tendon examination

Special attention should be paid to the examination of tendon sheaths and linings, e.g. the tendons of tibialis anterior and tibialis posterior and of peroneus longus and peroneus brevis as they pass around the ankle joint, for evidence of tenosynovitis or tendon nodules (Fig. 6.6a, b).

Signs of synovitis may include:

– pain in the tendon sheath on movement,
– local linear swelling in the line of the tendon,
– increase in heat,
– sponginess and crepitations on active contraction of the tendon.

Growth discrepancies

The limbs should be assessed for length, any discrepancy noted and further measurements taken in order to identify the source of the discrepancy. The feet should be measured and a tracing of the external dimensions of the foot can provide a crude indication of foot asymmetry.

Posture and gait

The posture of the child with juvenile chronic arthritis is frequently affected by a number of lower limb changes including flexion contractures of the knees and hips, limb length discrepancies, joint deformity and pain. Generally posture may also be altered as a result of cervical flexion and tilting of the hips and shoulders. Similarly, as posture is affected, the pattern of gait may also be altered as a result of growth discrepancies, muscle weakness, joint synovitis and flexion contractures. For example, hip synovitis and contractures may result in hip flexor weakness and this results in a backward thrust of the trunk and pelvis in an attempt to lift the leg forward.

The examination of the posture of a child with a suspected rheumatic disorder should

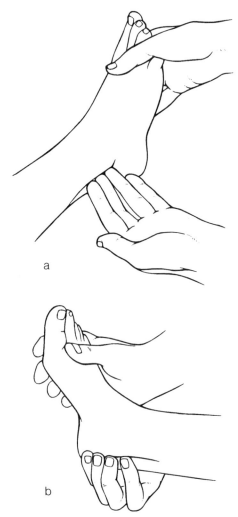

a

b

Figure 6.6   a, Technique for palpation of peroneal tendon sheaths behind the lateral malleolus. b, Technique for palpation of tendon sheath of tibialis posterior behind and below medial malleolus.

not differ significantly from the non-rheumatic child. However, signs of excessive flexion and asymmetry should always be looked for. Similarly when observing gait special attention should be paid to:

– evidence of fluidity of gait,
– signs of joint stiffness,
– loss of propulsion,
– development of a functional equinus,
– excessive use of the upper body to compensate for lower limb stiffness,
– increased muscle tone or muscle spasm, e.g.

tibialis anterior spasm in an attempt to immobilise the subtalar joint,
- variations in base of gait and/or stride length.

Footwear

Examination of the child's footwear should not be overlooked as it provides an accessible insight into the dynamic foot. Signs of abnormal sole wear should be noted as well as distortions of the shoe uppers. Often this valuable information helps to focus such investigations and provides supporting evidence for other clinical findings.

Podiatric treatment

Juvenile chronic arthritis

The general prognosis is good in that approximately two-thirds of children may expect to achieve permanent remission, unlike many adults with rheumatoid arthritis who usually experience ongoing progressive joint destruction. The one exception to this general rule is the adolescent female who is positive for rheumatoid factor and present with nodules; she will tend to develop the same joint problems as an adult would with rheumatoid arthritis. The long-term prognosis for these cases is generally worse in terms of the severity of the disability.

In children with juvenile chronic arthritis all joints should be moved through a full range of motion on a regular daily basis. During periods of acute synovitis the child may be advised to rest the affected limb or to undertake gentle passive exercise. However, prolonged rest may result in irreversible joint damage. Exercise programmes should be developed in order to improve musculature which will help in the stabilisation of joints. Perhaps the most valuable contribution podiatry can make is to limit any abnormal joint motion which may arise as a result of compensatory mechanisms.

Many healthy asymptomatic children may present with a number of minor biomechanical problems which do not seriously affect the limb or its function in the short term. This situation may change when the minor biomechanical problems are amplified as a result of an additional compromising factor, e.g. overweight, over-use or intrinsic joint damage. It is the latter of these factors which places the limb at such risk. For example, many children over the age of eight will still function with their feet in an abnormally pronated position. When the subtalar joint is weakened as a result of a destructive arthritis, the joint will be less able to withstand the excessive abnormal forces placed upon it. The resultant effect is rapid progressive deformity. Therefore it is imperative that the foot should be maintained in a sound biomechanical position so that it is more able to withstand the possible effects of internal joint damage.[2] This may necessitate putting the child into orthoses prior to the development of any serious deformity. This form of preventative therapy still requires to be fully evaluated. Many children will present with either a limb length discrepancy which may need to be accommodated or with a muscular ankle equinus which will need to be 'stretched out'.

In addition to functional orthoses, older children may require a more accommodative form of orthosis in order to protect and to cushion a painful plantar metatarsophalangeal area. Similarly, digital silicone orthoses may assist joint stability or may provide soft tissue protection from footwear. Rest splints and splints aimed at reducing and minimising deformity are commonly used in lower limbs and to date this therapy is undertaken by orthotists and rheumatologists.

The importance of well-fitting footwear should be emphasised in a positive light as patient cooperation will help relieve discomfort and will eliminate one of the contributory factors to deformity. Many 'sports shoes' with their high technology materials, greater forefoot width and depth allowance and their peer group acceptability provide a footwear solution which is acceptable to both patient and therapist.

A final treatment principle which should always be adhered to is that footcare should not be delivered in isolation and must always be seen in the context of an overall treatment programme. This necessitates good and effective interdisciplinary communication if the podiatrist is to make a valued and effective contribution to podopaediatric rheumatology.

Septic arthritis

The treatment of acute septic arthritis is outside the current scope of practice of podiatry. The podiatrist's role is to ensure that the patient has the earliest referral if irreversible joint damage is to be prevented.

Connective tissue diseases

The principles of treatment remain the same as for chronic juvenile arthritis. In addition to these much can be done to maintain the integrity of the vulnerable tissues by means of:

1. Health education: (a) advice about the adverse effects of low temperatures on tissues; (b) advice about the care of tissues and the inter-relationship between trauma and tissue ulceration.
2. Eliminating or minimising the effects of abnormal biomechanical stresses on the tissues.

Pain as a symptom of joint disease in children

Podiatrists predominantly employ a clinical method of diagnosis which relies very heavily on the patient's history, presenting symptoms and clinical examination. Therefore it is important that something should be known about the validity of the child's report of pain as a measure of the clinical state of the disease. It was thought that children's reports of pain would increase with age and that the relationship would take into account increased cognitive development.[3,4] It has been reported that pain is a valid indicator of the clinical state which may be used in the management of chronic juvenile arthritis.[5] In children with pauci-articular disease, younger children reported greater pain than older children. In very young children, where reliable reports of pain cannot be obtained, subjective reports from parents have not been found to be significantly biased by their obvious involvement.

References

1 JRA Criteria Sub-Committee Criteria for the classification of Juvenile Rheumatoid Arthritis. *Bull Rheum Dis* 1973; 25: 712–19.
2 Root ML, Orien WP, Weed JH. *Normal and Abnormal Function of the Foot*. Clinical Biomechanics Corporation, 1977.
3 Laaksonen AL, Laine V. A comparative study of joint pain in the adult and juvenile rheumatoid arthritis. *Ann Rheum Dis* 1961; 20: 368–70.
4 Scott RJ, Ansell BM, Huskisson EC. Measurement of pain in juvenile chronic arthritis. *Ann Rheum Dis* 1977; 36: 186–7.
5 Ross CK, Lavigne JV, Hayford JR, Dyer AR, Pachman KM. Validity of reported pain as a measure of clinical state in juvenile rheumatoid arthritis. *Ann Rheum Dis* 1989; 48: 817–19.

Further reading

Andersson Gare B, Fasth A, Andersson J, Bergulund G, Ekstrom H, Eriksson M, Holmquist L, Ronge E, Thilen A. Incidence and prevalence of juvenile chronic arthritis: a population survey. *Ann Rheum Dis* 1987; 46: 277–81.
Ansell BM. *Rheumatic Disorders in Childhood*. Butterworth, 1980.
Ansell BM, Schaller JG, Rudge S. *Colour Atlas of Paediatric Rheumatology*. Wolfe Medical Publishing, London (in press).
Benjamin CM. Review of UK data on rheumatic diseases – 1 juvenile chronic arthritis. *Br J Rheumatol* 1990; 29: 231–3.
Cassidy JT, Petty RE. *Textbook of Paediatric Rheumatology*, 2nd ed. Churchill Livingstone, 1990.
Kelly WN, Harris ED, Ruddy S, Sledge CB (eds). *Clinical Pharmacology in Rheumatic Diseases Section VI. Textbook of Rheumatology*. WB Saunders, 1990.
Lang BA, Shore A. A review: the current concepts on the pathogenesis of juvenile rheumatoid arthritis. *J Rheumatol* 1990; Suppl 21: 1–15.
Langman RE (ed) *The Immune System*. Harcourt Brace Jovanovich, 1989.
Logigian MK, Ward JD. *Pediatric Rehabilitation. A Team Approach for Therapists*. Little, Brown and Company, 1989.
Tachdjian MO. *The Child's Foot*. WB Saunders, 1985.
Yale I, Yale J. *The Arthritic Foot*. Williams and Wilkins, 1984.

7 General Medicine

Christopher Steer and Maureen O'Donnell

The pattern of childhood disorders identified in a particular community is influenced by climate, geography, socio-economic status and notably by the prevalence of malnutrition and reservoirs of disease, particularly diarrhoeal and respiratory infection. In the past few decades many countries have witnessed dramatic reductions in childhood mortality and morbidity achieved by improved standards of nutrition and hygiene and by the introduction of immunisation and antibiotics. This has allowed greater input and attention to the early diagnosis and management of less common disorders, e.g. congenital malformations, neonatal disorders, epilepsy, cerebral palsy, mental handicap and disorders of the endocrine, lymphoreticular and immune systems. Improved understanding of genetic mechanisms and the pathophysiology of disease has also led to the wider application of preventative and screening techniques, e.g. antenatal diagnosis in pregnancy utilising chorionic villus biopsy or amniocentesis (for alpha feto protein and chromosome analysis) and neonatal Guthrie testing (for phenylketonuria, galactosaemia, hypothyroidism). 'Gene probe' techniques using enzymes to cleave DNA have also allowed for the first time the identification of specific gene loci, e.g. for muscular dystrophy and cystic fibrosis. This allows early and specific diagnosis in fetal and postnatal life and may yield important clues to the underlying mechanisms operating in some diseases. Although vast resources are being invested to assist in some of these developments this should not obscure the fact that in global terms, malnutrition and infection remain the most significant contributors to childhood disease.

In podiatric practice a large number of children will be seen with abnormalities of the feet determined by intrauterine and genetic influences. These disorders will be considered first, followed by discussion of systemic disorders, e.g. immune system, haematological system, which may influence management of the foot.

Congenital anomalies

Congenital anomalies may be classified as *malformations* (defective formation of tissue and organs), *deformations* (defects caused by unusual forces acting on otherwise normal tissue), and *disruptions* (defects caused by breakdown of previously normal tissue).

Malformations

Such defects in morphogenesis may be single, affecting a single structure in an otherwise completely normal child, or multiple where several structural abnormalities are present due to the same underlying cause. A *syndrome* is said to occur when a recognisable pattern of malformation is identified usually with multiple features and again with a single presumed specific cause.

Major malformations affecting, for example, major organ systems such as brain, heart, kidney or viscera are identified in approximately 2% of children at birth although this figure reaches 5% when allowance is made for diagnosis in later childhood.

Minor malformations are identified in approximately 4% of children at birth and by definition such malformations rarely require treatment and mostly affect the skin and appendages, e.g. sacral dimples, simian creases, clinodactyly of fifth fingers, syndactyly of second and third toes, extra nipples and pre-auricular sinuses.

The underlying mechanism in malformation syndromes may involve defective tissue and organ formation due to abnormal cell shape, inappropriate cell matrix (collagen), vascular insufficiency, or defective programming of cell regression and death during development.

The aetiology of various congenital defects is outlined in Table 7.1. Genetic mechanisms and examples are described more fully in the following pages.

'Teratogens', agents thought to mediate abnormality by direct action during pregnancy, are listed in Appendix II. In general, teratogens have more harmful effects when they influence fetal development in the early stages of pregnancy. Harmful pregnancy influences are easiest to blame for fetal and neonatal abnormality but it should be remembered that in many instances these are difficult to prove unequivocally against a background where the causes of approximately 40% of fetal abnormality are at present not known.

Deformations

Deformations are caused by abnormal mechanical forces acting on normal tissue. The majority involve the musculoskeletal system and are secondary to intrauterine moulding. This may be due to 'crowding' caused by such conditions as oligohydramnios (lack of liquor amnii), congenital uterine abnormality (e.g. bicornuate uterus), chronic leak of liquor, persistent breech presentation, twins, or uterine tumours. Neuromuscular imbalance or paresis due to spina bifida cystica, spinal muscular atrophy, or dystrophia myotonica may also impair fetal movement and normal joint and muscle development.

Intrauterine 'positional deformity' of variable severity secondary to the above may cause relatively simple anomalies, e.g. talipes (equinovarus or calcaneovalgus), congenital dislocation of the hip, or scoliosis. However, multiple severe anomalies may occur as in 'Potter's syndrome', usually secondary to oligohydramnios caused by renal agenesis in the fetus: in such cases the fetus is subjected to severe compression resulting in severe talipes, multiple joint contractures, plagiocephaly, torticollis and hip dislocation.

Disruptions

Disruptions represent rare sporadic events where previously normally formed or forming tissues 'break down', for example as a result of 'entanglement' in aberrant uterine amniotic bands. This results in uterine reduction de-

Table 7.1 Recognised aetiology of congenital defects in newborn infants (Nelson and Holmes, 1989)[1] (N = 1549 from 69 227 births)

Chromosome abnormalities	10.1%
Single mutant gene disorders	3.1%
Familial disorders	14.5%
Multifactorial disorders	23.0%
Teratogens	3.2%
Uterine factors	2.5%
Twinning	0.4%
Unknown	43.2%

formity or 'amputation', most often involving the extremities but, in rarer cases, the head or thorax (Fig. 7.1).

Genetic considerations

Defects in morphogenesis and many other disorders are mediated by interactions between environment and genetic endowment. Such effects may be obvious at birth and may manifest as a congenital abnormality or may only become evident with time as a consequence of growth or environmental factors. The three principal genetic mechanisms are single major gene disorders, chromosomal abnormalities and polygenic (multifactorial) inheritance.

Single gene inheritance

Genes located on the X chromosome are known as X-linked genes and those on the autosomes as autosomally linked genes. Chromosomes are arranged in pairs, one of each pair being derived from each parent, with comparable gene determinants located at the same position. The pairs of genes are known as 'alleles' and normally function together. Gene mutation is said to occur when changes in gene structure arise and produce an abnormal characteristic. When a mutant gene produces an abnormality despite the presence of a normal 'allelic' partner, this is regarded as a dominant pattern. A mutant gene which only produces an abnormality when mediated by a 'double dose' (i.e. one from each partner) represents a recessive pattern. In X-linked recessive disorders the abnormal gene is situated on the X chromosome. In the female, the presence of the normal allele on the other X chromosome protects her from the disease but

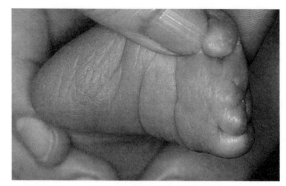

Figure 7.1   Toe 'amputation' secondary to intrauterine bands.

she is a carrier. However, in affected males the abnormal gene on the X chromosome is not balanced by the appropriate allele on the Y chromosome, and he manifests the disease state. In X-linked dominant disorders the above mechanism also applies but the female carrier also shows manifestations of disease albeit less severe than in the male. In addition certain disorders are found almost exclusively in females and apparently are lethal early on in utero in affected males. It is not yet clear whether these are X-linked dominant or autosomal dominant disorders although the former is suspected.

Autosomal dominant disorders

More than 1000 disorders result from this mode of inheritance. As previously stated the abnormal gene responsible for disease is carried on one of the autosomes only. Each offspring has a one in two chance of inheriting the gene and manifesting the disease. The degree of severity or 'expression' of disease may vary considerably from one affected individual to another. In certain examples of dominantly inherited disorders 'new' cases arise from spontaneous gene mutation within the ovum or sperm (e.g. up to 80% of individuals with achondroplasia, an autosomal dominant disorder, have normal parents). The risk of a similar mutation affecting subsequent offspring is low but the individual arising from the new mutation will still pass the disorder on to 50% of their offspring. A selection of examples of more than 1000 conditions mediated by autosomal dominant inheritance,

many of which affect the extremities, are listed in Appendix III.

Autosomal recessive disorders

Whereas autosomal dominant disorders tend to cause gross structural defects and clinically obvious abnormalities, recessively inherited disorders are in addition commonly implicated in biochemical disorders. In recessive inheritance neither parent shows any sign of the disease but the risk of offspring being affected is 1 : 4 whilst the risk of a child being a carrier is 1 : 2. Many individuals carry abnormal genes but the risk of a spouse carrying similar genes is usually small unless there is consanguinity as, for example, in first cousin marriages. Examples from the 700 or so known autosomal recessive mediated disorders with a special emphasis on disorders of the extremities are listed in Appendix IV.

X-linked disorders

As noted these disorders are carried by the female on the X chromosome and therefore manifest in 50% of male offspring while 50% of daughters perpetuate the carrier state. A selection from the 100 or so recognised X-linked disorders is listed in Appendix V with special emphasis on disorders of the extremities.

Major structural chromosomal abnormalities

Modern cytogenetic techniques permit direct visualisation of human chromosomes including the identification of heterochromic 'bands' alternating with lighter non-staining areas. These bands are ascribed special numbers in order to facilitate the detection of loss (deletion) of even a small part of a chromosome or the addition of extra genetic material. Such changes occur during sperm and ovum formation (gametogenesis) during meiosis (see Chapter 1).

Diseases carried by chromosomal abnormalities result from changes in the total number of autosomes or sex chromosomes or from alterations in chromosome structure resulting from deletion or interchange of chromosome material from one chromosome to another – *translocation*.

Approximately one in 150 newborn infants has a chromosome abnormality, distributed as in Table 7.2.

Table 7.2   Incidence of chromosome abnormalities

Down's syndrome (21 trisomy)	1 in 600–800 overall
Edwards' syndrome (18 trisomy)	1 in 8000
Patau's syndrome (13 trisomy)	1 in 20 000
Turner's syndrome (XO)	1 in 10 000
Klinefelter's syndrome (XXY)	1 in 1000
Poly-X syndrome (XXX etc.)	1 in 1000
XYY syndrome	1 in 1000
Balanced structural rearrangements	1 in 520
Unbalanced structural rearrangements	1 in 1700
Fragile X males	1 in 2000
Fragile X females	1 in 1000

The more common disorders will be outlined here. For more detailed description the reader should refer to a detailed 'Atlas' such as Smith.[2, 3]

Chromosome abnormalities affecting the autosomes

Trisomy syndromes. Down's syndrome is mediated by an extra no. 21 chromosome and is the best recognised and most common chromosomal abnormality. A high correlation exists between increasing maternal age and the non-disjunction during meiosis resulting in an extra chromosome in the conceptus. Approximately 5% of cases are due to translocation, i.e. centric fusion between chromosome 21 and chromosomes 13, 14 or 15. Important features of Down's syndrome are summarised in Table 7.3 along with the principal abnormalities noted in the less common trisomic syndromes. In contrast to Down's syndrome most infants with trisomy 13 and 18 die in early infancy and usually within the first few months although longer survivors are occasionally reported. Long-term management includes early diagnosis and sympathetic counselling; and antenatal care in future pregnancies is important.

Autosomal deletions. Chromosomal deletions are associated with a number of clinical syndromes and have been described affecting the short (p) arms of chromosomes 4, 5, 11, 18 and the long arm (q) of chromosomes 9, 13, 18, 21 and 22. Mental retardation is invariable, mostly in association with facial dysmorphism. A variety of abnormalities of the hands and feet occur and include syndactyly, clinodactyly, short metacarpals and metatarsals and dysplastic nails. The commonest deletional disorder affecting the short arm of 5 (5p−) has been dubbed the 'cri du chat' syndrome on account of the high pitched mewing cry noted in the newborn period. Other features include microcephaly, hypertelorism, micrognathia, prominent epicanthic folds, antimongolian palpebral fissures and occasional congenital heart disease. Such individuals are frequently happy with an engaging outgoing personality.

Abnormalities affecting the sex chromosomes

Abnormalities of the sex chromosomes constitute approximately half of all chromosomal abnormalities detected in the newborn period. The physical abnormalities encountered vary considerably but nearly all affect gonadal function in some form. Features of the commoner syndromes are summarised in Table 7.4.

Polygenic (multifactorial) inheritance

'Polygenic' inheritance refers to genetic defects which are thought to be caused by the cumulative action of a number of genes. Whether a given polygenic disorder manifests or not is also influenced by environmental factors and whether a given 'threshold' for expression of a disorder is reached. This has led to use of the term 'multifactorial' inheritance. When a particular family member is affected, the risk of first degree relatives (sons and daughters) also being affected is increased. The commoner recognised multifactorial disorders are listed in Table 7.5.

As stated several reference atlases (e.g. *Smith's Recognisable Patterns of Human Malformations* and *Recognisable Patterns of Human Deformation*[2, 3]) are available for perusal in cases where children are encountered and where a congenital disorder is suggested but not immediately recognised by the clinician. Computerised databases are also becoming available where a given selection of physical abnormalities may be entered and where a

Table 7.3 Trisomy syndromes

	21 trisomy (Down's)	18 trisomy (Edwards')	13 trisomy (Patau's)	8 trisomy	9 trisomy
General	Mental retardation Hypotonia	Severe mental retardation Low birth weight	Severe mental retardation Apnoea Seizures	Mental retardation Short stature	Mental retardation
Head and face	Brachycephaly Mongolian slant of eyes Prominent epicanthic folds Brushfield's spots (speckled iris) Prominent malformed ears Flat nasal bridge Short broad neck	Micrognathia Low set malformed ears Prominent occiput	Microcephaly Midline scalp defects Cleft lip and palate Microphthalmia	Prominent brow Low set ears High arched palate Micrognathia	Microcephaly Deep set eyes Prominent ears 'Fish mouth' Micrognathia
Extremities	Simian crease Short broad hands Hypoplastic mid phalanx of fifth finger Widely spaced great toes Abnormal dermatoglyphics	Flexion deformity of fingers Short dorsiflexed big toes 'Rockerbottom' feet or talipes equinovarus Abnormal dermatoglyphics	Polydactyly Hypoplastic or hyperconvex finger nails Simian crease Flexion deformities of fingers Abnormal dermatoglyphics Retroflexible thumb	Deep flexion creases on palms and soles	Clinodactyly Digital and nail hypoplasia Syndactyly Simian crease Abnormal dermatoglyphics
Some other features	Congenital heart disorders Intestinal atresia Hypothyroidism Conductive deafness	Congenital heart disorders Cleft lip and palate Tracheo-oesophageal fistula	Congenital heart disorders. Polycystic kidneys Omphalocoele	Congenital heart disorders Limited joint mobility Patella dysplasia	Congenital heart disorders Congenital dislocation of the hip Urinary tract anomalies

number of differential diagnoses are generated from the program. These approaches considerably enhance the ability to make an early diagnosis and to arrange appropriate counselling and treatment.

Growth and growth disorders

Normal growth is mediated by increases in cell number and size, defined as hyperplasia and hypertrophy. Whilst early embryonic growth results mostly from cellular hyperplasia, subsequently the balance between hyperplasia and hypertrophy varies considerably. Postnatal growth is influenced by a given child's genetic endowment, adequate nutrition and normal hormonal function. In early infancy the rate of growth is rapid compared to later with a doubling of length and a 2–3 fold increase in weight within the first year. Growth rates of up to 2 cm per month in the first year decline to 5–6 cm per year in later infancy until the pubertal growth spurt, when acceleration to peak rates of up to 12 cm per year may be encountered.

In order to define and to identify disorders of growth in an individual, access is required to appropriate population standards. Such standards are presented in the form of 'growth charts' prepared from longitudinal and cross-sectional data in appropriate populations. Probably the most widely used in the UK are those prepared by Tanner and Whitehouse[4]

Table 7.4   Abnormalities of the sex chromosomes

	Turner's syndrome 45 XO and Mosaics	Klinefelter's syndrome 47 XXY	Poly-X Female 47 XXX etc	Fragile X Sites	Y Polysomy 47 XYY etc.
Incidence	1/10 000 females	1/1000 males	1/1000 females	1/1000 females 1/2000 males	1/1000 males
Features include:	Short stature Primary amenorrhoea and infertility due to ovarian dysgenesis Webbing of neck and shield chest Down-turned mouth Micrognathia Downward slanting of palpebral fissures Increased incidence of cardiac defects Congenital lymphoedema Short metacarpals or metatarsals Hypoplastic/ hyperconvex nails	Long limbs with low upper to lower segment ratio Impaired spermatogenesis Eunuchoidism Gynaecomastia Increased incidence of mental retardation Ulceration of skin over anterior lower legs	Mental deficiency Variable short stature and facies within syndromes Clinodactyly Overriding toes and multiple joint dislocation in 'Penta X' syndrome	Mental deficiency Hypotonia Lax joints Mild cutis laxa Large ears Macro-orchidism	Tall stature Aberrant often anti-social behaviour Increased skeletal length versus breadth in skull vault, hands and feet

from the Institute of Child Health in London. Charts most commonly referred to are those for height and weight and also for height and weight velocity represented in centile form.

The 97th and 3rd centiles are conventionally taken as the upper and lower limits of normality representing plus or minus two standard deviations from the population mean. There is an increased likelihood of identifying significant pathological causes of short stature in children whose dimensions plot below the 3rd centile. When serial measurement identifies an individual whose measurements are crossing centile lines, or in whom growth velocity is persistently low, active further investigation is indicated.

It is important to ascertain the pattern of growth over time in order to identify and to categorise growth disorders in children. For example, infants and children with a congenital growth disorder show persistent deviation from the normal curve from early on, whilst those with an acquired disorder progressively decline from a normal point on the growth curve.

Attention to detail and care in measurement technique is central to early and adequate diagnosis of growth disorders. A wide range of accurate and reliable equipment is now available. Careful positioning for measurement of height, ensuring bare feet and correct alignment of the spine and head, is essential. Errors

Table 7.5   Polygenic (multifactorial) disorders

Ankylosing spondylitis	Hirschsprung's
Atopy	disease
Congenital cardiac defects	Perthes disease
Isolated cleft lip and palate	Psoriasis
Isolated club foot	Pyloric stenosis
(talipes equinovarus)	Schizophrenia
Congenital dislocation of hip	Spina bifida complex
Diabetes mellitus	and anencephaly

caused by diurnal 'shrinkage' in stature due to intervertebral compression may be avoided by measuring and charting at a standard time of day and by stretching the spine slightly by upward pressure on the mastoid process during measurement.

In certain situations it may be useful to determine bodily proportions, e.g. the relationship of trunk length to leg length. The former may be determined by measuring sitting height and leg length (subischial) by subtracting this value from total height. Patients with variants of short limb dwarfism, e.g. achondroplasia, may have normal sitting height but markedly reduced subischial leg length, whereas patients with pubertal delay frequently demonstrate a disproportionately long leg length compared to sitting height.

Body weight should be carefully recorded and charted under standard conditions and ideally with the patient in underclothes only. Body weight should always be interpreted in the context of height. For more exact assessments of body fat stores some centres also assess skin fold thickness by using special callipers.

Assessment of skeletal maturity may be undertaken by measuring bone age, utilising a standard radiograph of the left wrist in order to identify centres of ossification. Used in conjunction with a known chronological age and measured height, final adult height can be predicted. Final height is obviously achieved once epiphyseal fusion has occurred.

Finally, accurate knowledge of parental height is essential in the evaluation of stature. In order to produce a parental height target range, respective parental heights should be incorporated in the child's growth chart as centile equivalents with appropriate corrections to allow for intersex differences and to produce a final 'mid parent' height.

Factors affecting growth: the role of hormones

Normal growth is sustained by an adequate nutritional intake, adequate sensory stimulation (psychogenesis), satisfactory general health, by genetic endowment and by hormonal influences. Hormones producing significant effects on growth are growth hormone, insulin and insulin-like growth factors (somatomedins), thyroxine, parathyroid hormone, calcitonin, cortisol and the sex steroid group. Hormonal effects are closely inter-related and apart from important effects on growth, they are also vital in maintaining the internal milieu, for withstanding stress, i.e. trauma, infection, starvation and psychological stress, and for normal reproductive function.

Output of given hormones from effector (endocrine) glands is influenced by the level of a trophic hormone released from the anterior pituitary gland or by changes in the level of a given circulating hormone metabolite. Inhibition is achieved by negative feedback mechanisms. The pituitary gland is under direct control of the hypothalamus. This is the site of specialised neurons which secrete regulatory peptides which themselves control the release or inhibition of individual pituitary hormones via a specialised hypothalamic/pituitary 'portal system'. The principal hypothalamic regulatory peptides and their target anterior pituitary hormones are listed in Table 7.6.

Table 7.6 Hypothalamic regulatory peptides and their target anterior pituitary hormones

Hypothalamic regulatory peptide	'Target' anterior pituitary hormone
Growth hormone releasing hormone	Growth hormone (increases)
Growth hormone release inhibiting hormone (somatostatin)	Growth hormone (decrease)
Luteinising hormone releasing hormone	Luteinising hormone and follicle stimulating hormone (increase)
Thyrotropin releasing hormone	Thyroid stimulating hormone (increases and thence increases thyroxine)
Corticotrophin releasing hormone	Adrenocorticotrophic hormone (increases and thence increases cortisol)

It is difficult to summarise specific hypothalamic effects on the individual regulatory peptides. However, these have been fairly clearly demonstrated for growth hormone and are summarised in Table 7.7.

Table 7.7   Growth hormone releasing hormone

Increased by	Decreased by
Increased dopaminergic activity	Non REM sleep
Increased noradrenegic activity	Deprivation
Increased serotoninergic activity	Malnutrition
REM sleep	Head trauma
Hypoglycaemia	Asphyxia
Anxiety/stress	
Exercise	
High protein intake	
L dopa	
Clonidine	

Growth hormone itself has a peripheral lipolytic and anti-insulin effect whilst promoting skeletal growth, protein synthesis and cell proliferation via the intermediary effects of insulin-like growth factors.

The principal effects of other 'target hormones' are summarised in Table 7.8 (parathormone and calcitonin, adrenaline and noradrenaline are included although there appears not to be any direct control via the hypothalamic/pituitary axis).

Causes of growth failure

The causes of growth failure and short stature are summarised in Table 7.9 and discussed further below.

1. Children with genetically determined short stature are small from the outset and grow parallel to but below the third centile. Growth velocity is normal and a normally timed pubertal growth spurt occurs with ultimately the attainment of a short adult height similar to their parents. Bone age is always appropriate for chronological age and on examination there is no evidence of malabsorption or of any particular 'syndrome' and there is no biochemical abnormality detectable on investigation. At present the role of growth hormone therapy is being assessed in this group of children even though they are not known to be growth hormone deficient ('small normal'). It is not yet clear whether final attained height will be increased with such treatment.

2. Several chromosome disorders are described more fully in an earlier part of this chapter and it is worthy of note that many are associated with short stature and growth failure. Probably the most important chromosome disorder presenting with short stature in paediatric clinics is Turner's syndrome (XO constitution). This disorder involves absence of an X chromosome or other abnormalities including partial deletions of fragments of an X chromosome, translocation and mosaic forms with incomplete physical stigmata of the full syndrome. The overall incidence of Turner's syndrome varies between 1 : 3000 to 1 : 10 000 female births. The classical form of this disorder presents with short stature, ovarian dysgenesis producing primary amenorrhoea and absent secondary sexual characteristics with dysmorphic features. In most affected children, growth failure becomes obvious by the time of school entry. Poor growth may be exacerbated by hypothyroidism and by deficient growth hormone production which may possibly be related to lack of adequate oestrogenic stimulation.

Due to the occurrence of 'atypical' forms, Turner's syndrome should always be considered in girls who present with short stature, particularly since it has been shown that linear growth may be promoted with anabolic steroid therapy combined with growth hormone treatment. Puberty is also induced artificially with appropriate hormone replacement.

3. Intrauterine growth retardation (IUGR) may result from several factors, notably maternal smoking, excessive intake of alcohol during pregnancy (producing the fetal alcohol syndrome) and placental insufficiency, particularly when it is associated with chronic pre-eclampsia and hypertension. Intrauterine infections (see above) and chronic antepartum bleeding may also be implicated. Frequently neonates with multiple congenital abnormalities show evidence of poor intrauterine growth and there are a small number of low birth weight dwarf syndromes, e.g. de Lange 'Amsterdam' dwarfism (Fig. 7.2), Seckel's 'bird headed' dwarfism and the Russell–Silver syndrome, in which there is symmetrical, longstanding intrauterine growth retardation.

Many newborns with IUGR have poor glycogen stores and therefore they are particularly susceptible to neonatal hypoglycaemia. Although such cases show 'catch-up' growth, often in quite dramatic fashion over the first

Table 7.8 Examples of specific hormone effects

Peptide hormones	Effector glands	Principal actions
Thyroxine	Thyroid	Increased oxygen consumption, protein synthesis. Growth and differentiation and glucose utilisation
Parathyroid	Parathyroid	Mobilises calcium by increased bone resorption and by decreased urinary excretion
Calcitonin	Parafollicular cells of thyroid	Decreases calcium mobilisation by inhibiting resorption in bone
Insulin	Islets of Langerhans in pancreas	Promotes uptake of glucose by cells (gluconeogenesis) and storage of protein and lipid
Cortisol	Adrenal cortex	Increased glucose production; protein catabolic effect in muscle, skin and connective tissues
Adrenaline/ noradrenaline	Adrenal medulla	Mediate 'fight and flight' response
Androgens	Adrenal cortex and testes	Mediate male secondary sexual characteristics and spermatogenesis
Oestrogens	Ovaries	Mediate ovulation and secondary sexual female characteristics
Progesterone	Ovaries and placenta	Mediates ovulation and maintenance of endometrium

Table 7.9 Causes of growth failure

1. Genetically determined short stature
2. Chromosome disorders
3. Intrauterine growth retardation
4. Skeletal dysplasia
5. Constitutional delay in growth and puberty
6. Malnutrition and psychosocial deprivation
7. Chronic system disorders, e.g. gut, renal and cardiovascular systems
8. Endocrine disorders, e.g. hypothyroidism and growth hormone deficiency

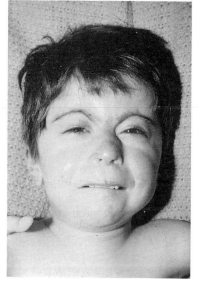

Figure 7.2 Typical facial appearance of Amsterdam (de Lange) dwarf.

two months of life, this is difficult to predict with certainty and is less likely to occur with long-standing IUGR and does not occur at all in the low birth weight dwarf syndromes.

4. Skeletal dysplasias represent a group of disorders in which development of cartilage and bone are defective, resulting in disproportionate 'short limbed' short stature with abnormalities in the size and shape of limbs, skull, pelvis and spine. The most widely known is the dominantly inherited condition achondroplasia in which severe limb shortening makes the diagnosis obvious at birth. In certain of the rarer dysplasias (osteochondrodysplasias), now numbering more than 40,[3] diagnosis may be more difficult and may be aided considerably by detailed radiological examination.

Many subtypes of the osteochondrodysplasias are incompatible with survival beyond early life, e.g. achondrogenesis, fibrochondrogenesis, thanatophoric dysplasia and asphyxiating thoracic dystrophy of Jeune, whilst other types, such as hypochondroplasia, represent a less severe variant of achondroplasia with more normal growth of the face and cranial bones. Osteochondroplasias affecting the spine, e.g. spondyloepiphyseal and spondometaphyseal dysplasia, may only become apparent and cause delay in linear growth in later infancy.

No specific treatment is available to correct the underlying osteochondroplastic disorder although orthopaedic and orthotic support may be necessary, for example in order to treat kyphoscoliosis and to stabilise valgus feet.

5. *In children who exhibit signs of constitutional delay* in growth and puberty, short stature is secondary to a slower than normal rate of maturation. Height *and* bone age are usually delayed by 18 months to 4 years and pubertal onset is delayed until the bone age is appropriate. The exact cause of this condition is unclear although a family history of a similar growth pattern is often obtainable. Final adult stature is eventually reached in the late teens and is appropriate for the target 'mid parent' height. The development of secondary sexual characteristics occurs normally. Growth velocity is normal for bone age in such individuals and only occasionally is treatment indicated for amelioration of psychosocial difficulty caused by peer group pressures. In this situation anabolic steroids are sometimes prescribed.

6. *Malnutrition* is the most important cause of growth failure on a global scale with, at current estimates, 60% or so of the world's children being undernourished. Catch-up growth and restoration of bowel integrity occur rapidly with correction of environmental deficiency and infection. Psychosocial deprivation in developed countries has also been shown to affect growth and a Scottish study demonstrated potentially reversible growth hormone deficiency in areas of particularly severe deprivation.[5] Poor growth is frequently accompanied by psychological maladjustment and behavioural abnormality and in many cases may only realistically be remedied by altering the child's environment by means of statutory measures. This may result in dramatic catch-up growth and in changes in demeanour. Regular careful physical examinations including charting of height and weight are essential features in the monitoring process of any child in whom chronic psychosocial deprivation is suspected.

7. *Chronic disorders* of any major organ system are well recognised causes of growth failure.

Important examples include malabsorptive disorders such as coeliac disease (gluten enteropathy) associated with sub-total villous atrophy of the small bowel lining, or cystic fibrosis in which pancreatic malabsorption and chronic respiratory infection are implicated. Adequate early diagnosis and treatment lessen the impact of these disorders on growth. Similar degrees of growth failure are sometimes seen in late diagnosed cases of chronic inflammatory bowel disorder due, for example, to ulcerative colitis or Crohn's disease. In long-standing severe congenital heart disease, tissue hypoxia, chronic cyanosis and cardiac strain frequently accompany growth failure. Catch-up growth following successful cardiac surgery is not invariable. Chronic gastrointestinal, pulmonary, and cyanotic heart disease may all produce the phenomenon of 'clubbing' affecting the fingers and toes. Bulbous swellings of the terminal phalanges are associated with loss of nail angulation and fluctuation of the nail base; occasionally this is encountered as a benign familial (dominant) disorder (Fig. 7.3).

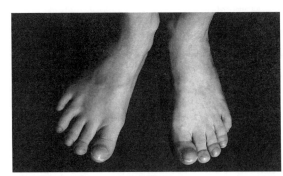

Figure 7.3 Toe clubbing due to pulmonary disease (cystic fibrosis). Note nail angulation.

Chronic renal disorders, in which there is a significant fall in glomerular filtration and reduced availability of calories and protein, are associated with poor growth. This may be complicated by renal calcium loss and by secondary hyperparathyroidism (renal osteodystrophy), and may be accompanied clinically by impaired bony remodelling.

8. *Endocrine (hormonal) mechanisms.* Ovarian dysgenesis in Turner's syndrome and severe psychosocial deprivation mediate their effects

on growth via these mechanisms. The remaining endocrine disorders which significantly affect growth are growth hormone deficiency, hypothyroidism and excessive cortisol production.

The principal causes of growth hormone deficiency are summarised in Table 7.10.

Table 7.10 Causes of growth hormone deficiency

Congenital	Other
Autosomal recessive type	Neoplasm of
Autosomal dominant type	hypothalamus or
Idiopathic type	pituitary
Associated with pituitary	e.g.
hypoplasia/aplasia	craniopharyngioma
Associated with midline	Irradiation
defects, e.g. cleft palate,	Meningitis
septo-optic dysplasia,	Encephalitis
holoprosencephaly	Histiocytosis
	Birth asphyxia
	Skull trauma
	Hypothyroidism
	Haemochromatosis
	Severe psychosocial
	deprivation

Estimates of the prevalence of growth hormone deficiency vary considerably and many authors consider this to be an underdiagnosed condition. A figure of 1 : 3000–4000 would seem to be appropriate at present. Even with congenital growth hormone deficiency, growth failure velocity measurements below the third centile may not become apparent until late infancy. However, there is progressive deviation of the growth curve away from the population mean; secondary behavioural difficulties and poor peer group integration often ensue, particularly in male school age children. Features in addition to growth velocities of less than 4 cm per annum include normal body proportion (particularly limbs), crowding of the midfacial structures, increased skinfold thickness, micropenis and delay in bone age. The voice may be high pitched. Growth hormone provocation tests, using clonidine or insulin-induced hypoglycaemia, fail to induce satisfactory growth hormone release and thereby confirm the diagnosis. Bone age is usually significantly delayed. Other screening provocation tests for growth hormone release have included post exercise testing, early sleep

sampling, arginine infusion and glucagon. Any patient found to be growth hormone deficient should undergo careful radiological evaluation of the hypothalamus and pituitary region in order to exclude surgically remediable lesions or to confirm a congenital defect. Effective and safe synthetic growth hormone preparations are now available as replacement therapy and are administered by daily subcutaneous injections. Early diagnosis and treatment is associated with the best long-term outcome and in optimum circumstances a target height significantly above the third centile can be achieved. In such cases where growth hormone deficiency is part of a multiple pituitary hormone deficiency, the clinical picture may be more complex and additional therapy may be required, e.g. thyroxine, cortisone acetate and at puberty gonadotrophins in boys and oestrogens in girls. In rarer cases where there is coexisting posterior pituitary dysfunction, treatment with DDAVP (desmopressin) will readily maintain satisfactory fluid and electrolyte balance and reverse diuresis.

Growth failure is an important clinical feature of hypothyroidism. Untreated congenital hypothyroidism (Fig. 7.4) is now rare

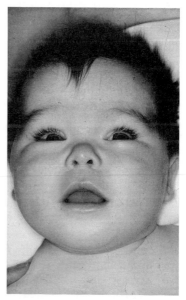

Figure 7.4 Typical facial appearance in congenital hypothyroidism (cretinism).

following the introduction of neonatal Guthrie screening for this disorder. Acquired hypothyroidism secondary to an autoimmune disorder presents with fall-off in intellectual capacity, weakness, constipation and significant fall-off in growth velocity. Body proportions are usually normal with a stocky muscular appearance; this condition is seen more frequently in girls. Other features include hoarseness of the voice, dryness and thickening of the skin, dry brittle hair, delayed dentition and asymmetrical, non-nodular thyroid enlargement. Diagnosis is confirmed by demonstrating decreased levels of serum thyroxine and tri-iodothyronine and elevated levels of thyroid stimulating hormone (TSH). Skeletal radiographs will reveal significant delay in epiphyseal maturation. Rapid resolution of signs, with significant catch-up growth, occurs following replacement treatment with thyroxine.

Steroid excess due to medical treatment or to increased endogenous secretion of cortisol or ACTH, e.g. due to tumours, causes growth failure by inhibiting growth at tissue level. No defect in growth hormone or insulin-like growth factor levels has been demonstrated. Clinical signs, in addition to fall-off in growth velocity, include truncal obesity, glucose intolerance, hirsutism, vascular fragility and skin thinning. Because of these effects, steroid therapy should be reserved for treatment of a limited number of medical disorders in childhood and when long-term treatment is required, alternate day regimens produce less suppression of normal hypothalamic function.

Removal of offending glucocorticoid or ACTH secreting lesions is usually followed by a period of catch-up growth in situations where such lesions are the underlying cause of steroid excess.

Disorders of the immune system

Intact and properly functioning skin and mucous membrane and the action of cilia form the primary barriers to invasion by infectious agents. Subsequent defence is mediated by the immune system whose main functional components are listed in Table 7.11.

Table 7.11   Components of the immune system

Lymphocytes	T cells: 'Helper', 'suppressor' and 'killer' subtypes
	B cells: Immunoglobulin synthesis (IgG, IgM, IgA, IgE)
Lymphokines	
Complement system	
Phagocytes	Polymorphonuclear leucocytes
	Macrophages
	Mononuclear cells

Disorders of different parts of the immune system tend to present with different and distinct clinical syndromes.

Lymphocyte populations

Stem cells of the lymphoreticular system differentiate into two major cell lines known as 'T' (thymus derived) cells and 'B' ('bursa' or bone marrow derived) cells. One of the most important differences between B and T cells is the ability of the former to synthesise various classes of immunoglobulin. The major functions of these different lymphocyte populations are summarised in Table 7.12.

Table 7.12   B and T cell function

Properties of B cells
Major immunoglobulin synthesis (e.g. protection against common major bacteria)
Viral neutralisation on initial exposure
Local mucosal protection in gut and respiratory tract
Initiate macrophage killing
Initiate vasoactive amine (e.g. histamine) release from mast cells and basophils

Properties of T cells
T helper function
T suppressor function (modulation of immune response)
T killer function (initiation of cytotoxic processes)
Containment of infection with agents such as mycobacteria, Herpes group viruses, Epstein–Barr virus, fungal and protozoal infection
Allograft rejection
Graft versus host disease

Table 7.13   Immunoglobulin subtypes

Class	Molecular weight	Main biological role
IgG	140 000	Complement fixation and neutralising antibody
Serum IgA	160 000	Polymer formation
Secretory IgA	370 000	Mucosal surface protection and polymer formation
IgM	900 000	Complement fixation and polymer formation. Agglutination; opsonic activity
IgD	160 000	? Biological role
IgE	197 000	Skin and mast cell fixation; elimination of parasites Anaphylaxis

Close cooperation between T and B cells is necessary for mounting an immune response – to include neutralisation with specific immunoglobulin and the initiation of further processes such as phagocytosis by macrophages and polymorphs. Such cooperation is augmented by a cascade of complement protein factors in the case of B cells and for T cells by recently discovered proteins known as 'lymphokines', the best known of which are migration inhibition factors and the interleukins

B cell secretory products (immunoglobulins) are divided into five main classes each of which is synthesised by a specific cell line. Immunoglobulins are active against staphylococci, streptococci, pneumococci and *Haemophilus influenzae* and may initiate adequate initial protection against some viral diseases such as varicella and hepatitis although they are less effective in containing established viral disorders. B cells also mediate immediate hypersensitivity reactions such as those seen in allergic rhinitis and asthma. The main subtypes of immunoglobulin are summarised in Table 7.13.

Immune deficiency diseases are summarised in Table 7.14.

Disorders affecting the T cell system carry a poor prognosis compared with disorders of the B cell system whilst 'combined' deficiency states are the most difficult to treat and have the poorest outcome.

Primary B cell disorders

The commonest disorder in this group is *panhypogammaglobulinaemia* which is usually inherited as an X-linked recessive disorder (Bruton type) although sporadic and recessive types have also been described. Children present in early infancy with repeated infections due to

Table 7.14   Disorders of the immune system

Panhypogammaglobulinaemia (Bruton type)
Selective specific IgA or IgM deficiency
Common variable immunodeficiency

DiGeorge syndrome
Nezelof syndrome

Severe combined immunodeficiency
Ataxia telangiectasia
Chronic mucocutaneous candidiasis
Wiskott–Aldrich syndrome

Complement deficiencies
Chronic granulomatous disease
Myeloperoxidase deficiency
Chédiak–Higashi syndrome
Leucocyte motility and cidal effects (glucose-6-phosphate dehydrogenase deficiency, glutathione synthetase deficiency, Kartagener's syndrome, Shwachman's syndrome, hyperimmunoglobulin E syndrome)

Secondary immunodeficiency states
Adenosine deaminase and nucleoside phosphorylase deficiency
Nephrosis
Protein losing enteropathy
Protein/calorie malnutrition
Steroid therapy
Other immunosuppressant therapy
Viral infections including HIV virus and acquired immune deficiency syndrome

Pneumococcus, Staphylococcus aureus and *Haemophilus influenzae*. System involvement includes recurrent conjunctivitis, sinusitis and pulmonary infections frequently with bronchiectasis and pulmonary heart disease. There is an increased incidence of autoimmune disorders and malignancy. Other problems include eczema, chronic viraemia and encephalitis. Investigations reveal low serum levels of all the principal immunoglobulins. Treatment involves early rigorous treatment of bacterial infections and replacement immunoglobulin therapy intramuscularly or intravenously.

Selective immunodeficiencies of IgA and IgM are rare. In IgA deficiency, inherited as a recessive or dominant disorder, the principal symptoms are chronic diarrhoea and recurrent respiratory infection. There is also an increased incidence of immune mediated disorders, especially systemic lupus erythematosus and juvenile chronic arthritis. Deficiency affects both serum and mucous membrane (secretory) production of IgA although rare examples of isolated deficiency of the secretory component have also been described. Treatment is symptomatic but immunoglobulin therapy may be harmful because of possible sensitisation to small amounts of exogenous IgA in this preparation. Children with selective IgM deficiency usually die from rapid onset of uncontrolled septicaemia; this may be preceded by signs of atopy and by splenomegaly. Treatment is symptomatic; no specific replacement therapy is available.

The term 'common variable immunodeficiency' is sometimes used to define deficiency states with a mainly B cell component and little or no T cell defect. The clinical picture is milder than Bruton type disease, occurs later and affects both sexes. B cell abnormalities are prominent early on, whilst T cell abnormalities tend to develop over time. Children with this disease are prone to malabsorptive disorders such as disaccharidase deficiency and non-caseating granulomas of skin. Treatment utilises a combination of early vigorous antibiotic therapy and careful immunoglobulin replacement.

Primary T cell disorders

When T cell function is compromised without coexisting B cell deficits the infections encountered are mainly fungal or viral. Isolated T cell disorders are very rare but may be seen in patients with DiGeorge syndrome in which there are associated abnormalities of the thymus (thymic aplasia) with hypoparathyroidism, and abnormalities of the heart and aortic arch. Hypocalcaemia associated with stubborn candidiasis and absent thymic shadow on chest radiograph are suspicious features and the diagnosis may be confirmed by assay of parathormone activity and studies of T cell

function. Treatment is symptomatic although thymic transplantation has been used with success in some infants. In the similar syndrome of thymic aplasia and defective T cell function (Nezelof syndrome), parathyroid and cardiac abnormalities are not seen.

Combined T cell and B cell disorders

The commonest disorder in this group is *severe combined immunodeficiency*. This disease shares the signs and symptoms of the individual deficiency states already discussed and is often accompanied by progressive wasting, alopecia, excess seborrhoeic activity and increased skin elasticity. Associated haematological abnormalities include anaemia and thrombocytopenia. *Pneumocystis carinii* pneumonia is common. In addition to intensive supportive therapy, bone marrow transplantation from donors matched for major histocompatibility antigens may prove beneficial.

In *ataxic telangiectasia*, a condition characterised by progressive neurological deterioration particularly involving the extrapyramidal system and cerebellum, a number of immunological abnormalities may be observed. These include IgA and IgE deficiencies and deficiencies in DNA repair manifested by progressive chromosomal breakages and predisposition to lymphoma formation. Recurrent sinupulmonary disorders may precede the onset of neurological abnormality and the development of cutaneous and ocular telangiectases which are typical of this disorder. The inheritance is autosomal recessive and treatment is by supportive measures only. Intellect is usually spared although the neurological disorder inevitably leads to a wheelchair existence often with malignancy as a terminal event.

Children with chronic *mucocutaneous candidiasis* involving skin, nails and mucous membranes may manifest progressive loss of immune competence, along with endocrine abnormalities such as hypoparathyroidism, hypothyroidism and hypoadrenocorticism. Characteristic abnormalities include T cell dysfunction and selective deficiency of IgA. Such individuals may be managed with amphotericin, ketoconazole and local applications of clotrimazole although response is variable.

Wiskott–Aldrich syndrome presents with thrombocytopenia, chronic suppurative middle ear disease and eczema. Laboratory assessment reveals small platelets, reduction in IgM and elevation of IgA and IgE; T cell dysfunction of moderate severity may also be present. Treatment is supportive and has included marrow transplantation.

Disorders of the complement system

Approximately 10% of the globulin fraction of serum is made up of heat labile protein components known as 'complement' and 'complement control proteins'. These proteins act as the principal mediators of the inflammatory response and are important in defence against infection. The 'classical' complement pathway consists of 11 separate proteins; there is a further alternative system with constituents designated as B, D and P. Complement C3 is a component of both pathways. The cumulative effect of an activated complement system, triggered by antigen antibody combination, includes viral neutralisation, opsonisation, induction of granulocytosis, leucocyte chemotaxis, endotoxic inactivation and microbial lysis.

Congenital deficiencies of all the components of the classical complement system and deficiency of factor D of the alternative pathway have been described. The most common clinical sequel is recurrent bacterial infection, e.g. septicaemia, pneumonia, meningitis, sinusitis, bronchitis and bronchiectasis. Management of these fortunately rare disorders is supportive, with attention to the early diagnosis and management of infection; regular plasma infusions may be effective in isolated C5 deficiency but have not proved valuable in other forms of complement deficiency.

Disorders of the phagocytic system

The phagocytic system consists of polymorphonuclear leucocytes and monocytes. When monocytes leave the circulation they develop into macrophages within many organ systems or migrate into areas of inflammation. Polymorphs are usually marginated in the circulation or stored in bone marrow in order to be rapidly released in response to infection and acute inflammation. At sites of inflammation neutrophils adhere to capillary walls and migrate into surrounding tissues by diapedesis. Bacteria are prepared for phagocytosis by a process of opsonisation which involves complement and the action of specific immunoglobulin antibody to neutralise surface virulence factors on a given micro-organism.

Disordered phagocytic function is the main abnormality in *chronic granulomatous disease of childhood*. In this disorder there is defective oxidative metabolism within leucocytes which severely impairs normal function resulting in recurrent severe pyogenic infection in early infancy. Lesions include abscess formation in lymph nodes, gut and liver. Osteomyelitis is also seen and hepatosplenomegaly is invariable. Defective neutrophil function may be identified by means of the nitroblue tetrazolium (NBT) test, or tests for cellular chemiluminescence. Early aggressive and appropriate antibiotic therapy is important; occasionally granulocyte transfusions may be indicated in resistant cases and surgical drainage procedures are often necessary. Isolated lack of myeloperoxidase enzyme in leucocytes may also impair phagocytic activity but unlike chronic granulomatous disease this usually presents with recurrent fungal disease.

Chédiak–Higashi syndrome (autosomal recessive) presents in early infancy with oculocutaneous albinism, recurrent infections and neurological problems such as mental retardation, pyramidal and cerebellar dysfunction and peripheral neuropathy. Abnormal granules are demonstrated in leucocytes and all other marrow derived cells. Polymorph function is significantly impaired although the exact mechanism responsible is not fully understood. This disorder progresses to cause anaemia, leucopenia and thrombocytopenia with death from infection or malignancy before teenage.

Rarer disorders associated with defects of leucocyte motility or bactericidal ability include glucose-6-phosphate dehydrogenase deficiency, glutathione synthetase deficiency, Kartagener (immotile cilia) syndrome, Shwachman syndrome (pancreatic insufficiency and metaphyseal chondrodysplasia), and the hyperimmunoglobulin E syndrome of Job.

Secondary immunodeficiency disorders

Deficiencies of adenosine deaminase and nucleoside phosphorylase are biochemical defects which result in immunodeficiency because of an inability to catabolise purine. This leads to accumulation of inosine and guanosine and then to products which have toxic effects on lymphocytes. Adenosine deaminase deficiency presents with features of combined immunodeficiency disease and nucleoside phosphorylase deficiency with isolated T cell defect. The diagnosis may be confirmed by measurements of appropriate red cell enzyme levels. Management is supportive.

Non-specific loss of immunoglobulin resulting in hypogammaglobulinaemia and susceptibility to infection may occur in protein-losing deficiency states such as nephrotic syndrome or protein-losing enteropathy and protein calorie malnutrition. Other important considerations include the use of immunosuppressive agents, e.g. steroids, cyclophosphamide or other anti-cancer agents and irradiation, all of which significantly impair the immune response. Patients in this predicament should always be closely monitored for infection and treated 'expectantly' when this is suspected.

Viral infections, e.g. intrauterine infection with rubella or cytomegalovirus, may influence the differentiation and normal function of B and T cells as may Epstein–Barr virus infection in postnatal life. However, the most important disorder to be considered is the profound disturbance in T cell function resulting from infection with human T cell lymphotrophic virus (HTLV 3) now known as human immunodeficiency virus (HIV). Infection with this agent results in the acquired immune deficiency syndrome (AIDS).

Childhood AIDS was first described in 1982 and by 1990 more than 1300 cases were reported to Centres for Disease Control in the United States with more than 500 cases reported in Europe alone and more than 2000 cases worldwide. It has been estimated that on a global scale paediatric AIDS cases may number several million by the turn of this century. Approximately 80% of children contract AIDS following transplacental infection with a falling proportion becoming infected via contaminated blood or blood products. Recent studies suggest a seropositive rate of between 0.01 and 0.02% in European women, with materno-fetal transmission rates estimated to be 10–30%.[6] Passively acquired maternal anti-body is thought to be cleared from the infant's circulation by approximately 18 months of age thus limiting the usefulness of antibody screening in this age group. Definitive diagnosis depends upon the detection of viral antigen; typical immune dysfunction includes elevated levels of IgG, IgM and IgA (polyclonal hypergammaglobulinaemia), thrombocytopenia, anaemia and a reversal of the normal greater-than-one ratio of helper to suppressor T cells. As the disease progresses further T cell dysfunction manifests as a lymphopenia of CD4 lymphocyte subsets, abnormal responses to mitogens and decreased production of interferon and interleukin-2.

The mean age of diagnosis of AIDS children is at present about six months although the trend is for increasing numbers of older children with milder disease to be reported. Early symptoms include recurrent respiratory infections, failure to thrive with persistent diarrhoea, candidiasis, pyrexia of unknown origin and generalised lymphadenopathy. Opportunistic infection with *Pneumocystis carinii* presents with fever, cough and tachypnoea associated with significant hypoxia. Another troublesome respiratory disorder is lymphocytic interstitial pneumonitis which is usually accompanied by parotid gland enlargement, finger clubbing, hepatosplenomegaly and generalised lymphadenopathy.

Progressively severe candidiasis involving the mouth, pharynx and oesophagus compounds the nutritional difficulties in AIDS children who often develop terminal wasting disorder accompanied by enteropathic bowel changes and further opportunistic infection with *Cryptosporidium*, *Salmonella* and atypical *Mycobacteria*. A significant proportion of children also show signs of nervous system involvement manifested by regression in milestones and by signs of pyramidal tract dysfunction. Other signs of multisystem involvement include cardiomyopathy, hepatitis and nephropathy.

At present AIDS is an irreversible disorder and management is supportive with the emphasis on family management since the mother may already be dead or ill from AIDS herself. Such treatment includes optimising nutritional status, treatment of recurrent bacterial infection (with monitoring of respiratory flora), and treatment of anaemia and thrombocytopenia and regular gammaglobulin infusions. Pneumocytis pneumonia is treated with co-trimoxazole or pentamidine and oxygen therapy and some centres practise regular prophylaxis with inhaled pentamidine to head off infection. Invasive or severe candidal infection is treated with Amphotericin B, ketoconazole or fluconazole. Acyclovir is indicated for the management of herpes virus group infections. Specific anti-viral therapy with AZT, (azidothymidine) inhibits viral replication and may slow the progression of AIDS. However, it is not curative and newer drugs such as dideoxycytidine and dideoxyinosine are under clinical trial.

Until a specific cure or immunisation techniques become available the emphasis is on prevention by thorough screening of blood donors and blood products and by appropriate counselling with respect to intravenous drug abuse and 'safe sex' whatever the gender of the participants. There are very few cases of proven HIV infection following needle stick injury from an infected patient although recently a single case report documented HIV infection in a dental patient thought to have been infected by her dentist. Clearly professionals involved in managing infected patients should take all necessary precautions to avoid self-contamination with virus laden blood. Other general measures include the washing of potentially infected linen at 95 °C for 10 minutes; designated infected waste to be disposed of separately and incinerated. Disposable equipment should be used whenever possible and where reuseable equipment is employed this should be heat sterilised by autoclaving or where appropriate by gas sterilisation using ethylene oxide. Although HIV seroconversion following needle stick injury is very uncommon, guidelines for staff should include the following:

1. Staff with infections such as herpes simplex or eczema should not care for AIDS patients.
2. Cuts and abrasions should be covered with waterproof dressings and disposable plastic aprons and latex gloves should be worn when exposed to blood and saliva. Eye protection should be worn if splashing into the conjunctiva is possible.
3. Safe handling and disposal of sharps should be undertaken to avoid needle stick injury. Re-sheathing of needles after use should be avoided in order to reduce the risk of finger needle stick.

A sharps container conforming to Department of Health standards, e.g. 'CIN BIN', should be used and subsequently incinerated. All specimen containers and request cards should be appropriately labelled as 'biohazard' and spillages of blood or blood stained secretions should be mopped up with 1% sodium hypochlorite (10% bleach diluted 1 : 10) and the area in question should be left covered in disinfectant for 30 minutes before wiping clean using disposable gloves. Any inoculation incidents should be 'milked' to encourage bleeding and then washed immediately with soap and water. Splashes of blood into the eye should be irrigated with copious amounts of water or saline (see also Miller et al.[7]).

Disorders of the blood and lymphatic system

Anaemia in childhood

Anaemia is defined as a reduction in the red cell volume or haemoglobin level below normal for age. Below a total haemoglobin level of 8 g/dl pallor becomes evident on inspection of the skin and mucous membranes. Nail changes include koilonychia and with severe degrees of anaemia decompensation occurs with lethargy, loss of appetite, splenomegaly, exertional dyspnoea, tachycardia, systolic murmurs and cardiac failure. It has been suggested that even moderate degrees of anaemia or poor iron stores may be implicated in defects of attention, alertness and learning in infants and children.

The two principal aetiological groups are disorders where there is inadequate red cell haemoglobin production and those where there is excessive red cell or haemoglobin destruction (haemolysis). Anaemias are designated macrocytic when the mean red cell volume exceeds 100 fl and microcytic when less than 75 fl.

Anaemia secondary to defective red cell or haemoglobin production

Causes are summarised in Table 7.15.

Normal newborns have relatively high haemoglobin and packed cell volume (haemocrit) and during the first few months of life there is a progressive decline to values of 9–10 g/dl. During this period of physiological adaptation to extrauterine life, erythropoiesis in marrow is quiescent but resumes thereafter. Such 'physiological anaemia' does not usually require active treatment although it may be exacerbated in preterm infants by frequent blood sampling and by deficiency of folic acid and vitamin E, when corrective intervention may become necessary.

Congenital (Blackfan–Diamond) and acquired pure red cell anaemias are extremely rare. The congenital type represents a genetic abnormality presenting with marked pallor in early infancy with profound normochromic, sometimes macrocytic, anaemia in which there is a deficiency of red cell precursors in an otherwise normal bone marrow. Serum iron levels are increased although iron binding capacity is reduced. Management is troublesome and involves repeated blood transfusions and steroid therapy; occasional spontaneous remissions are seen although the prognosis is otherwise poor. A similar acquired anaemia may be observed in older children but its aetiology is at present uncertain, although viral infections may have been implicated. A similar specific defect in erythropoiesis may sometimes complicate haemolytic anaemia (a so-called 'aplastic crisis').

Anaemia frequently accompanies chronic system infection, inflammation and advanced renal disease. This anaemia is usually normocytic and normochromic and is associated with defective erythropoiesis, reduced red cell life span, mild haemolysis and defective iron metabolism. Serum iron levels are low and iron binding capacity is unchanged. Serum ferritin is often elevated. In this group of disorders management is that of the underlying disease, the signs and symptoms of which usually predominate.

In the rare *megaloblastic anaemias*, the red blood cells are large with a mean cell volume greater than 100 fl and variable in shape with, in certain cases, concomitant neutropenia and

Table 7.15 Defects in red cell production

Congenital hypoplastic anaemia (Blackfan–Diamond syndrome)
Acquired hypoplastic anaemia
Anaemia secondary to chronic renal disease, infection and inflammation
Megaloblastic anaemia secondary to malabsorption, folate and B12 deficiency
Microcytic anaemia secondary to iron deficiency, lead poisoning and thalassaemia trait

thrombocytopenia. Folic acid deficiency may be demonstrated in some cases, associated with prematurity, malabsorption, phenytoin, methotrexate and occasionally long-term co-trimoxazole therapy. Vitamin B12 deficiency and megaloblastic anaemia may also be associated with malabsorption or intrinsic factor deficiency in older children. Clinical manifestations in megaloblastic anaemia vary and may be accompanied by other signs of nutritional deficiency such as marasmus, kwashiorkor and nervous system dysfunction such as ataxia and hyporeflexia in B12 deficiency. Diagnosis is readily made by determining red cell morphology in the presence of low levels of either folate or B12 and response to specific replacement therapy is usually dramatic.

Iron deficiency anaemia is the most commonly encountered haematological disorder of infancy and childhood. Optimal iron intake in early infancy invites an input of 10–15 mg per day and when iron rich foods are not well represented in the diet, anaemia frequently ensues particularly between the age of nine months and two years. This situation may be exacerbated by occult blood loss from the gastrointestinal tract caused by peptic ulceration, oesophagitis due to gastro-oesophageal reflux, polyps, haemangiomas and cow's milk protein intolerance. Such disorders may also cause sufficient blood loss to be the primary cause of anaemia. Characteristically the anaemia is microcytic with a mean cell volume of less than 70 fl with hypochromic cells which vary considerably in size and shape (anisocytosis). Ferritin stores are low and mean cell haemoglobin concentrations are markedly reduced. Bone marrow examination shows hypercellularity and hyperplasia of erythroid cells. Iron deficiency anaemia is usually easy to differentiate from the beta thalassaemia trait (where blood film changes may be similar) by demonstrating characteristic elevations of abnormal haemoglobin (haemoglobin F and haemoglobin A2) in the latter. Lead poisoning may be mistaken for iron deficiency on blood film unless basophilic stippling of red blood cells characteristic of lead toxicity are noted.

Treatment consists of removing the underlying cause of blood loss, if present, and in all cases by the administration of iron. Response to treatment is usually brisk with a reticulocyte response demonstrable in blood within a few days and with restoration of normality within two to three months. Blood transfusion is only indicated for severe anaemia, particularly when it is accompanied by infection, and this should be undertaken carefully because of the dangers of cardiac decompensation.

Anaemia secondary to excessive destruction of red blood cells (haemolytic anaemias)

Causes are summarised in Table 7.16.

Table 7.16 Defects causing haemolytic anaemia

Hereditary spherocytosis
Hereditary elliptocytosis
Paroxysmal nocturnal haemoglobinuria
Glucose-6-phosphate dehydrogenase deficiency
Pyruvate kinase deficiency
Sickle cell anaemia
Other haemoglobinopathies – including the
   thalassaemias, Rhesus isoimmunisation
   (erythroblastosis foetalis)
Autoimmune haemolytic anaemias

In this group of disorders the normal red cell survival time of 100–120 days is significantly reduced due to abnormal destruction of red blood cells. Bone marrow output of relatively immature red cells, known as reticulocytes, increases to values exceeding 2–3% and the products of haemoglobin degradation cause jaundice. The haemolytic process also predisposes to biliary calculi owing to accumulation of bile pigment. Plasma levels of 'free' haemoglobin rise along with elevations in levels of binding proteins, known as haptoglobins.

Children with haemolytic anaemias may also be subject to episodes of bone marrow failure, known as aplastic crisis, when the number of reticulocytes falls and when there is a marked reduction of red cell precursors in marrow. This results in an acute and potentially life threatening exacerbation of the underlying anaemia.

Hereditary spherocytosis and elliptocytosis are dominantly inherited disorders where red cell membrane dysfunction results in abnormally shaped and fragile erythrocytes. These abnormal cells are prone to lysis and sequestration in the spleen. Such disorders may present with neonatal jaundice (hyperbilirubinaemia) and anaemia or more usually with repeated episodes of childhood anaemia associated with mild jaundice, normally coloured urine and splenomegaly (acholuric jaundice). Diagnosis is confirmed by blood film examination and by red cell osmotic fragility studies. Splenectomy is usually curative but should be delayed when clinical circumstances allow because of the considerable risk of primary pneumococcal peritonitis in aplastic patients. When splenectomy is undertaken, these children should always receive regular prophylactic penicillin and periodic pneumococcal immunisation.

Paroxysmal nocturnal haemoglobinuria is a condition also thought to be associated with abnormalities of the erythrocyte membrane. Affected children present with episodes of haemolysis which are particularly prominent during sleep. These episodes are thought to be complement induced. Associated features include thrombocytopenia, leucopenia, thromboembolic phenomena and risk of infection. Diagnosis may be confirmed using the acid serum or Ham test or by demonstrating reduced levels of red cell acetylcholinesterase. Treatment is supportive.

Glucose-6-phosphate dehydrogenase deficiency is an X-linked recessive disorder in which activity of this enzyme within red blood cells is markedly reduced. This disease is particularly prevalent in Africa, Middle and Far East and in the Mediterranean. Although severity may vary considerably, the syndrome is one of potentially severe episodic haemolytic anaemia induced by infections or drugs or alternatively, a chronic haemolytic anaemia with normally shaped erythrocytes. Implicated drugs include sulphonamides, antimalarials, naphthaquinolones, aspirin, phenacetin, nitrofurantoin, nalidixic acid, chloroquine and a notorious dietary trigger is the fava bean. Occasionally neonates with this disorder may present with moderately severe neonatal jaundice. Diagnosis is suggested by the presence of marked haemoglobinaemia and haemoglobinuria with anaemia and reticulocytosis and may be confirmed by demonstrating reduction in enzyme activity to levels of 10% or less.

Treatment is supportive and may involve blood transfusions for marked falls in haemoglobin. A similar, less severe haemolytic syndrome may result from red cell deficiency of *pyruvate kinase enzyme*, a disorder usually mediated by recessive inheritance.

Recessive autosomal genes for *sickle cell* disease have been identified on chromosomes 11 and 16, responsible for defective synthesis of unstable haemoglobin S susceptible to physiochemical distortion when exposed to low oxygen concentrations. Heterozygotes who carry this gene are common in Africa, the Mediterranean and the Middle and Far East and are said to carry the 'sickle cell trait'. In this situation 30–45% of the circulating haemoglobin is represented by haemoglobin S. Haemolysis occurs only very rarely and life expectancy is normal. A degree of protection is afforded against falciparum malaria. In contrast, homozygotes suffer from true sickle cell anaemia which is usually detectable clinically by haemoglobin electrophoresis during the latter part of the first year of life, as fetal haemoglobin disappears from the circulation. Other typical blood findings include the presence of sickle cells on film, reticulocytosis, 'target cells' and 'Howell–Jolly' bodies indicating functional hyposplenism. Such children have chronic reduction in haemoglobin to values of 5–9 g/dl accompanied by mild jaundice. A variety of acute problems may occur including 'painful' crisis caused by splenic or osseous infarction without a significant fall in haemoglobin level. Aplastic crisis, haemolytic episodes, megaloblastosis and troublesome obstructive jaundice all occur. These children are prone to infection notably with tetanus and salmonella organisms, the latter causing troublesome chronic osteomyelitis. Ankle ulceration is typical. Treatment is supportive for painful crisis by using appropriate analgesia, warmth, antibiotics and by maintenance of adequate fluid balance. Other sequels of multisystem involvement include hemiplegia, nephrosis, pulmonary and splenic infarction and functional hyposplenism with recurrent sepsis.

Analogous but milder forms of haemolytic anaemia are associated with other unstable haemoglobins, e.g. haemoglobin C, D and E. In haemoglobin M disease dominantly inherited defects in haemoglobin synthesis result in methaemoglobinaemia which may mimic congenital cyanotic heart disorders. In contrast to other forms of methaemoglobinaemia treatment with methylene blue or ascorbic acid is of no benefit.

The *thalassaemias* represent a group of haemoglobinopathies with separate defects of the specific (alpha, beta, gamma, delta) haemoglobin chain. The most common disorder is beta thalassaemia which involves impaired production of the beta chain. The recessive gene for this disorder is prevalent from areas around the Mediterranean coastline and in the Middle East and Arab countries.

Heterozygotes with *beta thalassaemia* are designated as cases of beta thalassaemia minor, or beta thalassaemia trait. Characteristically there is chronic low grade hypochromic/microcytic anaemia. Signs of overt haemolysis are usually absent and the serum iron is frequently elevated. There may be modest elevations of HbA2 and HbF. For the purposes of genetic counselling when prospective parents both carry the beta thalassaemia trait the risk of offspring suffering from the much more troublesome thalassaemia major is 1 : 4 and of being 'trait' sufferers 1 : 2.

Homozygotes for this disorder suffering from *beta thalassaemia major* usually present with severe progressive haemolytic anaemia during the second half of the first year. Regular blood transfusions are necessary where there are also attendant problems of iron deposition (siderosis) in liver, pancreas and cardiac muscle. Survival is unusual beyond 20–30 years. Characteristic blood changes include severe hypochromic microcytic anaemia with levels as low as 5 g/dl without transfusion. Bilirubin and serum iron levels are elevated and red cells contain up to 70% of fetal haemoglobin although values decline over time. Inexorable haemosiderosis may be reduced to a certain extent by using chelating agents such as desferrioxamine. Splenectomy may be indicated when there is massive splenomegaly or in cases of secondary hypersplenism where red cell breakdown is exacerbated by splenic overactivity. Again in such cases penicillin prophylaxis and regular pneumococcal immunisation is mandatory.

The commonest immune mediated anaemia is *Rhesus* isoimmunisation where maternal antibody is found against Rhesus positive fetal red cells in Rhesus negative mothers. Sensitisation is necessary from a previous pregnancy or miscarriage. The degree of severity varies but marked degrees of haemolysis may cause intrauterine death due to severe anaemia and cardiac failure (hydrops foetalis). Hydrops is now uncommon following the introduction of screening programmes and treatment of at-risk mothers with protective anti-D immunoglobulin. Affected newborns are monitored closely and are managed with early phototherapy or exchange transfusions. Affected babies yield a positive Coombs test denoting the presence of maternally derived immunoglobulin or components of complement on the red cell surface. A similar mechanism is responsible for *autoimmune haemolytic anaemias* in which infection or drug therapy is thought to induce a process whereby the immune system mistakes red cells as foreign and attempts to degrade them. Some cases are associated with pre-existing disease such as systemic lupus erythematosus, lymphoma or known immunodeficiency. Although many cases are thought to be idiopathic with no specific cause identified, infections, particularly viral infections, may be trigger factors as may drugs. Implicated drugs include antimalarials, sulphonamides, penicillin and other antibiotics and antituberculous drugs, aspirin, phenacetin, many organic chemicals, thiazides, barbiturates and amphetamine. Onset may be acute, with a fairly short disorder lasting a few weeks, or as a chronic disorder lasting over months or years. Anaemia is usually severe with a positive Coombs test and reticulocytosis. Specific red cell agglutinating antibodies can sometimes be demonstrated. Occasionally these antibodies are designated 'cold agglutinins', associated clinically with haemolysis on exposure to cold environments – the best recognised trigger being *Mycoplasma pneumoniae*. Management of autoimmune anaemias is usually by blood transfusion during the acute stages combined with steroid therapy. In refractory cases other immunosuppressants such as cyclophosphamide or azathioprine may be indicated or splenectomy may be undertaken.

Primary disorders of the leucocytes

Several genetic disorders of leucocyte function affecting immune competence have already been discussed in the section dealing with chronic granulomatous disease and associated conditions.

Neutropenia refers to a reduction in circulating neutrophils to a level less than 1500/mm^3. This commonly occurs following viral infections, brucellosis and infection with typhoid organisms and is usually self-limiting with resolution occurring over weeks. In the context of acute severe bacterial infection, neutropenia has a different prognosis and usually implies overwhelming infection and poor host response. Other associations include juvenile chronic arthritis, systemic lupus erythematosus and immune mediated neutropenia. In all these disorders the defect is chronic and more difficult to treat. Occasionally in older children neutropenia may be cyclical with bouts lasting on average one week every two to four weeks. Drug induced neutropenia may be caused by sulphonamides and phenothiazines and a recessively determined lethal type of early onset has also been described. Lastly, reduction in neutrophil numbers may be a feature of pancytopenia and leukaemia (see below).

In all cases of neutropenia secondary infection is a major risk and vigorous antibiotic therapy and close monitoring is necessary. This disorder is easily detected by examining total white cell numbers and morphology. In chronic disorder it may be worthwhile trying intravenous gammaglobulin.

Childhood leukaemia represents the most common form of childhood cancer and accounts for approximately one-third of all newly diagnosed neoplastic disorders. The most common type in childhood is acute lymphoblastic leukaemia followed by acute 'non-lymphoblastic' types (myeloblastic, monocytic, myelomonocytic and erythroleukaemia), followed by chronic myelocytic type. Childhood leukaemia usually presents with progressive pallor and anaemia accompanied by the onset of generalised purpuric spots and spontaneous bruising with ulceration and bleeding from the gums. There may be superimposed signs of sepsis frequently with enlargement of the liver, spleen and lymph nodes. Blood examination reveals either a very markedly raised or sometimes markedly reduced white cell count with a preponderance of immature white cell forms (depending on the leukaemia type). There is anaemia of variable degree usually with marked thrombocytopenia, i.e. reduction of platelets. Diagnosis is confirmed by bone marrow examination which usually shows almost total replacement with either immature lymphocytes or myelocytes. Lumbar puncture may reveal cerebrospinal fluid evidence of meningeal involvement. Further investigations include chest X-ray, infection screening and membrane marker analysis for prognosis – for example of the lymphoblasts designated as 'common', 'T cell', 'B cell' or 'null', the 'common' type carries the best prognosis. Adverse clinical factors at onset include very high white cell counts, age under one year, mediastinal or central nervous system (CNS) involvement, or non-lymphoblastic type of cell involvement. Drug treatment includes induction of remission with a combination of, for example, prednisolone, vincristine and asparaginase. This may be followed by cranial irradiation and intrathecal methotrexate to reduce the risk of subsequent nervous system involvement. Maintenance is usually sustained with combinations of oral mercaptopurine and methotrexate and periodic reinduction courses of vincristine and prednisolone. Treatment, which is best restricted to specialist centres, continues for two years with regular monitoring for disease progress and drug side effects being mandatory. Supportive care includes close monitoring for treatment for infection in necessarily immunocompromised children. Anaemia and thrombocytopenia are corrected with transfusions of packed cells or platelets. Care should be taken to diagnose and to treat opportunistic infection briskly, e.g. due to herpes viruses, measles and *Pneumocystis carinii*. Skin sepsis may occur without any normal pus formation or signs of acute inflammation (redness, local heat, pain and swelling). Empirical antibiotic treatment should be given at a low clinical threshold. Specific immunoglobulin, e.g. measles or herpes varicella zoster, may sometimes be of considerable value in exposed patients.

Drug protocols are continually being refined and have resulted in dramatic changes in overall prognosis in childhood leukaemia, particularly the acute lymphoblastic type. In this disorder the five year survival has risen from a few per cent to 60% or more within the past twenty years. Relapses, e.g. in testes, CNS or in blood, bode ill for eventual survival. Bone marrow transplantation is being assessed in treatment and requires an HLA compatible donor sibling, total body irradiation and subsequent treatment with potent immunosuppressant drugs. The main treatment hurdles are infection risk, graft rejection and recurrence of leukaemia.

The pancytopenias

Marrow aplasia or replacement of haematopoietic tissue with other elements results in reduction or in complete cessation in formation of all formed blood elements or pancytopenia. The combined clinical manifestations are anaemia, haemorrhage due to thrombocytopenia, and susceptibility to infection due to neutropenia. Genetically determined aplastic anaemia (Fanconi syndrome) is inherited as an autosomal recessive disorder. Many affected children have associated physical abnormalities such as microphthalmia, absent radii and thumbs, microcephaly, short stature and renal and cardiac abnormalities. In early infancy such children present with bruising followed by frequent infections which are due to leucopenia and progressively severe anaemia. Investigation reveals severe pancytopenia in peripheral blood and strikingly hypocellular marrow. Treatment includes antibiotic therapy, blood transfusion and anabolic steroids together with relatively low dose conventional steroid therapy. Side effects from life saving long-term androgen therapy include masculinisation, liver cysts and hepatoma so that bone marrow transplantation may need to be considered.

Acquired aplastic anaemia with similar blood and marrow findings may follow presumed damaged bone marrow after exposure, for example, to the antibiotic chloramphenicol. Other recognised potential toxic agents include ionising radiation, methotrexate, 6-mercaptopurine, benzene, phenylbutazone, sulphonamides and carbamazepine. Certain infections such as Epstein–Barr virus or hepatitis A are occasionally causative.

Diagnosis is confirmed by identifying sig-

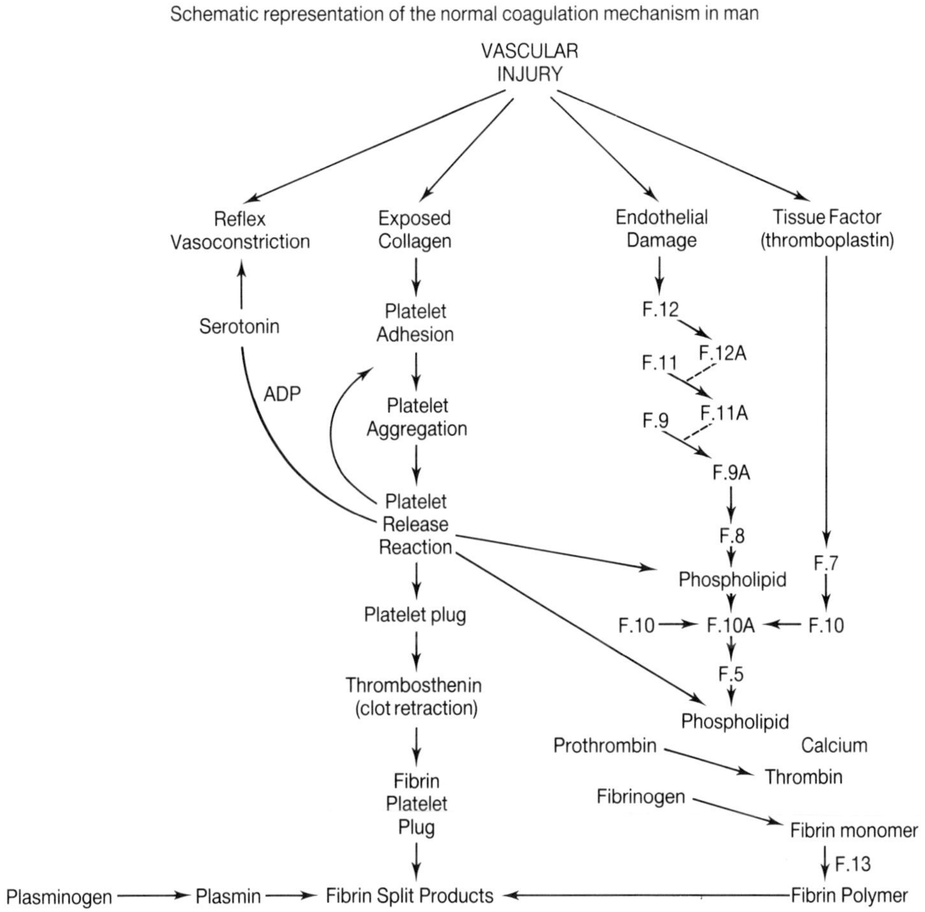

Schematic representation of the normal coagulation mechanism in man

Figure 7.5   Schematic representation of the normal coagulation mechanism in man.

nificant pancytopenia in blood film and by marked hypocellularity of marrow. Treatment is supportive with early antibiotic therapy together with blood or platelet transfusions and removal from exposure to the proposed causative agent where possible.

In the acquired aplastic anaemias the overall prognosis is poor and treatment with androgens is ineffective in the long term. A small number of children have been managed successfully with marrow transplantation. A similar clinical picture may be encountered in patients with marrow replacement due to neuroblastomas or osteopetrosis.

Disorders of haemostasis

Haemostasis is normally maintained by a complex mechanism involving local reactions of blood vessels, altered platelet activity and the interactions of protein 'coagulation factors' circulating in the blood. After vascular injury there is active vasoconstriction followed by mobilisation of platelets and clotting factors as shown schematically in Fig. 7.5.

In the first phase of normal coagulation thromboplastin is formed by the interaction of plasma, platelets and extracellular fluid; this facilitates conversion of prothrombin to thrombin in the presence of calcium ions. Thrombin then converts soluble fibrinogen into a stable fibrin clot (polymer) which interacts with platelets to form a firm plug. Factors 8, 9, 11 and 12 act through a so-called 'intrinsic' system to activate factor 10 whereas in the 'extrinsic' system this factor is directly activated by factor 7 (proconvertin). Fibrin lysis is mediated by a substance known as plasmin

Table 7.17   Examples of commonly used tests of haemostasis

Test	Assesses
Tourniquet test	Platelet function. Vascular stability of small vessels
Platelet count/platelet function test	Platelet number and function
Bleeding time	Platelet function and vascular stability of small vessels
Clotting time	Whole coagulation mechanism
Thrombin time	Conversion of fibrinogen to fibrin polymer
Prothrombin time	Adequacy of factors 2, 5, 7 and 10
Partial thromboplastin time	Adequacy of factors 8, 9, 11 and 12

Table 7.18   Haemostatic disorders

Condition	Abnormality
Haemophilia A	Factor 8 deficiency
Haemophilia B (Christmas disease)	Factor 9 deficiency
Other factor deficiences	Factors 11 and 12
Von Willebrand's disease	Factor 8 deficiency and reduced platelet adhesiveness
Parahaemophilia (Owren's disease)	Factor 5 deficiency
Haemorrhagic disease of the newborn	Reduced activity of factors 2, 7, 9 and 10
Congenital afibrinogenaemia	Absent fibrinogen
Idiopathic thrombocytopenic purpura	Reduced platelet number and function

which is derived from its serum precursor plasminogen.

Assessment of coagulation disorders is aided considerably by utilising several diagnostic tests outlined in Table 7.17. These tests are complementary to history and physical examination; a careful family history is also important since several coagulation disorders have a genetic basis.

The principal disorders manifesting with increased bleeding tendency are listed in Table 7.18. Only the commoner disorders are now discussed.

The haemophilias are X-linked recessive disorders and represent the commonest and most troublesome coagulation disorders. Types A and B are clinically indistinguishable and are secondary to factor 8 and 9 deficiency respectively. Clinical severity depends upon the degree of factor depletion, which becomes clinically progressively severe at levels below 5% although signs are not necessarily apparent in the newborn period. Certain neonates with these disorders do present with, for example, prolonged bleeding times from the umbilical cord or circumcision sites. With increased activity haematomas develop in response to minor trauma, affecting joints and muscles. Multiple painful haemarthroses are followed by progressive joint deformity. Other complications include prolonged bleeding from trivial lacerations, haematuria and intracranial haemorrhage. Diagnosis may be expected from the family history and will certainly be confirmed by demonstrating a prolonged partial thromboplastin time and low factor levels. Management is by minimising trauma in early infancy, avoiding exposure to aspirin and expeditious specific factor replacement using specially formulated concentrate. It is important to achieve 50% of factor levels as soon as possible and to maintain these at a level greater than 5% for more than three days after any specific bleeding event. Other local measures to reduce bleeding include the application of cold compresses and careful pressure. Initial immobilisation should be followed by gentle remobilisation in the event of haemarthroses in order to reduce the risk of ankylosis. Careful screening of factor concentrate should hopefully avoid contamination of blood products with HIV virus which has led to tragically avoidable cases of AIDS in patients with haemophilia. Careful genetic counselling is mandatory in this disease; antenatal diagnostic techniques are now available utilising chorionic villus biopsy.

Von Willebrand's disease is inherited in autosomal dominant mode. In this disorder factor 8 deficiency is compounded by defects in platelet adhesiveness. Clinical presentation is usually with epistaxis, bleeding from the gums, prolonged oozing from cuts and increased bleeding after trauma or surgery. Management is similar to that of haemophilia.

Haemorrhagic disease of the newborn is now rare following the widespread use of the prophylactic vitamin K1 in neonates. Such treatment reduces the risk of depletion of factors 2, 7, 9 and 10 seen in a minority of newborn infants and potentially exacerbated by the absence of vitamin K from the breast milk. In affected babies bleeding becomes evident from the second day of life typically as umbilical cord bleeding, melaena, haematemesis and rarely fatal intracranial haemorrhage. Prothrombin time is prolonged. Treatment involves the administration of parenteral vitamin K1 and support of the circulation with replacement transfusion when necessary.

Congenital afibrinogenaemia is a rare, recessively inherited disorder associated with unexpectedly prolonged bleeding following trauma or surgery. Thrombin time is prolonged. Management is supportive and also involves the administration of replacement fibrinogen.

Thrombocytopenic purpura is characterised clinically by small haemorrhages into the superficial layers of the skin inducing purple discoloration. Tiny extravasations are designated petechiae and more extensive 'bruised' areas as ecchymoses. Bleeding may also occur into mucous membrane, brain or viscera. As already stated platelets are essential integral components of the normal clotting mechanisms. Following damage to small blood vessels platelets accumulate at the site of injury forming a platelet fibrin plug. Adhesion of platelets is favoured by contact with collagen, by endogenous adenosine diphosphate (ADP) and thromboxane. Thrombocytopenia is said to exist at platelet counts of less than 150 000/mm^3 although purpura may not become a clinical problem until levels of less than 50 000/mm^3 are achieved.

The commonest platelet disorder in childhood is *idiopathic thrombocytopenic purpura* (ITP)

(Fig. 7.6), which is thought to be caused by sensitisation due to virus infection, following a latent period of two to three weeks. Antiplatelet antibodies can be demonstrated. Generalised ecchymoses and a petechial rash are typical with lesions, particularly prominent over the extremities. Other sites of bleeding include the gums, nasal mucosa and occasionally, early on during the disorder, intracranial haemorrhage. The platelet count is typically found to be less than 20 000/mm^3. The tourniquet test is positive and the bleeding time is prolonged beyond 10 minutes. Bone marrow examination reveals a normal or increased level of platelet precursor (megakaryocytes). Such examination is important to differentiate ITP from acute leukaemia and aplastic anaemia although patients with the latter disorder are more acutely ill.

Treatment of ITP includes the use of steroids which have been shown to reduce the severity and duration of the acute phase although such treatment does not reduce the incidence of chronic ITP. Intravenous gammaglobulin may also be effective although some clinicians reserve its use for chronic cases.

Splenectomy remains controversial because of its inherent risks in what almost invariably turns out to be a disorder from which children recover. One year after onset more than 90% of children have regained normal platelet counts.

Very occasionally thrombocytopenia may be drug induced; *Wiskott–Aldrich syndrome* (eczema, thrombocytopenia and susceptibility to infection) is described in a previous section. Another rare association of thrombocytopenia is aplasia of the radii and thumbs which may be coupled with congenital cardiac and renal abnormalities.

ITP should not be confused with *Henoch–Schönlein (anaphylactoid) purpura* (Fig. 7.7) which is a disorder in which vasculitic lesions affect small blood vessels, frequently following an upper respiratory infection. Boys are affected more than girls with peak incidence in the age range three to five years. Skin blood vessels are surrounded by cellular reaction of polymorphs and round cells and IgA deposits may also be seen. Other regions involved include brain, gut, joints and kidney. In distinction from ITP, skin lesions develop as small wheals or as red maculopapular lesions which occur in crops particularly over the pre-tibial

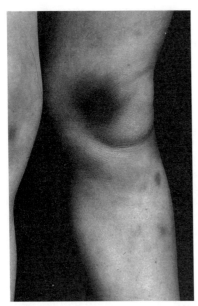

Figure 7.6 Typical ecchymoses in idiopathic thrombocytopenic purpura.

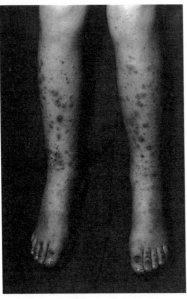

Figure 7.7 Typical rash of Henoch–Schönlein purpura.

areas, buttocks and extensor surfaces. Such lesions may develop petechial or purpuric qualities but frank ecchymoses are uncommon. Signs of multisystem involvement include abdominal pain, haematemesis, melaena, haematuria, hemiplagia, seizures and arthritis. Renal involvement is potentially the most serious complication and may lead to chronic renal failure. Diagnosis of Henoch–Schönlein purpura is usually made on clinical grounds and treatment is supportive. Steroid therapy is reserved for the more serious complications or for cases of particularly severe skin involvement.

Disorders of the lymphatic system

The mononuclear and phagocyte population of the spleen, liver and bone marrow act as an immunological filter mechanism for the blood circulating through them. A large number of foreign antigens invade the body via the skin, respiratory and gastrointestinal tracts and then enter the lymphatic system rather than the blood. In this situation the first line of cellular defence is represented in the lymph node system. Lymph nodes represent separate anatomical units distributed along lymphatic channels and are surrounded by a connective tissue capsule perforated at several points by feeding lymphatics which deliver antigens, lymphocytes and macrophages. Circulating lymph is actively 'filtered' within the node whose efferent vessel exits via the hilus containing sensitised B and T cells and antibody secreting plasma cells (see above). The outer part of the node is designated the cortex and contains lymphoid follicles which are centres of B cell activity. Antigenic stimulation causes primary follicles to become secondary follicles by enlarging to form pale staining germinal centres containing activated B cells, T cells, macrophages and reticulum cells. The paracortical areas between the primary and secondary follicles and the central medullary portion of the node are centres of T cell activity. This structure provides a suitable system for delivering and exposing antigens to the immune system. Following such immunological stimulation node size may increase tenfold within one week. After birth and following continuing exposure to environmental antigens the mass of lymphoid tissue steadily increases during childhood to reach its peak in early puberty. Palpable lymph nodes are a common finding in children compared to adults, particularly in the cervical, inguinal and axillary regions. It is unusual to find parallel enlargement affecting the popliteal, mediastinal or supraclavicular regions in the absence of significant pathology.

Normal lymph node enlargement in childhood rarely exceeds 2.5 cm diameter in the neck, axilla or inguinal region although enlargement above 2–3 mm should be treated with suspicion when affecting other areas. Other causes for concern are when lymphadenopathy affects more than two regions or when nodes are associated with local heat (inflammation), pain, erythema, fluctuance, 'rubberiness' or a tendency to mat together or to become adherent to surrounding tissues. The causes of generalised and significant lymphadenopathy are summarised in Table 7.19.

Table 7.19 Causes of generalised lymphadenopathy in childhood

---

Viral infections (Epstein–Barr, cytogemalovirus, HIV, rubella, varicella, measles, upper respiratory viruses)

Bacterial infection (tuberculosis, typhoid, staphylococcal or streptococcal bacteraemia)

Protozoal infection (toxoplasmosis)

Fungal infection (coccidioidomycosis)

Immune mediated disorders (systemic lupus erythematosus, serum sickness, drug allergy, juvenile chronic arthritis)

Storage disorders (Gaucher's disease, Niemann–Pick disease)

Neoplasia (leukaemia, lymphoma, Hodgkin's disease, neuroblastoma, histiocytosis X)

Localised, isolated 'regional' lymphadenopathy is most often due to infection. Nodes in inguinal and iliac groups drain the lower extremities, perineum, genitalia, buttocks and lower abdominal wall. A small number of moderate sized, discrete inguinal nodes are a common finding in children. Readily overlooked sources of infection producing such lymphadenopathy include insect bites, napkin dermatitis, injection site inflammation and low grade infected eczema or seborrhoeic dermatitis. It is important to differentiate between enlarged lymph nodes and other inguinal swellings such as ectopic testes, hernias and lipomas.

Lymphatic vessels collect lymph from almost all tissues and organs except the central nervous system, muscle and non-vascular structures such as cornea and cartilage. Essentially lymph represents extracellular fluid loaded with lymphocytes and material of molecular size which is too large to cross capillary endothelium. This fluid is first delivered into lymph 'capillaries' and is then carried to regional lymph nodes via larger thin-walled transparent lymph vessels. Eventually body lymph enters the thoracic duct and then the great veins via the right lymphatic duct.

When infection is not contained locally it may enter the lymphatic vessels as an *ascending lymphangitis* which is characterised by erythematous linear streaks along the course of a given group of lymphatics. This is usually followed by painful swelling of the appropriate regional nodes and may be followed by local oedema where there is associated lymphatic obstruction. Bacteraemia or septicaemia may ensue unless infection is treated promptly.

Lymphoedema refers to the diffuse pitting type of oedema which results from obstruction of lymphatic flow. The most common site is in the lower extremities where it may be accompanied by firm thickening of skin and by susceptibility to cellular infection. The commonest causes of acquired lymphoedema are post-inflammatory (lymphadenitis), surgical obliteration of nodes or lymph channels or post-therapeutic irradiation. Congenital pedal oedema is a feature of Turner's syndrome (Bonnevie–Ullrich syndrome).

Congenital (early onset) lymphoedema or *Milroy's disease* is an extremely rare, dominantly inherited disorder characterised by chronic pitting oedema of the lower limbs. Variability of genetic expression ranges from minimal ankle swelling to greatly enlarged feet, legs and thighs. Overlying skin is attenuated but otherwise normal and there is usually slow asymptomatic progression of oedema with time. Attempts to visualise lymphatics in involved areas have proved unsuccessful and the defect has therefore been thought to be due to an abnormality in lymphatic development rather than secondary to increased output of interstitial fluid. This defect is largely cosmetic with minor degrees of disability resulting in cases of gross lower limb oedema. Resection of subcutaneous tissue and skin autografts have been performed with variable results and the use of diuretics and bed rest are only temporarily and partially effective.

Obvious care should always be taken to differentiate lymphoedema from the commoner phenomenon of pitting oedema due to diseases such as hypoproteinaemia, hepatic, renal and cardiac failure and venous obstruction.

Podopaediatric management considerations

Patients with HIV

Broad outlines covering staff guidelines have already been given with regard to treating patients who have the AIDS virus. The psychological effects of this condition are enormous and the practitioner should be tactful but matter of fact when explaining to patients the precautions which must be carried out during treatments.

The aims during treatment are to prevent contamination of the environment and of the operator by the virus which is present in the patient's bloodstream or tissue fluids and to prevent cross infection of the patient from the environment or from the operator. It must be remembered that these patients' own defence mechanisms are impaired and thus extremely strict antiseptic precautions must be carried out.

When the podiatrist is working in a multiple treatment clinic the treatment area for the patient should be chosen with care. This is to avoid embarrassment to the patient and also to negate the possibility of cross infection to other patients. The treatment area should where possible be entirely separate. A dressing trolley should be marked clearly 'For restricted use' and reserved for this type of patient. The patient must be given the last appointment of the clinical session as this will enable a thorough postoperative disinfection of the unit, chair and floor to be carried out.

Prior to treatment, the chair unit and floor should be swabbed down with 70% isopropyl alcohol and allowed to dry. The floor area where the patient will stand, the foot and leg rests of the chair should all be covered with paper towels.

The dressing trolley should be covered with a sterile paper drape and all materials and drugs considered necessary for the procedure to be carried out should be placed on top of the sterile drape, e.g. a preoperative swabbing solution, full set of sterile instruments and a spare autoclave tray to receive used instruments. Taped to the dressing trolley should be a large plastic disposal bag. This preparation is carried out before the patient enters the treatment area.

The treatment of HIV patients is made easier when an assistant is available. When an assistant is not available the podiatrist should visually examine the patient's feet and make an assessment of the postoperative medicaments and dressings which are likely to be required and these should be placed on top of the dressings' trolley. In this way everything should be available for the complete treatment of the patient without the podiatrist having to leave the treatment area.

The following are procedure guidelines to be carried out during treatment (with or without an assistant).

Podiatrist

Protective clothing should be disposable whenever possible and should include:

- Paper gown and disposable plastic apron.
- Mask.
- Sterile disposable gloves (two pairs should be worn when the podiatrist is working single handed). Cuts or abrasions on the hands should first be covered with a first aid plaster.
- Goggles with side panels. These should be used when an open lesion is present and where there is danger of splash-back from irrigation of the wound.

Once treatment has commenced the operator should only touch equipment or material on top of the sterile drape. The operator has become 'dirty'.

Assistant

Protective clothing should be as for the podiatrist with the exception of the goggles. The assistant's role is to supply medicaments, to prepare dressings and to cut pads and dressing tapes. Once these have been prepared they should be placed on top of the sterile drape. The assistant remains technically 'clean' and may move outside the treatment area when anything further is required.

Treatment procedure

When working single-handed the outermost pair of gloves are removed after all nail work, reduction of callus and the cleansing of ulcers has been carried out. This is in order that medicaments in multi-application tubes are handled with non-infected gloves.

Postoperatively

All debris is placed in the disposable bag, e.g. gloves, gowns, apron and mask. Goggles if worn should be placed in a chemical sterilising solution. A clean pair of disposable gloves should be worn and the instrument tray transferred directly into the steriliser. Do not attempt to remove the blades, scrub instruments or put them into the sonic cleaner at this stage.

The patient should be escorted from the surgery and after the patient has left, the treatment area must be thoroughly cleaned. Heavy duty rubber gloves are needed for this purpose. All paper towels are removed from the floor and are placed in the disposal bag. The chairs, dressing trolley and floor are wiped over with 1 : 100 Clearsol solution. Once the instruments have been through the cycle in the autoclave they are placed in a detergent solution for a minimum of six hours. The plastic disposal bag containing all the debris is tied and placed inside another plastic bag, re-tied, and clearly labelled ready for incineration.

When the instruments are removed from the solution any blades are removed using a blade remover and are then placed in the sharps container. The instruments are then thoroughly rinsed, placed in the ultrasonic cleaner for 10 minutes and then re-sterilised.

Hospitals and various health authorities all have their own method of disposal for infected material and this method should be adhered to. These precautions should also be carried out for patients who have viral hepatitis.

When treating other high risk patients who are prone to infection, extra precautions must be carried out in order to prevent cross infection. Since the patients themselves are at risk from infection and not the practitioner, there is no need for certain of the measures mentioned above.

High risk patients would include patients with primary B and/or T cell disorders, disorders of the complement system and the phagocytic system. Any patient whose medical condition outlined previously makes him/her prone either to infection, or who has a reduced ability to fight infection, should be considered an 'at risk' patient and treated accordingly. Such patients are prone both to bacterial and to fungal infection and preventative measures should be taken wherever possible. Reference to the chapter on the diabetic child (Chapter 8) would be appropriate.

Haemostatic disorders

The child with a haemostatic disorder is a high risk patient. When carrying out routine treatments on such a child extra vigilance is necessary when reducing lesions. Areas should be under-reduced in order to prevent trauma to and bleeding of skin tissues. The use of local analgesia is contraindicated in such patients due to the inherent risk of bleeding. Therefore the use of treatments which require analgesia, unless carried out with medical management and hospitalisation, is precluded.

Bleeding into joints also occurs in the haemophiliac. In the lower limb the main joints that are affected are the knee and ankle joints but no joint is excluded and deformity of the joint may eventually occur. Haemarthrosis is evident by swelling, increased heat, pain and tenderness accompanied by discoloration of the affected joint. Immediate treatment is rest until the acute stage has passed and the aim is to prevent joint deformity occurring as much as possible. This is achieved by stabilisation of the joint and by a daily regime of exercises in a similar manner to the treatment of acute degenerative arthritis.

Disorders of the lymphatic system

Local infection of the foot should be treated promptly and efficiently in order to prevent the development of cellulitis, lymphangitis and lymphadenitis. In an otherwise healthy child local infection, when treated promptly, should pose no problem and the use of topical antiseptics should suffice. When the infection does not respond to treatment then the use of an appropriate antibiotic should be arranged with the patient's general practitioner.

A child who presents with swelling of the foot or leg should be referred immediately to his/her general practitioner when no causative factor such as trauma, infection or dermatitis can be established.

Chronic lymphoedema of the foot and lower limb caused by Turner's syndrome or Milroy's disease presents many problems to the practitioner, not least of which are problems with footwear. Due to the oedematous state of the feet many problems arise which are related to trauma from footwear. These include onychocryptosis, bursitis, fissures and recurrent infection due to abrasions.

Footwear advice is imperative but due to the puffy foot and in the child pitting oedema (in later life this oedema becomes fibrosed, there is little pitting and the skin becomes thick and coarse), this invariably presents a problem. In summer when it is possible to obtain a sandal which laces to the toe or which has adjustable straps, this is advantageous but winter footwear is more difficult. Certain trainers provide adequate room for the less oedematous foot but when suitable footwear is not available prescription for surgical footwear or for bespoke trainers is necessary.

Avoidance of trauma may be achieved to a certain extent by footwear which has adequate room. Nail problems, e.g. onychocryptosis, may be avoided by regular treatment of relaxed sulci with the use of packing and astringent solutions and with the obvious advice not to cut nails too short or not to cut down the sides. Often the lesser toes as well as the first toe are affected. Once infection is present it is slow to heal due to the pressure and the relative stasis in the area.

Lesions which occur in lymphostasis are typically hyperkeratotic or verrucoid in nature. These usually occur on the digits, dorsum of the foot and at the front of the ankle and are chronic and very difficult to clear.

The treatment of such a lesion starts with advice on washing the feet regularly with a soap containing a bactericidal agent and with the gentle use of a soft nail brush since such lesions are liable to become infected due to their fissured and fragmented nature. The use of keratolytic agents such as low percentages of salicylic acid preparations provide the best results in clearing these lesions. When these are profuse daily applications of a solution are preferable to ointments and reduction should be carried out at weekly or two weekly intervals.

Such treatment may eradicate the lesions but the patient must continue with thorough washing and soft scrubs to keep them at bay. The use of 60% salicylic acid may be used when the lesions are extremely crusted but a maximum of two applications is recommended. When using preparations containing salicylic acid the possibility of dermatitis occurring in the surrounding skin should always be borne in mind.

Treatment of fungal infections should be rigorous since such patients are particularly prone to infection both in the interdigital spaces and in the heel areas where there may be associated hyperkeratosis and fissuring. Prophylactic treatment should be initiated before or after infection with the use of proprietary foot powders.

The use of daily applications of emollients should be advised in order to maintain the viability of skin tissues. This routine is most important in the older child as the tissues become more and more devitalised due to the oedema.

Growth disorders

When there is a problem of growth the practitioner must be aware that bone development may be delayed by between eighteen months and four years. This fact must be taken into consideration when carrying out biomechanical assessment on the child as the usual developmental patterns in the leg and foot will be altered. For example in the foot, during the first six years of life, the head and neck of the talus undergo a valgus rotation in relation to the body of the talus so that by the time the child has reached six years of age talar torque should be complete. When talar torque is incomplete forefoot varus is said to exist. However, it would be premature to assume that this derotation had taken place by this age in children with a growth disorder. Similarly with a delay in the ontogeny of the calcaneus an erroneous diagnosis of hindfoot varus could be made.

This applies to all the various developmental patterns of the lower limb, e.g. the angle of inclination of the femur, the relationship of the femur to the pelvis, progressive genu valgum/varum patterns and tibial torsion measurements. It is important that such factors are taken into consideration before corrective orthoses are manufactured. In a child with delayed ontogeny there will still be considerable changes in foot posture over the age of six years. Orthotic devices should not be posted as there will be no allowance for the normal ontogenetic changes which are still occurring and this will cause abnormal foot postures to develop.

Conditions such as osteochondritis which tend to manifest themselves in certain bones within a specified time scale in the child's development, relating to the ossification timetable, may be delayed and this possibility must be considered when making a diagnosis.

Hypotonia and abnormal pronation

All children pronate when they first start to walk and this is considered to be normal by many authorities while others believe that all abnormal pronatory movements should be avoided. Unless there is reason for excessive pronation in infancy, such as hypermobile states, normal development should be allowed without interference. If by the age of three there is still excessive abnormal pronation it should not be allowed to persist as it may lead to chronic osseous deformity in adulthood.

In conditions such as Ehlers–Danlos syndrome and Down's syndrome supportive measures should be started as soon as possible. The heel counters of the child's footwear should be firm and may be extended along the medial side and the addition of a half or full Thomas heel is of benefit. Orthoses should be manufactured in order to stabilise the foot.

In Down's syndrome the feet are broad with a wide space between the first and second toes. Pes planovalgus tends to be severe due to the marked hypotonia of muscle. In addition to the above measures footwear should be of an inflare type in order to accommodate the broad forefoot and to allow spacing on the medial side of the foot.

Ehlers–Danlos syndrome has the additional problem of paper thin skin which is very loose, friable and liable to trauma with resulting scarring. The looseness of the skin is liable to cause friction from footwear particularly at the posterior aspect of the heel. Good fitting footwear is extremely important in order to minimise this problem.

Mismatched foot sizes

Different sized feet may be remedied in two ways. The first is for the podiatrist to manufacture an insert for each pair of shoes that the child owns. This is unsatisfactory since it does not lead to good shoe fitting in both width and length, but for the parent who may struggle financially it may be the only solution. The other is to buy shoes in odd sizes. When the difference in length or width fitting is considerable this is the only course open to parents. Financial help may be made available after discussion with the appropriate authorities. The podiatrist should determine if this is likely, before discussing the probability with the parents.

Clarks provide an odd shoe scheme whereby they will take a special order to supply shoes in odd sizes and fittings, but in a limited range of styles. At present a surcharge of 25% is made for shoes supplied under the scheme. For further details write to:

Odd Shoe Service
Clarks Shoes Ltd
Box 50
40 High Street
Somerset
BA16 0YA

References

1 Nelson, K, Holmes, L. Malformations due to presumed spontaneous mutations in newborn infants. *N Eng J Med*. 1989; 320: 19.
2 Graham JM. *Smith's Recognisable Patterns of Human Deformation*, 2nd edn. WB Saunders, 1988.
3 Jones KL. *Smith's Recognisable Patterns of Human Malformation*, 4th edn. WB Saunders, 1988.
4 Tanner JM, Whitehouse RH, Takaish M. Standards from birth to maturity for height, weight,

height velocity and weight velocity. *Arch Dis Child* 1966; 41: 613.

5 Vimpani GV, Vimpani AF *et al. Br Med J* 1977; ii: 427–30.

6 Mok J. Paediatric AIDS. *Mat Child Health* 1990; 15 (11): 349.

7 Miller D, Weber J, Green J. *The Management of AIDS Patients.* Macmillan Press, 1986.

Further reading

Asherson GL, Webster ADB. *Diagnosis and Treatment of Immuno-Deficiency Diseases.* Oxford, Blackwell, 1980.

Brook CGD (ed.). *Clinical Paediatric Endocrinology.* Blackwell, Oxford, 1989.

Clinics in Endocrinology and Metabolism Growth Disorders. London. WB Saunders Company 1986; 15 (3).

Esterly JR. Congenital hereditary lymphoedema. *J Med Genet* 1965; 2: 93.

Horowitz SD, Hong R. *The Pathogenesis and Treatment of Immunodeficiency.* Basel, S. Karger, 1977.

Hosking CS, Roberton DM. The diagnostic approach to recurrent infections in childhood. *Clin Immunol Allergy* 1981; 1: 631–9.

McKusick V. *Mendelian Inheritance in Man; Catalogs of Autosomal Dominant, Autosomal Recessive and X-Linked Phenotypes,* 5th edn. Baltimore, Johns Hopkins University Press, 1978.

Marshall WA. *Human Growth and its Disorders.* London, Academic Press, 1977.

Miller DR. *Blood Diseases in Infancy and Childhood.* Oxford, Blackwell Scientific Publications, 1984.

Nathan DG, Oski FA. *Haematology of Infancy and Childhood,* 4th edn. Philadelphia, WB Saunders, 1986.

Schroeder E, Helweg-Carson HF. Congenital hereditary lymphoedema (Nonne–Milroys–Meiges Disease). *Acta Med Scand* 1950; 137: 198.

Shannon KM, Ammann AJ. Acquired immune deficiency syndrome in childhood. *J Paediatr* 1985; 106: 332.

Tanner JM. *Foetus into Man. Physical Growth from Conception to Maturity.* Open Books, London, 1990.

Warkany J. *Congenital Malformations.* Chicago, Year Book Medical Publishers, 1971.

Willoughby MLN. *Paediatric Haematology.* Edinburgh, Churchill Livingstone, 1977.

World Health Organization. Acquired Immunodeficiency Syndrome. WHO/CDC. Case Definition for AIDS. *Wkly Epidemiol Rec* 1986; 61: 69–73.

8 The Diabetic Child

Heather Stirling, Christopher Kelnar and Maureen O'Donnell

Diabetes mellitus is a disorder caused by loss of function of the beta cells of the islets of Langerhans in the pancreas. These cells produce the peptide hormone insulin which is necessary for glucose metabolism. The symptoms and signs of childhood-onset (insulin-dependent) diabetes mellitus (IDDM) are due to a lack of insulin.

Insulin is an anabolic hormone which is necessary for adequate carbohydrate utilisation. The main stimulus for insulin secretion from the islet cells is a rise in blood glucose (hyperglycaemia). Insulin then decreases glucose output from the liver by inhibiting glucose production (gluconeogenesis) and glycogen breakdown (Fig. 8.1). Insulin also

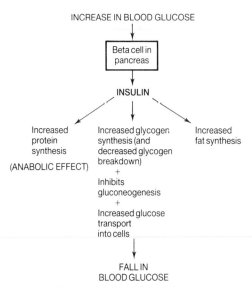

INCREASE IN BLOOD GLUCOSE

Beta cell in pancreas

INSULIN

Increased protein synthesis

(ANABOLIC EFFECT)

Increased glycogen synthesis (and decreased glycogen breakdown)
+
Inhibits gluconeogenesis
+
Increased glucose transport into cells

Increased fat synthesis

FALL IN BLOOD GLUCOSE

Figure 8.1 Physiological action of insulin.

increases the uptake of glucose by the liver and skeletal muscle; it stimulates protein, glycogen and fat synthesis. By a combination of all these measures blood glucose will return to normal levels.

A lack of insulin leads to a decrease in glucose utilisation and to an increase in gluconeogenesis, producing hyperglycaemia. Once the blood sugar rises above the renal threshold, glucose spills over into the urine (glycosuria). Glucose is a powerful osmotic agent and an osmotic diuresis is produced. Urine output is significantly increased leading to thirst, and when persistent, dehydration will occur. Lack of insulin also produces increased fat breakdown with a rise in 'ketones' in the blood.

There are marked geographical variations in the incidence of IDDM in children, with the highest reported incidence in Finland (28.6/100 000 per year) and the lowest in Japan (1.7/100 000 per year). This wide variation suggests the importance of environmental factors in the development of the condition.

In the British Isles in 1988, a national incidence rate of 13.5/100 000 per year in children aged under 16 years, i.e. 1600 new cases per year in the British Isles was recorded, with the highest incidence in Scotland (19.8/100 000 per year).[1] This is an increase on the previously reported rate of 7.7/100 000 per year in 1977.[2] There is an equal sex ratio. Peak age at diagnosis is 10–14 years, but a quarter of cases occur under the age of 5 years. The increased incidence at age 10–14 years reflects hormonal changes at the beginning of puberty that may exacerbate the islet cell damage. There is seasonal variation in the presentation of the disease with more cases being diagnosed in the winter months, particularly February and March.

In the United Kingdom 1 in 500 children under 16 years of age will have IDDM. Thus it is a common important disease in childhood with significant mortality and morbidity.

The development of diabetes in an individual is multifactorial, with both genetic and environmental factors playing a part. By the time the child with diabetes presents, approximately 90% of the islet cells will have already been destroyed. Finding the cause of this destruction and possible ways to prevent it are major areas of diabetic research.

Genetic associations with diabetes are well recognised, particularly with certain histocompatibility HLAs (human leucocyte antigens) such as HLA DR3, DR4, Dw3 and Dw4 which are located on chromosome 6. However, only 10–20% of individuals who carry these genes develop IDDM, so it seems that these genetic markers are associated with an increase in susceptibility for beta cell damage. Other 'trigger' factors must be important in the development of IDDM. Cellular immunological mechanisms are thought to be involved. Autoantibodies against islet cells are present in 80% of newly diagnosed diabetics and are likely to be the mechanism by which the islet cells have been destroyed. There is also an increased incidence of other autoimmune diseases in diabetic patients, particularly Hashimoto's thyroiditis and Addison's disease.

Environmental factors have been implicated as triggers, particularly viruses, e.g. mumps, Coxsackie B4 and B5, cytomegalovirus and rubella. Serological evidence of recent Coxsackie viral infections was found in one series.[3] The seasonal variation in presentation may be partly explained by the hypothesis that viruses are implicated in the increased insulin requirements leading to metabolic decompensation as well as the pathogenesis of IDDM, as viral infections are more common in the winter months.

The wide geographical variation in the incidence, particularly the increased incidence in north European countries, has led to the speculation that environmental factors, e.g. diet, may be important casual factors.

Presentation

Symptoms of IDDM are polyuria, polydypsia and thirst. The child may drink several litres of fluid per day and may develop nocturia. A previously dry child may start to wet the bed at night. Weight loss is common. Most parents or children will recognise there is a problem at this stage and the diagnosis should be made by the general practitioner testing the urine for glucose. The duration of symptoms at presentation is fairly short, three to four weeks on

average. However, when unrecognised, the child will go on to develop diabetic ketoacidosis (DKA) which is life-threatening. The child becomes severely dehydrated. Vomiting and abdominal pain are common and the child becomes drowsy and eventually comatose. The ketosis leads to disruption of the acid–base balance of the body with a marked metabolic acidosis causing rapid deep respiration (Kussmaul breathing). When untreated death would occur. Approximately 25% of children present with DKA.[4]

Diagnosis

The diagnosis is confirmed by finding a raised blood glucose level (normal range 4.5–7 mmol/l). At presentation blood glucose levels are often in the order of 20 mmol/l, but may be as high as 80 mmol/l. There will be glycosuria with or without ketonuria management.

In contrast to maturity-onset diabetes mellitus (MODM), juvenile-onset IDDM patients are dependent upon insulin for their treatment. The aims of management of a diabetic child are to maintain blood glucose concentrations as near as possible to those seen in a non-diabetic. There is increasing evidence that 'good control' in childhood may delay or diminish the frequency of complications in adult life.[5] However, it is vital to remember that the child must also have as normal a lifestyle as possible.

The basic principle of diabetic management involves balancing insulin dosage with dietary intake of carbohydrate and the patient's lifestyle, particularly in relation to growth activities and exercise.

Management of diabetic keto-acidosis (DKA)

The first most important step in treating DKA is to resuscitate and rehydrate the child using intravenous fluids (plasma if shocked, then normal (0.9%) saline, followed by dextrose/saline) aiming to correct the dehydration over 24 hours. It is important not to do this too rapidly as cerebral oedema may occur. Treatment with insulin is also required, and in DKA this is best given as a low-dose continuous in-

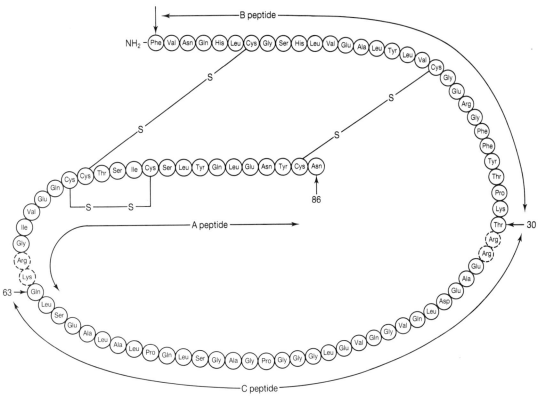

Figure 8.2   Structure of insulin molecule. Insulin is synthesised as a precursor molecule proinsulin, which undergoes splitting to form insulin and the peptide, C peptide. The insulin molecule consists of two amino acid chains linked together by disulphide bridges. C peptide can be measured in blood and is a useful marker of a patient's ability to produce insulin.

travenous infusion (0.05 units/kg/h). A drowsy vomiting child is in danger of aspirating and inhaling stomach contents so a naso-gastric tube is inserted and allowed to drain continuously. Oral fluids are withheld until vomiting has stopped and the child is alert. The child usually requires intensive treatment in this manner for 24–48 hours, and is then able to eat and drink and will be ready to be changed on to subcutaneous insulin treatment.

Insulin

Insulin can be extracted from ox or pig pancreas and purified by crystallisation and these were the main sources of insulin used to treat patients. Insulin is now made by recombinant DNA techniques using *E. coli* or semi-synthetically by enzymatic modification of porcine

insulin and has the same peptide sequence as naturally occurring human insulin.

All newly diagnosed patients and many established patients are now treated with this 'human' insulin. There are differences in the amino acid sequence of animal and human insulins, and many patients develop antibodies to beef or porcine insulins. Human insulin is less antigenic than the porcine or, in particular, the beef varieties, and this factor may be of importance.

Unfortunately insulin is inactivated in the gut by gastrointestinal enzymes and so is ineffective when taken orally. This means that it needs to be given by injection and is best given by the subcutaneous route, e.g. into the upper arm, thigh, abdominal wall or buttocks (Fig. 8.3).

The injections are given by means of a disposable syringe and needle, or via a pen device.

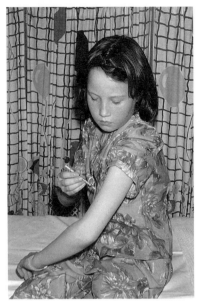

Figure 8.3 Nine year old girl administering her own insulin injection.

There are three main types of insulin which vary in the rapidity of their onset and in their duration of action.

1. The most rapid in onset is 'soluble' insulin, e.g. Actrapid, Velosulin, Humulin S. This has an onset of action within 30–60 minutes, has a peak action at 1–3 hours and a duration of action of 4–6 hours.
2. Intermediate-acting insulins such as isophane insulin, e.g. Insulatard, Humulin I, or insulin zinc suspensions, e.g. Monotard, have a more gradual onset 1–2 hours after injection, peak action at 4–12 hours and a duration of 12–24 hours.
3. Long-acting insulins with slow onset, e.g. Ultratard.

There are various insulin regimens in use. The majority of patients use a combination of the above insulins in order to try to maintain blood glucose levels within the accepted range for most of the day. Most children require twice daily insulin (before breakfast and before evening meal) in order to maintain optimal control although some very young diabetics may be managed on a once daily injection (pre-breakfast).

A typical regimen is to administer a combination of soluble and isophane insulins before breakfast and before the evening meal. The morning soluble insulin will have maximum effect over the course of the morning, the morning isophane over the afternoon, the pre-tea soluble working over the evening, and the pre-tea isophane during the night.

Other newer regimens involve the use of multiple injections often utilising a pen device. The pens carry cartridges of a single type of insulin. Small amounts of soluble insulin are given before each main meal, with a further injection of medium or long-acting insulin at bedtime (Fig. 8.4). This multiple injection regimen allows more flexibility in eating habits, and could lead to better control, but in many children the advantages are outweighed by having four injections each day. Newer pen cartridges are becoming available with mixtures of soluble and isophane insulins in a single cartridge.

The parents and the child, when old enough, need to be taught how to draw up insulins from the bottles, how to mix two types of insulin in the syringe if necessary, and how to administer the injection. An older child or adolescent will often prefer to do his or her own injections and this is to be encouraged. The majority of children will carry out their own injections by the age of 10–12 years, and some as young as 5 years will manage with supervision.

The injection sites must be constantly changed otherwise areas of fat hypertrophy or more rarely, lipodystrophy, will develop. Such lumpy areas are unsightly, but more importantly insulin absorption from such an area is erratic and may lead to marked swings in the blood glucose. Children like injecting into these areas as it is less uncomfortable, and so they need frequent encouragement to move their injection sites.

In non-diabetic individuals insulin output is dictated by blood sugar levels, but in the diabetic insulin levels are balanced by carbohydrate intake and exercise in order to maintain normoglycaemia.

Diet

Diabetic children do not require a special diet. However, they do need a healthy eating pattern. They have the same basic nutritional re-

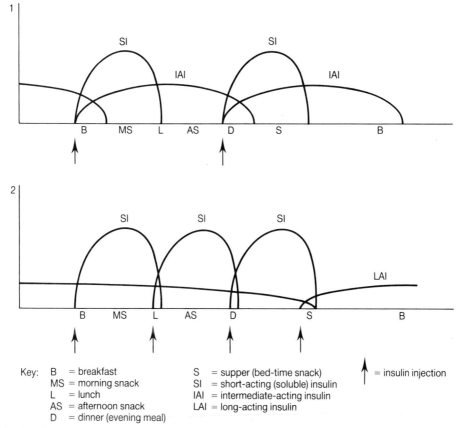

Key: B   = breakfast
       MS = morning snack
       L   = lunch
       AS = afternoon snack
       D   = dinner (evening meal)

       S   = supper (bed-time snack)
       SI   = short-acting (soluble) insulin
       IAI = intermediate-acting insulin
       LAI = long-acting insulin

       ↑ = insulin injection

Figure 8.4   Insulin regimens – timing of insulin action in relation to meals. 1, Two daily doses of short- and intermediate-acting insulins. 2, Insulin pen regimen: pre-meal short-acting insulin with long-acting insulin at bedtime.

quirements as their unaffected siblings and any dietary advice should be directed to establishing good eating habits for the whole family.

Diabetic children require carbohydrate as an energy source. In the past the proportion of energy eaten as carbohydrate was often restricted.[6] Regulation rather than restriction of carbohydrate intake is a better philosophy in this context.

Food may be divided into three categories:

1. Carbohydrate-free food, e.g. meat, cheese, most vegetables.
2. Highly refined carbohydrate-containing foods, e.g. processed foods and soft drinks, cakes, sweets, chocolate. These contain concentrated sucrose or glucose which is rapidly absorbed from the gut.
3. Other carbohydrate-containing foods in

which the carbohydrate is more steadily absorbed, e.g. whole foods with high fibre content such as dried beans, wholemeal bread and pasta.

Diabetic children may eat relatively unrestricted amounts of the first group of food, and should be discouraged from eating food from the second group. Ideally their daily carbohydrate intake should be based on foods from the third group although this may be difficult in practice. When a diet contains significant amounts of high fibre and whole foods, glucose absorption from the gut is more steady and leads to less marked rises in blood glucose following a meal. Blood glucose control is significantly better when unrefined foods are used in the diet compared to refined foods,[7] and carbohydrate diets based on high fibre whole foods, e.g. wholemeal bread, potatoes, beans, and fruit, can make a significant contribution to the blood glucose control of diabetic children. Guidance as to which foods are in which categories may be obtained from the BDA Food Values leaflet and book *Countdown*[8] which lists the carbohydrate content of manufactured foods.

The total amount of carbohydrate the child receives during 24 hours is most usefully based on an 'exchange' system. An exchange is a convenient measure of the carbohydrate content of foods.

One exchange = 10 g of carbohydrate.

As a guide to the daily carbohydrate intake the child receives 100 to 120 g + (10 g per year of age) per day.

Thus an eight year old child is likely to need, 100 to 120 + 80 g carbohydrate/day = 180 to 200 g/day, i.e. 18 to 20 'exchanges' per day.

The carbohydrate needs to be spaced at regular intervals throughout the day in order to balance the action of the insulin injections and to prevent unacceptably high glucose levels, i.e. hyperglycaemia, or low glucose levels, i.e. hypoglycaemia.

Most conveniently it is divided into three main meals and three snacks with a typical exchange pattern for an eight year old being:

Breakfast 3
Mid-morning snack 2
Lunch 4
Mid-afternoon snack 3
Evening meal 4
Supper 2
Bedtime snack

Typical exchange values would be:

⅓ pint fresh milk = 1 exchange.
Thick slice wholemeal toast (large) = 2 exchanges.
2 Weetabix = 2 exchanges.
1 small carton diet fruit yoghurt = 1 exchange.
Packet low fat crisps = 1½ exchanges.
1 medium apple = 1 exchange.

It is important to regularly review the child's carbohydrate intake taking into account the child's growth, particularly at the time of the pubertal growth spurt. An adequate calorie intake (with appropriate insulin) is necessary in order to provide a good growth spurt. After puberty carbohydrate intake can be decreased as necessary and this may be important to prevent obesity in the young diabetic adult.

Foods such as cheese or meat contain no carbohydrate and in carbohydrate terms they are 'free' foods. However, they may add significant calories to the diet due to their fat content so low fat varieties should be chosen.

Non-diabetic children will obtain approximately 45–50% of their total energy from carbohydrate. The aim should be to keep the diabetic child's carbohydrate intake at about the same level. When less carbohydrate is taken then more fat will be required for energy. The risk of disability or death from cardiovascular causes is increased in the diabetic so it is extremely important to avoid high fat diets, which have been implicated in the aetiology of cardiovascular disease. The healthy diet of a diabetic will provide adequate levels of protein, vitamins and minerals for these children. Just as in non-diabetic individuals, salt intake should not be excessive.

Home monitoring of glycaemic control

Diabetic children and their parents must have some means of knowing whether or not the balance of insulin and diet is correct and must not wait for symptoms of hypoglycaemia or hyperglycaemia to develop. The best way to know is to regularly measure the blood sugar level and this can be done easily at home using a fingerprick blood sample and reagent strips. The reagent strip changes colour according to the blood glucose level. These strips are simple to use and the colour change on the stick is matched to a chart either by eye or by one of the commercially available reflectance meters.

The children are recommended to check their blood glucose once a day, most usefully before meals and bed, and to vary the times of the test so that over the course of a week the blood sugar has been checked throughout the day and a profile of the results built up. A record of these should be kept so that it can be seen whether there are any particular times at which the blood sugar is running too high or too low.

The aim is to keep most of the tests in the region of 4–9 mmol/l. With this information the parents and child should be able to make sensible adjustments to the insulin or diet. The advent of home blood glucose monitoring has produced better control in both adults and children[9, 10] provided that the children and their families are educated and motivated to make appropriate insulin adjustments on the basis of the test results. In addition the child and parents need to be taught how to test the urine for ketones (using Ketostix – a reagent strip dipped in the urine), and this should be done when the blood sugar is >17 mmol/l or when the child is unwell, particularly if vomiting.

Glycosylated haemoglobin

Measurement of the blood glycosylated haemoglobin level (HbA1c) permits a longer-term assessment of blood glucose control. Glycosylated haemoglobin is the product of a non-reversible reaction between glucose and haemoglobin occurring in red cells in the peripheral circulation. The percentage of haemoglobin that is glycosylated is directly related to the blood glucose concentration that the red cells are exposed to during their life span. Thus a single measurement will reflect the average blood glucose concentration over the preceding 6–8 weeks. The glycosylated haemoglobin level from a non-diabetic individual is 4–6%; in a diabetic child levels of 8% reflect 'optimal' control, 8–10% reasonable control and levels >10–12% poor control. Thus information about longer-term control is obtained and this may point to chronic problems such as poor compliance with insulin regimen and/or diet, which may be due to underlying problems with basic knowledge or more commonly ongoing problems at home, school or in the psychological adjustment to the diabetes itself. A dietary record of perfect home glucose tests with a poor HbA1c result would suggest that the child is fabricating glucose results and the underlying reason needs to be sought. Combined with an accurate diary of blood glucose results, the HbA1c allows informed decisions about adjusting regimens to be made.

Hypoglycaemia

The complication of diabetes most feared by parents and children is hypoglycaemia, a 'hypo', when the blood sugar falls unacceptably low and usually causes symptoms. It is important that the child and parents recognise the symptoms and act appropriately, as without treatment the child may become unconscious and occasionally this may prove fatal. Hypoglycaemia occurs when there is an imbalance between the carbohydrate ingested and the insulin that has been taken, such that there is relatively too much insulin or too little carbohydrate. This will occur, for example, if the child takes the usual insulin but does not eat a full meal or snacks, or is very late in having the meal. A very energetic child should take extra carbohydrate in order to compensate for that used for the exercise and when they forget to do this they are likely to become hypoglycaemic.

Symptoms of hypoglycaemia usually occur when the blood glucose level falls below 2.5 mmol/l and these are partly due to the body's response to the low blood sugar. Counter-regulatory hormones such as adrenalin, glucagon, cortisol and growth hormone are produced, all of which have a role in raising the blood sugar level. In addition the adrenalin will produce tachycardia, sweating, pallor, dilated pupils – all of which are important signs of hypoglycaemia. When the blood sugar level is low, cerebral function becomes altered and manifests itself most commonly as drowsiness, confusion, aggression or weepiness. In addition some children will develop a grand mal convulsion during severe hypoglycaemia and this is extremely frightening for the parents. Children report feeling tremulous, sweaty or experiencing muscle jerks and with bizarre feelings and experiences during an episode. Only approximately half of children studied can confidently recognise a 'hypo',[11] thus placing a significant burden on carers to be alert to the possibility. About 10% of 'hypos' occur at night, causing worry to many parents. Such 'hypos' may be prevented if a late evening blood glucose level is checked, particularly after a very active day, and additional carbohydrate eaten before bed when the test is unacceptably low.

Severe symptomatic hypoglycaemia (defined as help needed from another person) occurs relatively frequently – almost half of the child diabetic population will experience this at some time,[12] with loss of consciousness or convulsions occurring in about 1 in 15 each year.[13] Mild occasional hypoglycaemia may be one of the prices to be paid for the achievement of good metabolic control but severe repeated hypoglycaemia should be prevented wherever possible. Brain growth is most rapid in children under five years of age and repeated hypoglycaemia in very young children may have deleterious effects on brain growth and function.

If the child (or parent) suspect hypoglycaemia rapidly acting carbohydrate should be immediately given: three glucose tablets, e.g. Dextrosol, or 50 ml glucose drink, 100 ml (not diet) Coca-Cola = 10 g carbohydrate, or glucose gel to be applied to the buccal mucosa (Hypostop). This should be repeated until the child feels better and then a snack of longer acting carbohydrate should be given. All diabetic children should carry glucose tablets in case of such an event. If the child is too drowsy to eat or drink, is unconscious or convulsing, give an injection of glucagon (1 mg intramuscularly or subcutaneously). This will cause breakdown of glycogen, so elevating the blood sugar. Blood glucose levels will rise within 10 minutes of giving glucagon[14] and once the child is conscious and able to drink further carbohydrate should be given by mouth. If there is no response to the glucagon, the child should be seen by a medical practitioner as an emergency (GP or hospital) as he or she will require intravenous dextrose. All families should have glucagon available for use at home, and should be instructed in its administration. Once recovered, precipitating events should be analysed to try to prevent recurrence. The commonest identifiable reason is unexpected or unexpectedly vigorous physical activity but disrupted eating habits or errors in insulin dosage are also important causes.

All diabetics should wear an identity SOS talisman alerting strangers to the possibility that they may be hypoglycaemic if they are found confused or unconscious.

Exercise

Children vary widely in the amounts of exercise they undertake, and indeed each individual child varies from day to day. Exercise is to be encouraged as in non-diabetic children. Vigorous exercise will increase the energy expenditure of the child who should be given extra carbohydrate prior to the exercise to compensate for this. One to two exchanges should be given prior to organised games activities or swimming and this should prevent hypoglycaemia during the activity. For very strenuous activities, e.g. hill walking, insulin requirements will decrease significantly (by a third to a half) and extra exchanges should be consumed at meal and snack times. The diabetic child should be encouraged to take part in all activities although a responsible adult should be present for swimming.

Complications of IDDM

After the isolation of insulin in 1922 it was hoped that young people developing diabetes would be able to have a full, normal life. However, in the 1940s it was becoming apparent that their life expectation was lowered and their quality of life impaired by the development of complications. The diagnosis of IDDM in a child has considerable implications for the long-term health of the individual, coupled with a poor prognosis. In 1978 one study[15] showed that within 40 years of diagnosis 60% were dead – 34% dying of renal failure or myocardial infarction, 30% were blind or severely visually handicapped, and 12% had gangrene or had lower limb amputations. Life expectancy was only 29 years. Many of these patients had their diabetes diagnosed in the early days of therapy and the care of diabetics has greatly advanced since then. However, complications in early adult life are a very real threat for these young patients and an understanding of their pathogenesis is necessary in order to try to prevent them.

Vascular complications

Vascular complications account for 75% of diabetic deaths. They may involve large and/or small blood vessels.

Large vessel disease

Atheromatous changes in large vessels are widespread and are earlier in onset than in non-diabetics. Ischaemic heart disease (angina or myocardial infarction) is five times more common in middle-aged diabetics than in the general population. Occlusion of large blood vessels with atheroma is common and may lead to gangrene of the feet.

Small vessel disease

In diabetics there is thickening of the basement membrane of the capillaries together with proliferation of the capillary endothelium, producing diabetic microangiopathy. This microangiopathy has wide-ranging effects, particularly on the kidney and eye (see below) but also on skin circulation especially the feet and may lead to gangrene with wedge-shaped infarcts.

There does appear to be a relationship between poor diabetic control and the development of microvascular complications[5] and good control should be encouraged to try to decrease the incidence of these complications.

Renal complications

Renal disease accounts for 30% of diabetic deaths under the age of 40 years.[15] The main pathological changes are glomerular lesions with thickening of the glomerular basement membrane and glomerular sclerosis which may be diffuse (70%) or focal (Kimmelstihl–Wilson lesions which are pathognomonic of diabetes). The main feature of diabetic nephropathy is the insidious development of proteinuria which may progress to nephrotic syndrome. Once proteinuria is established a gradual decline in renal function leads to chronic renal failure and hypertension. There is considerable interest in detecting proteinuria early – before it becomes detectable with routine laboratory tests or urinary dipstick. This 'microalbuminuria' seems to be an early predictor of diabetic nephropathy.[16] Diabetic children and adolescents have significantly higher albumin excretion rates compared to healthy matched controls, with 20% of children having levels exceeding the upper range of the controls and 5% of adolescents having levels above the levels reported to be predictive of diabetic nephropathy in adults.[17] Microalbuminuria in the at risk range is rare before puberty and is not due simply to the length of time the child has had diabetes. Thus it has

been postulated that screening for microalbuminuria should be performed in all diabetics over the age of 12 years as a marker for incipient diabetic nephropathy. However, detecting microalbuminuria does not necessarily prevent the development of nephropathy. Optimising diabetic control with intensive insulin regimens and early treatment of hypertension may reverse microalbuminuria and may reduce the risk of progression into overt nephropathy, but it is too early to know yet what effects such measures will have on the ultimate development of severe renal disease. Established chronic renal failure may need to be managed by dialysis or by transplantation.

Eye complications

Complications affecting the eyes occur in 20% of diabetics. Blindness is preventable. To detect changes the eye must be examined with the pupils dilated. The retina is affected by two main types of pathological changes.

1. *Background retinopathy* is due to increased capillary permeability and is characterised by haemorrhages and microaneurysms (seen as bulges in the capillary wall), which leak plasma to produce hard exudates. Background retinopathy is common but has surprisingly little effect on vision.

2. *Proliferative retinopathy* is due to capillary non-perfusion and usually occurs 15–20 years after the onset of IDDM. New vessel formation occurs chiefly near the optic disc, with venous irregularity, cluster haemorrhages and cotton wool spots (small deep retinal infarcts). Haemorrhage may occur in the vitreous fluid of the eye causing sudden blindness, followed by fibrosis with sudden retinal detachment and glaucoma. Once proliferative retinopathy occurs it will progress to blindness within five years in 50% unless treated. Argon laser therapy is effective in stopping progression of new vessel formation.

In addition diabetics are more susceptible to the development of cataracts (causing 20% of diabetic blindness) which occur at an earlier age than in non–diabetics.

Duration of diabetes seems to be important in the development of retinopathy and those diabetics with poor glycaemic control have a higher incidence of eye complications.[18] Genetic factors may increase the risk of development of retinopathy. The occurrence of eye complications prior to puberty is rare. It is vital that all diabetics have their eyes checked regularly from puberty onwards, and annual eye examinations with dilation of the pupils is recommended. Diagnosis and treatment of early changes may prevent visual handicap.

Neurological complications

Neurological complications develop in adult life in approximately 30% of diabetics. The commonest neurological complication is peripheral neuropathy which is predominantly sensory and presents as numbness, paraesthesia and loss of pain sensation. This is important as patients may not recognise that gangrenous changes are imminent as they will not develop the warning symptoms of pain. Single nerve palsies are less common but occur as a result of occlusion of the nutrient artery to the nerve – most often the third cranial nerve, ulnar nerve or lateral popliteal nerve. The autonomic nervous system may become affected and may lead to impotence in the male, nocturnal diarrhoea and postural hypotension. The autonomic nervous system is responsible for producing many of the warning symptoms of hypoglycaemia (pallor, sweating and tachycardia), and so patients with autonomic neuropathy are at risk of unexpected hypoglycaemic episodes.

Autoimmune thyroid disease

Children with IDDM have an increased incidence of auto-immune thyroid disease, particularly Hashimoto's thyroiditis, which most commonly manifests itself as hypothyroidism. Five per cent of diabetic children and young adults develop hypothyroidism.[19] Its onset is insidious and is easily missed, before poor growth, deteriorating school performance, lack of energy and excess weight gain become apparent. It is easily screened for with a measurement of plasma thyroid stimulating hormone (TSH), on a fingerprick sample, and the test should be performed yearly. Hypothyroidism is treated with a once-daily dose of oral thyroxine.

Prevention of complications

Complications in pre-pubertal children are extremely rare and seem to be related to very poor glycaemic control.[20] There is likely to be a connection between puberty, sex hormones and the development of microvascular disease. At present the only way to decrease the incidence of complications is by optimising diabetic control from the time of presentation. The devastating effects of some complications may be minimised when they are detected early, e.g. laser therapy for proliferative retinopathy, and all children should have annual blood pressure measurements, urine screening for infection and proteinuria, examination of skin state and inspection of feet, plasma TSH measurement, and from puberty onwards an annual eye examination.

Psychological effects

Not surprisingly most parents are devastated when their child is diagnosed as having diabetes, and will go through a period of 'bereavement' for loss of their healthy child: this will include appropriate emotions of anger, guilt and fear. The parents themselves may feel very isolated. The child too has to come to terms with injections and blood testing which are going to be part of the daily routine for the rest of their lives. Diabetic children will see themselves as 'different' to their friends, and will know they have to live their life with a new set of rules. They may be subject to teasing by their peer group. The child and the parents require considerable support not only around the time of diagnosis but continuing throughout childhood and into adult life. Children with any chronic physical problem are known to have an increased risk of psychiatric disorder. Up to 30% of diabetic children aged 9–18 years are described by their parents as having appreciable emotional or behavioural difficulties,[21] with 12% of the children considering themselves depressed. It is not only the poorly controlled diabetic children that have emotional problems and it may well be very stressful psychologically to constantly achieve good metabolic control.

Emotional and behavioural problems are

much more common at adolescence. Adolescents are by nature, rebellious individuals who are self-assertive and live 'for today', and it is unrealistic not to expect them to rebel against the rules that diabetes imposes upon them. Parents may find it more difficult to let go of their diabetic teenager and allow them to take full responsibility for their life and management of diabetes. The adolescents themselves may have very real, but probably unexpressed, fears, for example, of complications or of becoming hypoglycaemic whilst living alone. With understanding and support appropriate to their needs at differing ages and stages of development, the majority of diabetic children will mature into adults who are competent at looking after their condition and who can lead full lives.

Support

Diabetes is a demanding condition both for the child and for the family. It is a lifelong illness which demands regular uncomfortable treatment if the child is to keep well, and there is always the threat of complications. Monitoring of the condition is uncomfortable and a nuisance, and parents have to feel confident enough to make decisions based on the results of the tests they perform. Dietary restraints are imposed, both in content of the food eaten and the timing of when it is eaten. Even in the best-adjusted families, diabetes will impose some stresses on family life, including the parents and non-diabetic siblings.

A team approach is necessary in order to provide the best service for the diabetic child both in hospital and in the community. The majority of newly diagnosed diabetic children are admitted to hospital where they will meet not only the paediatrician, but also nursing staff and dietitians, who teach the basics of diabetic care. In some areas (notably Leicester) there is an extensive community-based system allowing newly diagnosed children (providing they are not keto-acidotic) to be managed at home with frequent visits by the above professionals. Whichever approach is taken, adequate time for explanation of the condition and for the teaching of both parents and child is vital as the foundations for the child's future health and well-being are being set.

Once the child is discharged from hospital the parents must not feel isolated and access to help and information should be available at all times. A community diabetic liaison nurse is very important as she will be able to visit the family at home, as frequently as necessary, and will provide not only practical but also emotional help. Contact with the paediatrician at the hospital should be encouraged whenever the parents are concerned and free hospital access for advice will prevent unnecessary hospital admissions. Many parents will turn to their general practitioner for help and advice, but most family doctors will have little experience of childhood diabetes and may be reluctant to give practical advice, although their knowledge of the family dynamics can contribute greatly to the management of the child. A child spends a large proportion of his time at school or nursery and it is important that the teachers understand enough about diabetes to feel happy having the child in their class. They particularly need to know how to manage hypoglycaemia. A child with diabetes should be able to take part in all school activities. The diabetic liaison nurse has an important educational role in schools and nurseries.

The family should be seen regularly; ideally children should be seen in a specialised children's diabetic clinic, or by a paediatrician with an interest in childhood diabetes.[22, 23] Initially these visits are frequent, but if all is well every three months should be sufficient. Opportunities should be available for the family to meet the dietitian, liaison nurses, dental hygienist and podiatrist whilst at the clinic. In many families who are experiencing significant emotional problems, the help of a child and family psychiatrist can be invaluable. Transfer of the child's care to an adult physician should occur when the child is physically and emotionally 'adult' enough to cope with an adult clinic. In practice this may range from 13 to 20 years! Whenever possible, joint clinics with the adult physician or some form of liaison will ease the change from paediatric to adult clinic and clinics designed specifically for adolescents, with their particular needs and difficulties, may be of benefit.

Information about financial allowances may be important and the family may be entitled to the daytime Attendance Allowance when the child is 2–12 years of age although this is not mandatory. Visits to hospital can be expensive and families may receive support from the Department of Social Security for these when their income is low. Advice from an interested social worker can be very helpful.

The family should be encouraged to join the British Diabetic Association (BDA) and can receive both information and support from this society. The BDA run children's holidays each year which are an ideal opportunity for the child to develop some independence away from home.

Support for the diabetic child and his family must have a team approach and must be well organised if the child is to obtain the maximum benefit.[23]

Podiatric management

The whole concept of the podiatric management of the young diabetic concerns the prevention of foot problems which result in skin manifestations of overload, friction and infection. Initially foot health education is the most important aspect in the management of the paediatric diabetic who presents with an asymptomatic foot. Maximum prophylactic footcare by the patient and by the podiatrist is essential in order to reduce the occurrence of minor foot problems which may ultimately develop into major problems.

Prevention of potential problems, by early diagnosis and management, is an integral part of the examination process. Presentation of any problem, no matter how minor it may appear, must be dealt with diligently.

Podiatric treatment of the diabetic patient is very much an interdisciplinary process with close liaison between the podiatrist, paediatrician/diabetologist, general practitioner, diabetic liaison sister and surgical shoemaker.

The podiatrist should be very aware of the complexities of the patient's condition. Consultations and discussions should take place regularly with the team with regard to treatment strategies since this is very relevant in the podiatric management of ulceration or when carrying out nail surgery.

Health education

It has been estimated that 20% of all diabetic hospital admissions are due to foot problems[24] and that these problems are often caused by a lack of awareness of preventative measures. It is the clinical experience of many podiatrists that the foot health education received by diabetic patients when they are first diagnosed is not comprehensive.

In most children the feet will be non-problematic but nevertheless foot health education must begin immediately. The degree of education will be dependent upon the age of the child at his/her first visit to the podiatrist. In certain cases it may well be education of the parent alone but there must be integration between the practitioner, child and parent.

Foot health education of the diabetic child is the same initially as that of the non-diabetic child but such education should be developed with the older child in order to relate to his/her condition. The methods of foot health education are discussed in the appropriate chapter and may be developed to suit the young diabetic.

Depending upon the home environment, levels of knowledge and skills of the patient or parent, basic first aid measures for minor cuts, blisters or fissures could be carried out by the patient or parent. A printed leaflet explaining the procedures to be followed should be provided by the podiatrist.

Empathy is critical to the podiatrist's relationship with the patient. The patient should not be admonished for not adhering to all the advice given and the practitioner should not show impatience but should try to motivate his patient towards good foot care.

Diabetic complications in the foot

Many of the complications of diabetes are manifested in the lower limb and may predispose to the development of foot lesions. In the young diabetic these complications are extremely rare before the age of puberty. The causes of foot problems are ischaemia, neuropathy, infection and trauma.

Vascular disease

In diabetes the progression of atherosclerosis is more rapid and more widespread distally in the lower limb than in the general population and severe vascular occlusion may occur at a relatively young age. In the lower limb the atherosclerosis is diffuse and in diabetics the more distal parts of the profunda femoris, popliteal and tibial arteries are more commonly affected than in non-diabetics. This carries a serious threat to the limb when the disease is severe due to the difficulties of distal reconstructive arterial surgery.

In long-standing diabetics calcification of the tunica media is a common feature. Although this may not have any great effect on the blood supply to the lower limb it must be borne in mind when blood pressure readings are being taken, as measurements will be less accurate due to lack of compression in the wall of the artery.

Microvascular disease also affects the lower limb and includes proliferative changes in arterioles and arteries and also thickening of the capillary basement membranes. In the lower limb such changes have been seen in skin, nerve and muscle tissue. Microvascular disease may be responsible for small areas of necrosis in the foot but it is unlikely to be responsible for larger ulcerated or gangrenous patches.

Such vascular changes result in the lower limb being at risk from ischaemia, ulceration, gangrene, rampant infection and possible loss of limb.

Neuropathy

Peripheral neuropathy in the diabetic patient is highly variable. There is an increasing prevalence and incidence of diabetic neuropathy related to the duration of the diabetes. The prevalence of neuropathy appears to be related to diabetic control levels. In poor control there is more rapid deterioration. Neuropathy is one of the major causes of foot lesions in diabetics.

In children and adolescent patients with IDDM, studies have shown deterioration in motor, sensory (peripheral) and autonomic function.[25-28] Microvascular complications were also noted.

In diabetic children polyneuropathy is rarely mentioned although it is stressed as a frequent complication of diabetes mellitus in adults. Although symptomatic neuropathy is rare in diabetic children several studies have reported decreased nerve conduction velocities. A sharp increase in the prevalence of reduced conduction velocities may be found in the mid-teens but there is also evidence of a reduction in younger children.[29]

The most common form of diabetic neuropathy is sensory impairment – a distal, symmetrical polyneuropathy which is predominantly sensory. This sensory impairment may be patchy but it usually follows a stocking and glove distribution and is characterised by loss of ankle reflexes and vibration sense. Perception of light touch, sharp and blunt discrimination, temperature and pain may be diminished or absent. This type of neuropathy is slowly progressive and makes the foot very susceptible to injury due to the patient's inability to perceive pain. Initially the patient will be unaware that sensory changes are taking place and may complain of a variety of symptoms ranging from a dull ache, burning sensation, tingling, coldness or numbness to pain initially starting in the toes and forefoot.

Motor involvement has important effects on foot function mainly in the small intrinsic muscles of the foot particularly with extensor digitorum brevis, the interossei and the lumbrical muscles. This affects the anti-buckling mechanism related to the long flexors and extensors and results in toe deformities and in particular, claw toes. Eventually joint degeneration and soft tissue contractures will occur and the joints will become fixed. This fixation predisposes to the formation of callus and possible ulceration related to pressure from footwear. In the diabetic patient this may be associated with sensory neuropathy and severe tissue damage is probable.

Autonomic neuropathy usually occurs hand in hand with somatic neuropathy but it is uncommon to find autonomic neuropathy in the absence of somatic neuropathy. Such neuropathy affects the vasoconstrictor nerve fibres and sudomotor nerve fibres and thus peripheral circulation and thermoregulation to the lower limb are affected. There are also abnormalities in sweating.

These deficiencies are manifested by a loss of sympathetic tone to the peripheral vessels, abnormal reactions to temperature changes, i.e. increased and prolonged vasoconstriction to cold which may lead to local hypoxia of superficial tissues, venous shunting, increased venous capillary pressure and oedema. There is also a failure in vasodilation in response to injury and this may lead to reduced healing. Production of sweat in the lower limb is reduced (upper body is increased) leading to dry devitalised skin, loss of elasticity with the increased risk of skin fissures and possible changes in the pH of the skin with reduced resistance to infection.

Major nerve lesion (mononeuritis)

The nerve most commonly involved in the lower limb is the common peroneal. Onset is usually gradual. Presenting symptoms are usually pain and weakness (asymmetrical), but there is little sensory loss. There is no association with this neuropathy and somatic or autonomic neuropathy. Prior to the onset of the symptoms diabetic control is often found to have been poor. Usually the symptoms remit spontaneously within a period of six to eight months when there is good control of the diabetic state.

Infection and trauma

The commonest site for infection in diabetics is in the foot and it is one of the most difficult problems to deal with in podiatric practice. Despite good foot health education and vigilance by the patient and podiatrist infection may develop.

Prevention of infection is of the utmost importance since healing will be retarded and the infection may well spread. This is particularly relevant when the blood supply is reduced. The vascular supply may be adequate to maintain the viability of the tissues when the skin is intact but may be insufficient to allow healing of small wounds. When neuropathy is present the patient may have been unaware of a wound and may have continued to walk on it thus allowing infection to develop and causing further spread of the lesion.

Diabetics have an increased susceptibility and a decreased resistance to infection. This may be due to abnormal cellular and humoral responses to inflammation, particularly when there is impairment of the blood supply, autonomic neuropathy and a decrease in the efficiency of the repair process.

The predisposing factor for infection is primarily trauma combined with ischaemia and neuropathy. Trauma should be minimised as much as possible. The role of the podiatrist is to prevent the development of major lesions. This is brought about by good foot health education, by treatment of nail and skin problems which may damage the integrity of the skin and by prevention of foot deformities which will lead to the development of pressure areas within the foot and ultimately to the formation of these lesions.

Podiatric assessment of the young diabetic

The assessments which the podiatrist is able to undertake will range from the very basic foot examination with the child seated on the parent's lap, to extensive vascular, neural and biomechanical assessment in the older child. Such examinations should be introduced gradually as the child becomes older, is able to communicate more rationally with the practitioner, and has had time to build up a rapport with the podiatrist. Intellectual ability should also be considered. Children under the age of eight are unsuited to prolonged sensory testing. The practitioner must use his experience and common sense in order to determine the suitability of the patient to undergo various degrees of assessment.

The results of the tests should always be accurately recorded, even when the vascular and nerve supply is 'normal'. There should be a set pattern for the examination procedures and an adequate case treatment record card which allows for extensive assessment records, either yearly or half yearly depending upon the results of the tests; e.g. when neuropathy is present then six monthly assessments are recommended. There should also be provision for treatment plans, treatments initiated, biomechanical assessments and for progress reports. A section for medical history is imperative and should constantly be updated. When the podiatrist is employed within a hospital department records should be included within the patient's folder.

The following are tests which should be carried out by the podiatrist certainly no later than the early teens and preferably earlier.

Vascular assessment of the lower limb

The following physical tests are mandatory:

1. *The pulses*, e.g. popliteal, anterior and posterior tibial and dorsalis pedis, must be assessed.
2. *Temperature* of the feet related to the ambient temperature, and temperature gradient must be noted.
3. Assessment of the *colour* of the feet and legs for variations from the normal.
4. Assessment of *capillary refill* time.
5. *Elevation dependency test*.
6. *Venous filling* time.
7. Presence or absence of *pain*, i.e. intermittent claudication or rest pain. Differentiation must be made between vascular and neurological pain.
8. Presence or absence of *oedema*.

Such standard physical examinations may be carried out by the podiatrist irrespective of the clinical setting. Specialised equipment may also be used to assess vascular competence but such equipment is frequently only available in specialised clinics or in hospital departments. Visual and physical examination of the patient is extremely important but when diagnostic equipment is available it should be used in conjunction with the above tests allowing quantitative measurements to be obtained.

One difficulty involved in using specialist equipment is that it may frighten young patients. It is also time consuming to use and it is possible that the clinician may rely too heavily on technology and may overlook obvious clinical signs.

Further specialised tests include the following.

Ankle systolic blood pressure may be obtained by using a Doppler flow probe and a blood pressure cuff placed just above the ankle. Small cuffs are available for the digits.

Diabetic patients have a higher pressure gradient between the toe and the ankle than non-diabetics. The pressure should be recorded from the posterior tibial and the dorsalis pedis arteries. Such pressures are recorded in absolute terms and as the ratio of the ankle/brachial pressure (pressure index; PI). In normal subjects the PI is >0.9. These pressures are a valuable guide to the viability of the blood supply to the foot and provide an estimation of healing of ulcers. The practitioner must always be aware of falsely high ankle pressure measurements which result from calcification of the vessel wall. This should be suspected when the ankle/brachial index is greater than 1.3.

Plethysmography is a non-invasive technique which works on the strain gauge principle and records limb segment volume changes with each cardiac cycle. It gives a printed read-out from which the practitioner can ascertain whether there is a normal pulse contour, a restricted pulse contour, a mildly, moderately or severely obstructive contour or absent pulsations. This equipment has good diagnostic potential. Photoplethysmography is also available.

Thermography provides a pictorial representation of the surface temperature of the foot and of the lower limb and will demonstrate hot or cold spots in the foot. It is a useful tool to investigate the many facets of peripheral vascular disease and is painless, safe and non-invasive. Low skin temperatures are usually indicative of vascular insufficiency but higher local temperatures indicate a state of inflammation which may be due to underlying infection, joint disease or malignant melanoma. A photographic system is supplied which allows instant recording of the thermograph for diagnostic and documentation purposes.

Neurological assessment of the lower limb

Physical examination of the child may be very difficult depending upon his concentration span. Therefore examinations must be carried out as quickly and as efficiently as possible and only when the child is considered capable of cooperation. Since sensory function has been shown to be disturbed early in the course of diabetic neuropathy large fibre modalities, i.e. vibration and proprioception, should be the first to be tested. These may be abnormal but may be asymptomatic in the absence of other signs of neuropathy.

Vibration may be tested with a tuning fork, but this has many disadvantages and whenever possible a biothesiometer should be used. This system will produce quantitative measurements. Vibratory sensation should be recorded on the dorsum of the interphalangeal joint of the first toe, on the medial aspect of the first metatarsophalangeal joint (MPJ) and on the malleoli.

Proprioception should be tested at the first MPJ and at the ankle. A Romberg test should be carried out in order to detect any early sensory ataxia and the gait should also be observed.

Small fibre function, i.e. light touch, sharp and blunt discrimination (superficial pain), deep pain and temperature, is then determined.

Light touch is easily assessed with a cotton wool ball ensuring that the quality of touch by the operator does not vary. This test and the following should be carried out in a set pattern, working distally to proximally and medially to laterally. Ideally all results should be clearly recorded on a foot chart with the dermatomes clearly mapped.

Sharp and blunt sensation testing should be carried out with a Neurotip. This should be done with care in order to eliminate dermal involvement.

Deep pain threshold is determined by squeezing the tendo Achillis just proximal to its insertion.

Temperature sensation may be tested by means of two test tubes, one containing cold water and one hot.

These tests are difficult to standardise and are qualitative in nature. Both motor and sensory nerve conduction velocity equipment is available for testing but examination is painful even when surface electrodes are used thus making this form of testing unsuitable for children. Temperature discrimination may be assessed in children by using two thermo-stimulators operating on the Peltier principle where the smallest temperature difference that the patient may be aware of is determined.

Autonomic neuropathy should be assessed by examination of the skin. Excessive dryness in a child or adolescent is very unusual unless there is a coexisting eczema or juvenile plantar dermatosis. Dryness in the lower extremity in the diabetic adolescent (excluding other skin conditions) is likely to indicate an absence of sweating related to diabetic neuropathy.

Decreased areas of sweating may be studied by the use of starch–iodine powder which will change colour when in contact with sweat. Thermography may also be used in the diagnosis of autonomic function.

Motor function is determined by appropriate tests for muscle weakness. The development of clawing of the lesser toes may be an indication, but the practitioner should bear in mind other factors such as restrictive footwear or biomechanical abnormalities which may predispose to this condition.

Biomechanical assessment of the lower limb

This is an essential part of the podiatrist's examination procedure. Full biomechanical assessment cannot be carried out in the young child and therefore techniques should be varied according to age. This type of examination is necessary in order to prevent or to reduce deformities developing which will lead to areas of friction or pressure. Ultimately such areas may be the site of ulceration or gangrene in later life.

Studies have shown that when an ulcer was present on the plantar aspect of the foot that it corresponded to an area which carried a high load. When available, equipment should be used to determine high load areas before complications have become established. Steps may then be taken, by the provision of a suitable orthosis or by adaptation of footwear, to redistribute load on the foot.

When sophisticated equipment is not available then the *Harris and Beath* mat is a very simple method of interpreting pressures. The mat may be used to obtain a simple footprint (either in the static or dynamic mode) and the

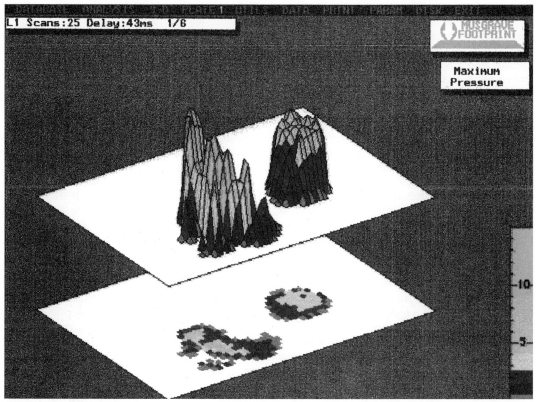

Figure 8.5 Musgrave Gait Analysis system – diagram of loading of the foot. The original colour diagram has been reproduced in black and white.

shape of the contact area, and provides a visual interpretation of low and high pressure areas.

The *Musgrave Force Plate* is a fully computerised gait analysis system and consists of 2048 transducers housed within a footplate which can measure static and dynamic pressures and provides excellent quantitative records of loading of the foot. It can identify total load and gives a colour related to pressure diagram of the loading of the foot. The data may be displayed sequentially and will therefore show function to a certain extent (Fig. 8.5).

The *Penny and Giles electro-goniometer* is portable, easy to use and does not interfere with joint function. It is comfortable for the patient and provides accurate and rapid measurements of limb movement which may be displayed on a digital indicator or recorded on a compact data recorder. This piece of equipment will measure extension and flexion with abduction and adduction. The advantage of the electro-goniometer is that it may be used to measure angles during the gait cycle and it may also be used in conjunction with a force plate. The main joints of the foot where angles can be easily measured with this instrument are the ankle and the first MPJ. The degree of range of motion may then be related to foot function and linked to areas of high pressure.

The *Shockmeter* measures shock loading on the foot. It quantifies impact at heel strike by measuring acceleration of the ankle during walking or running. By measuring the frequency spectrum of the measured acceleration it is possible to define a shock factor. Clinically it may be used for assessing the shock produced by the patient during the gait cycle and thus be related to any limitation in joint movement. The shockmeter may also be used to quantify the shock absorbing capacity of different sole structures in footwear or simply to examine the shock loading of various materials placed in the shoe which are used in the manufacture of orthoses.

Quantitative equipment may be used in order to verify the clinician's observations and to obtain objective, quantitative information. Improvements in the patient's gait may also be scientifically evaluated and related to various treatment regimes.

The prevention of deformities is of paramount importance in the young diabetic. When existing deformity can be arrested or corrected trauma will be minimised on high pressure areas and thus too the potential for development into ulcerative or gangrenous patches. The main deformities to be found in the forefoot of the young diabetic which are correctable are lesser toe and hallux deformities, and in the hindfoot, pronation, for whatever reason.

It may be difficult to explain to both parents and children the need for corrective and preventative measures in a foot which is asymptomatic. When toe deformities are obvious there is no problem but conditions such as forefoot varus are not obvious and thus explanation and advice are extremely important before preventative measures are initiated.

Prevention of cross infection

All possible measures should be taken in order to prevent the spread of infection. Although this is carried out routinely in any treatment area or during any treatment, when treating high risk patients such as diabetics extra precautions are always essential.

The operator's and patient's chairs should be thoroughly swabbed prior to the commencement of treatment. The use of prepacked sterile paper towels for the leg rests is advisable when the patient presents with open lesions, otherwise non-sterile paper towels are satisfactory.

Preparation of the operator's hands prior to treatment is of major importance in reducing cross infection and several surgical scrubs are available for this purpose. Alternatively the operator may wear disposable surgical gloves provided they are removed from the box just prior to use. Studies have shown such gloves to have a lower count of pathogens than the skin of the hands. When the patient has any infected lesion, fungal, viral or bacterial gloves should be worn in order to prevent cross infection from the patient to operator.

The skin of the patient's feet should be thoroughly swabbed in order to reduce the bacterial population. A 1% aqueous solution of chlorhexidine gluconate is suitable for this purpose provided that there are no open areas present. Care must be taken when using any dilute solution of antiseptic preparation as prolonged storage will lead to its contamination. *Pseudomonas* has been found in seven day old skin swabbing solutions. When this bacteria is introduced to an open area, even a small crack in the skin, it can have disastrous consequences particularly when dealing with patients who have a lowered resistance to fighting infection. On any open area a sterile solution should be used for cleansing. When an open wound has to be cleansed on a regular basis, frequent use of an antiseptic could alter the normal skin commensal population, could contribute to bacterial resistance, and might lead to overgrowth of more virulent organisms such as the *Pseudomonas* species. In this event cleansing of the wound should be by mechanical means using sterile gauze and a sterile solution of sodium chloride, 0.9% w/v. This solution is not antiseptic but is ideal for irrigation of ulcers as it is non-toxic and non-irritant. It is available as Normasol in 25 ml and 100 ml sachets.

Removal of soiled dressings and swabbing of the feet should be carried out by means of disposable forceps and a non-touch technique. Similarly, if the operator touches any contaminated material during treatment then the gloves should be replaced (if dealing with an open lesion), or hand or gloves rewashed in an antibacterial skin cleanser if carrying out routine treatment.

Sterilisation of instruments must be by autoclave. Chemical sterilisation is not acceptable. Instruments must be thoroughly cleansed prior to their sterilisation in order to remove organic material and to reduce the number of bacteria. The operator must wear gloves when handling dirty instruments in this manner. Ultrasonic cleansers are available for this purpose and are a worthwhile investment.

Prepacked single low adherent sterile dressings are essential in the treatment of ulceration and soiled dressings and debris should be kept well away from the operating area.

The most common skin problems found on the foot in the diabetic child are similar to those found in the non-diabetic population of the same age group. These common foot problems do not normally present any difficulties in their treatment, unlike in the long-term adult diabetic patient. However, a more rigorous treatment regime and follow-up is carried out in order to prevent possible complications which may arise due to the diabetic state.

Fungal infections

The most common site for fungal infection is in the toe webs with possible spread to the dorsum of the foot. It is often associated with hyperidrosis. Onychomycosis is infrequently encountered in the younger child but its prevalence increases with age.

More diabetics than non-diabetics present for treatment of fungal infections but this is not a true indication that diabetics are more at risk from fungal infections but more that they seek advice for foot problems rather than self-diagnosis and by initiating home treatments. Clinically there appears to be no significant difference in the prevalence of fungal infections relating to dermatophytes, between diabetics and the general population.

However, *Candida albicans* is more prevalent in diabetics than non-diabetics. High glucose concentrations appear to favour skin growth of *Candida*. *Candida albicans* affects skin, particularly in the interdigital spaces, and nails especially at the base of the nail plate under the eponychium. When such an infection affects the latter site, treatment may be protracted due to its inaccessibility to topical applications of fungal preparations.

The following are examples of fungi which may produce fungal infections in the foot:

Microsporum canis, cookei and *ferrugineum*   onychomycosis

Microsporum gypseum   tinea pedis

Trichophyton ajelloi, gourvilii, kuryangi megninii and *veruccosum*   onychomycosis

Trichophyton mentagrophytes, rubrum, interdigitale and *tonsurans*   onychomycosis and tinea pedis

Epidermophyton floccosum   onychomycosis and tinea pedis

The healthy child and adult have a high level of immunity to fungal infections. This natural resistance is of a non-specific type and depends upon genetic factors, age, nutrition and hormone balance. Another factor is the mechanical barrier of intact skin and surface secretions, i.e. fungicidal fatty acids in sweat and in sebaceous material. When the skin is degraded in any way, is thin and devitalised, is hyperidrotic, fissured or blistered then the likelihood of infection becoming established is enhanced. Hence the value of foot health education. The underlying cause, e.g. hyperidrosis, accidental abrasion, abrasion due to footwear, or stresses on the skin from a biomechanical foot problem, has to be treated in conjunction with the fungal infection.

Once established the management of this type of infection is in most instances relatively easy when it is a skin infection. Onychomycosis is more resistant to treatment. Ideally skin and/or nail scrapings from the infected area should be taken and should be sent to mycology in order to confirm the diagnosis and for identification of the precise species of fungi present.

Widespread or intractable fungal infections are often best treated systemically by the diabetologist/dermatologist. Most localised infections are treated with topical preparations. Before commencing the treatment of a fungal infection of the feet the patient must be strongly advised about the importance of personal hygiene: washing of the feet, hosiery and the care of potentially infected footwear, i.e. the use of fumigating agents. It is also necessary to explain to the patient that treatment will be protracted and must be carried out diligently in order to prevent regression of the condition.

Onychomycosis (tinea unguium) is very difficult to eradicate with topical applications of antifungal preparations since the infection affects the nail bed and the nail itself acts as a barrier to the penetration of the medicament.

The nail may be thinned down as far as possible and then painted with an antifungal solution, or an antifungal cream may be applied with occlusive dressings in order to enhance penetration of the medicament by keeping the nail soft. Alternatively the nail may be surgically avulsed. The nail bed must be carefully cleared of infected modified nail tissue still adhering after removal of the nail and a fungicidal cream applied. Healing usually occurs at around seven days, but applications of an appropriate fungicidal preparation should be applied twice daily by the patient until total regrowth of the nail has occurred. During this time it may be necessary for the podiatrist to reduce callus-like tissue from the exposed nail bed at two to three weekly intervals in order that infection is totally eradicated before the new nail covers the exposed bed.

When local analgesia is contraindicated, medical avulsion may be attempted with the use of 40% urea cream.[30] In this procedure the surrounding skin tissue is occluded with a dressing such as Tegaderm or Opsite wound dressings. The urea cream is applied thickly to the nail plate (after thinning the nail as much as possible without pain to the patient). The cream and nail plate are then covered with the same material which was used to protect the surrounding skin and the dressing is then firmly secured with tubular gauze which is left in situ for one week. Frequently a further application is required for complete avulsion of the nail. The same procedure as for surgical avulsion is carried out until new nail growth is complete. Although this is a painless procedure it is not always successful in obtaining complete avulsion of the nail plate.

Regardless of which method is used, treatment is very protracted and the degree of success variable. When the treatments described are not sufficient to clear the infection, or when there is recurrent infection of the nail, then avulsion with phenolisation should be considered. Systemic treatment of the fungal infection, with or without local applications of a fungal preparation, may also be considered by the child's physician.

Most other dermatophytes including tinea pedis may be treated successfully with topical preparations. It is extremely important that such infections are treated quickly and efficiently in order to prevent superimposed secondary bacterial infections.

There are many excellent fungicidal preparations available in a variety of forms. Topically they may be applied as creams, ointments, lotions, aerosol sprays or powders.

Lotions are generally chosen for application to large and hairy areas. Ointments are best avoided on moist surfaces because of their occlusive properties. Dusting powders have no place in the treatment of fungal infections unless they are used in conjunction with creams or lotions. Powders used alone are ineffective in fighting fungal infections but may be used routinely after infection has cleared as a prophylactic measure, or on areas at risk which are not actually infected by fungi. Powders may also be dusted inside hosiery and footwear which are in contact with infected skin.

Creams, ointments, lotions and sprays should be thinly and evenly applied to the affected areas at least twice daily. Treatment should be continued for a minimum of one month after the disappearance of all signs of infection in order to prevent relapse. When a patient is susceptible to fungal infection continued daily use of powder is advisable.

Certain preparations of fungicides also contain hydrocortisone which causes vasoconstriction and which will reduce inflammation. These are used in combination with antifungal preparations in the treatment of eczematous areas secondarily infected with fungi or in tinea pedis accompanied by inflammation and they should be used for the first few days only until the inflammation has subsided and should be applied sparingly. Great care is advised when using steroid containing preparations on infants or children where extensive areas of the lower limb are involved or where prolonged treatment is necessary. Long-term continuous use of corticosteroid therapy should be avoided in infants. Adrenal suppression may occur even without occlusion.

Other antifungal agents are dispensed in conjunction with a bactericidal agent and may be used effectively where there is a mild superimposed bacterial infection. Certain fungicidal agents are in themselves effective on some Gram-positive and Gram-negative bacteria.

Conversely many antibacterial drugs possess fungistatic or fungicidal properties.

Antifungal agents

The choice of agent depends upon the nature of the infecting organism, the state of the substrate and the site.

Fungicides which are available for use in podiatry in the UK are drugs on the General Sale List (GSL) and Pharmacy List (P). Topical applications of Prescription Only Medicines (POM) drugs may be used by patients and may be applied by podiatrists when prescribed by that particular patient's consultant or general practitioner.

When an adverse reaction to any of the topical fungicides occurs its use should be discontinued immediately and a drug from another group should be chosen. Oral antibiotic therapy is also available where the medical practitioner considers this to be essential.

Bacterial infections

Other than onychocryptosis, only minor superficial bacterial skin infections caused by trauma are normally seen in the diabetic child. After puberty deeper infections and ulcerations may be encountered depending upon the diabetic state of the patient. The practitioner must always be alert to the possibility of osteomyelitis developing in the presence of infection.

Prevention and prophylaxis should be the watchwords when dealing with the diabetic child since when ulceration develops, although the lesion may be cleared with thorough and aggressive management, the area involved is prone to further problems in the future. Foot health education and regular examination of the developing foot is essential in order to minimise the risk of major foot problems occurring.

The most common site for ulceration is on the dorsal interphalangeal joints (IPJs) of the lesser toes particularly when deformity is present. Hence the need for correction of such toe deformities at an early age. Ulceration here is due to pressure from the upper of the shoe onto the prominent IPJs. Interdigital ulceration is less common in young people as are apical lesions, but when toe deformities are allowed to develop these areas are also prone to pressure and possible ulceration, particularly when footwear is restrictive in either length, breadth or depth.

This also applies to the development of ulceration on the plantar aspect of the foot when high pressure areas are allowed to continue due to a biomechanical problem. Biomechanical examination is essential and when high pressure areas are found these should be rectified by the manufacture of an appropriate orthosis.

The clinician may not have any prior warning that ulceration is likely to develop and it may or may not occur on an area which already has callus formation. The first sign of underlying ulceration is usually the presence of a haematoma below the callus. On the dorsum of the foot ulcers may develop rapidly and without prior callus formation when the cause is related to ill-fitting new shoes which have been worn for long periods. Footwear must be examined frequently to ensure that it is of the correct fit, size, shape and style and also for signs of abnormal wear. Any source of pressure or likely cause of friction must be eliminated.

When gross deformity of the feet is present, surgical or bespoke footwear may be necessary. For the young diabetic certain types of footwear available would be aesthetically unacceptable. Rather than provide shoes which the patient would probably only wear when attending the clinic, the answer for the young patient is bespoke trainers. For this age group such trainers are much more acceptable and will be worn constantly. Prescription of these trainers may include soft uppers, extra toe depth or cushioning insoles.

Regardless of whether the infection is minor or not, vigorous therapy must be initiated immediately in order to prevent major problems such as cellulitis, deep tissue or bone infection occurring. Fissures, blisters or abrasions should be treated immediately in the appropriate manner. A limited staphylococcal infection in the child who has no vascular deficiency may be treated with local applications of antiseptic dressings. The use of antiseptics is preferable to topical antibiotics but certain antiseptics may have toxic effects on open areas and may delay healing. In order to avoid particular micro-organisms from becoming established antiseptics should be used on a rotational basis. The antiseptics of choice are polynoxylin, chlorhexidine and povidone iodine preparations. Prior to swabbing of the infected area a swab of the wound should be taken and this should be sent to a bacteriology department in order to identify the precise organisms present and their sensitivity. Where necessary, appropriate antibiotic therapy may then be commenced. Progress must be closely monitored.

When, in the adolescent diabetic, a deeper infected ulcer presents, immediate oral antibiotic therapy should be initiated in order to control and to clear the infection and so prevent further loss of tissue. Diabetic control must be assessed and urine should be examined for sugar and ketones and the blood sugar level determined. When control is poor, established lesions will take longer to heal and when infection is present diabetic control will be affected. Therefore a vicious circle is set up.

In the case of a deep infected lesion, curettage of the ulcer base after removal of overlying debris is a more reliable method of identifying *all* the pathogens present than simply using a superficial swab which will not necessarily pick up all the organisms present in the wound. When bone involvement is suspected or where healing of the ulcer is static then referral for X-ray is recommended.

In conjunction with oral antibiotic therapy probably the best method of management of diabetic ulceration is with modern wound dressings (sometimes referred to as environmental dressings or interactive dressings). The use of traditional dressings combined with antiseptics is now less in favour for the management of this type of wound because fibres from cotton gauze or cotton wool may remain on the wound surface and stimulate a foreign body reaction, retard the healing process and act as a focus for infection. They also allow leakage of exudate and therefore create a portal of entry for bacteria. Such dressings are also difficult to remove from the wound surface since the dried out exudate tends to adhere to the surface of the wound and this will cause trauma to the new granulation tissue which is forming.

The ideal dressing should provide the opti-mum environment for wound healing. Previously it was believed that a dry wound was essential in order to prevent further infection of the lesion and to allow healing to occur. It has now been shown that epidermal cells need a moist surface over which they are able to migrate. When the surface of the wound is dry the epidermal cells bury deeper in order to find a moist area across which they may migrate. This delays the healing process and may contribute to scar formation. Modern dressings eliminate the need for the body to produce a dry protective area over the ulcer and allow a more rapid migration of epidermal cells across the wound surface and a quicker rate of healing.

Therefore ideal wound dressings should maintain a moist environment at the wound/dressing interface. However, removal of excess wound exudate from the surface is important as within this exudate micro-organisms, dead cells and toxins will also be removed.

Such dressings should also allow gaseous exchange of oxygen, carbon dioxide and water vapour but should be impermeable to the passage of bacteria through the dressing. There is a degree of controversy at present as to the value of totally occlusive dressings which do not allow the passage of oxygen. Certain researchers have found that there is a more rapid formation of capillaries and granulation tissue with an anaerobic environment and due to the occlusion, prostaglandin synthesis is inhibited and there is therefore a reduction in pain. A great deal of thought must be given before the application of occlusive dressings in the diabetic patient. When there is existing vascular disease, particularly of the micro-circulation, and even the remotest possibility of the presence of anaerobic bacteria, they should not be used.

Thermal insulation has also been shown to be important in the healing process in order to provide the optimum temperature for mitosis to occur. Therefore dressings should provide thermal insulation (in addition the patient should wear wool socks and leather shoes in winter and the podiatrist can provide thermoplastic insoles which will help to retain heat).

The ideal dressing should also be: (i) free from particulate contaminants, (ii) sterile at the point of application to the wound surface, (iii) non-adherent to the wound, (iv) non-staining to the wound surface thus allowing evaluation of progress, (v) capable of providing some protection to the area of the ulcer, (vi) safe to use, (vii) cost effective and (viii) acceptable to the patient.

Modern wound dressings may be classified as follows.

Semi-permeable polymeric films are sterile, thin, transparent, hypoallergenic adhesive films which allow the passage of gases and water vapour but not bacteria. As they may trap excessive wound exudate under the film they should not be used on heavily exudating wounds. Their main use is in shallow ulcers with slight exudate but they may adhere slightly on removal. Usually they require a conventional dressing on top to protect and to insulate the wound.

Products available in this category are: Bioclusive, Dermafilm, Dermoclude, Ensure-it, Ioban-2, Omiderm, Opraflex, Opsite, Polyskin, Tegaderm, Transigen and Transite. Certain of these dressings have been modified in an effort to control exudate.

Hydrocolloids are adhesive flexible wafers comprising two layers. An outer protective waterproof layer which is bonded to an inner layer of hydrocolloid particles and a hydrophobic polymer. When this inner layer is in contact with wound exudate the exudate is absorbed, swells, liquefies and forms a soft moist yellowish gel over the wound surface (which should not be confused with slough) and may have a strong odour. When the dressing is removed the gel separates causing no trauma to tissues. These dressings allow rapid débridement of necrotic tissue. Apart from Biofilm, they are all occlusive dressings and produce an anaerobic wound environment. Therefore most of them are contraindicated when anaerobes are present in the wound.

Products available in this category are: Biofilm, Comfeel, Granuflex, Intrasite, Tegasorb and Varihesive.

Dextranomers are hydrophilic agents which absorb wound exudate and carry debris and bacteria away from the wound surface and may be used on sloughy, infected exudating wounds. Some (in the form of beads or granules) are difficult to apply to the foot and the dressing should never be allowed to dry out. Rinsing away the soiled beads in the case of Debrisan may be difficult for the podiatrist and uncomfortable for the patient. Dressings should be changed daily.

Products available in this category are: Bard Absorption Dressing, Debrisan range and Iodosorb (incorporating iodine).

Alginates are manufactured from brown seaweeds and may be produced in the form of alginate rope or as flat absorbent pads. The rope is used on deeper cavities. The alginates are indicated only for use on exudating wounds, never for dry wounds or for those covered with hard necrotic tissue. As they have no adhesive surface they require supplementary dressings when the wound is heavily exudating. They may be used on infected wounds but are not the dressing of choice. When in contact with wound exudate the dressing forms a gel which moulds to the shape of the cavity and produces an ideal moist environment. The gel is easily removed with sodium chloride solution 0.9%. Any fibres which remain are broken down eventually into simple sugars and are absorbed by the body.

Certain products available in this range are also deodorising. Available products are: Kaltocarb, Kaltoclude, Kaltostat Fortex, Sorbsan range and Tegagel.

Polyurethane foams are flat sheets of polyurethane foam, the undersurface of which is treated and is hydrophilic. The outer surface is untreated hydrophobic and does not allow the strike through of exudate. Some possess a carbon layer which controls offensive odours. These are indicated in the treatment of medium to heavily exudating infected wounds and may be left in situ for a period of up to seven days. The dressing should not be left for extended periods on dry shallow wounds as the drying exudate may cause adhesion between the dressing and the wound. The dressing has high thermal insulation properties.

Products available in the category are: Allevyn, Coraderm, Lyofoam and Silastic foam.

A combination of two of the above may be used in the management of ulceration depending upon the size and the stage of the ulcer.

The products within each category have slightly different characteristics and it is important that the practitioner is aware of the differences and characteristics of each dressing and the manufacturer's instructions for use.[31] The choice of dressing can be very confusing due to the large number available and the many new dressings currently marketed.

When managing ulceration detailed notes should be entered in the patient's record card at each visit. These should include: (i) site, size and depth of the ulcer, (ii) the nature and quantity of the exudate, (iii) state of the base of the ulcer and (iv) a description of the edges, (v) the degree of inflammation and pain present, (vi) reaction of the patient and lesion to the treatment regimes and (vii) the therapeutic advice given to the patient. Precise records are essential.

Nail conditions

Onychocryptosis is the most problematic and the most painful nail condition experienced by adolescents. This condition may be dealt with conservatively without recourse to nail surgery when it has been caused by trauma, poor nail cutting or nail picking.

When the problem is recurrent or where it is the result of involution, onychogryphosis, onychauxis or onychorrhexis, then the best course of action is nail surgery either by partial or by total avulsion of the nail. The nail is likely to continue to give problems and in later life could well be a constant source of infection or ulceration to the patient.

Neither local analgesia nor phenolisation is contraindicated in diabetics provided that the status of the circulation is good and that there is no evidence of neuropathy.

Corn and callus

The main aim of treatment is to minimise the formation of areas of increased keratin production. The first step when corn or callus is present in a child or adolescent is to determine the cause. It is most likely to be due to footwear or to a biomechanical problem. Once the cause is established it should be eliminated. Frequently this is more easily said than done,

particularly with plantar callus. Any areas of pathologically thickened plantar callus should be reduced carefully by minute dissection. There is evidence to suggest that removal of heavy plantar callus reduces the high pressures on overloaded areas. It is essential that such areas are regularly reduced in order to prevent possible underlying ulceration and infection occurring. Care must be taken not to over-reduce as this could lead to further traumatisation of the tissues with the possibility of consequent infection.

Verrucae

This is the most common viral infection of the skin in children and adolescents. Preventative measures would include advice on not walking barefoot in gymnasia or swimming pools and not exchanging footwear with friends. The use of special socks to wear in swimming pools may be recommended in order to minimise possible infection.

The types of treatment which are available for diabetic children are the same as for the non-diabetic population. Physical, chemical or astringent treatment may be used. Pyrogallol and monochloroacetic acid should be avoided as these drugs may penetrate deeply into the tissue and may cause severe reactions and breakdown of tissue. Chemical and astringent treatment may be used on the younger child but cryosurgery is contraindicated because of the pain factor. Adolescents should be able to tolerate cryosurgery. Another alternative which may be used on the adolescent is electrosurgery, either coagulation desiccation or fulguration. Since this procedure requires local analgesia the criteria for its use must be carefully evaluated. Astringents are very slow acting on verrucae and since treatment may be prolonged by their use they are best reserved for the very nervous child or for the diabetic who has neuropathy and vascular impairment.

Necrobiosis lipoidica diabeticorum (NLD)

NLD is a rare condition but it is slightly more frequent in children particularly in severe congenital diabetics. The condition presents as raised reddish-yellow papules which are usually evident over the tibial areas but which may occur on the soles of the feet. Treatment is advice in order to avoid trauma to the lesion thus lessening to the possibility of ulceration.

Charcot joints

Charcot joints occur as a result of diabetic neuropathy and are rare in children and uncommon even in the teens unless there is extensive sensory loss. In the younger patient joint changes are more likely to be seen in the tarsal and metatarsal joints and less commonly seen at the ankle or knee joints.

There are many other conditions which affect the skin and subcutaneous tissues but the conditions discussed here are considered to have particular relevance to the podiatric treatment of the diabetic child.

References

1 Metcalfe MA, Baum JD. Incidence of insulin dependent diabetes in children aged under 15 years in the British Isles during 1988. *Br Med J* 1991; 302: 443–7.

2 Bloom A, Hayes TM, Gamble DR. Register of newly diagnosed diabetic children. *Br Med J* 1975; 3: 580–3.

3 Banatvala JE *et al. Lancet* 1985; 1: 1409.

4 Karjalainrn J, Salmela P, Ilonen J, Surcel H, Knip M. A comparison of childhood and adult type 1 diabetes mellitus. *N Engl J Med* 1989; 320: 881–6.

5 Tchobroutsky G. Relation of diabetic control to development of microvascular complications. *Diabetologia* 1978; 15: 143–52.

6 Birkbeck JA, Truswell AS, Thomas BJ. Current practice in dietary management of diabetic children. *Arch Dis Child* 1976; 51: 568.

7 Kinmouth AL, Angus RM, Jenkins PA, Smith MA, Baum JD. Whole foods and increased dietary fibre improve blood glucose control in diabetic children. *Arch Dis Child* 1982; 57: 187.

8 *Countdown*. British Diabetic Association.

9 Walford S, Allison SP, Gale EAM, Tattersall RB. Self-monitoring of blood-glucose improvement in diabetic control. *Lancet* 1978; 732–5.

10 Baumer JH, Edelsten AD, Howlett BC, Owens C, Pennock CA, Savage DCL. Impact of home blood glucose monitoring on childhood diabetes. *Arch Dis Child* 1982; 57: 195–9.

11 MacFarlane PI, Smith CS. Perceptions of hypoglycaemia in childhood diabetes mellitus: a questionnaire study. *Practical Diabetes* 1988; 56–58.

12 Daneman D, Frank M, Perlman K, Tamm J, Ehrlich R. Severe hypoglycaemia in children with insulin-dependent diabetes mellitus: frequency and predisposing factors. *J Pediatr* 1989; 115: 681–5.

13 Bergada I, Suissa S, Dufresne J, Schiffrin A. Severe hypoglycaemia in IDDM children. *Diabetes Care* 1989; 12: 239–44.

14 Aman J, Wranne L. Hypoglycaemia in childhood diabetes. Effect of subcutaneous or intramuscular injection of different doses of glucagon. *Acta Paediatr Scand* 1988; 77: 548–53.

15 Deckert T, Poulsen JE, Larsen M. Prognosis of diabetics with diabetes onset before the age of 31. *Diabetologia* 1978; 14: 363–70.

16 Viberti GC, Jarrett RJ, Mahmud U, Hill RD *et al.* Microalbuminuria as a predictor of clinical nephropathy in insulin-dependent diabetes mellitus. *Lancet* 1982; i: 1430–2.

17 Dahlquist G, Rudberg S. The prevalence of microalbuminuria in diabetic children and adolescents and its relation to puberty. *Acta Paediatr Scand* 1987; 76: 795–800.

18 Dornan T, Mann JI, Turner R. Factors protective against retinopathy in insulin-dependent diabetics free of retinopathy for 30 years. *Br Med J* 1982; 285: 1073–7.

19 Court S, Parkin JM. Hypothyroidism and growth failure in diabetes mellitus. *Arch Dis Child* 1982; 57: 622–4.

20 Sorensen E, Aagenaes O. Diabetic complications in a prepubertal adolescent. *Arch Dis Child* 1988; 63: 1397–8.

21 Close H, Davies AG, Price DA, Goodyer IM. Emotional difficulties in diabetes mellitus. *Arch Dis Child* 1986; 61: 337–40.

22 Allgrove J. Improved diabetic control in a district general hospital. *Arch Dis Child* 1988; 63: 180–5.

23 British Paediatric Association. The Organisation of services for children with diabetes in the United Kingdom – report of a BPA Working Party.

24 Besman AN. Foot problems in the diabetic. *Compr Ther* 1982; 8(1): 32–7.

25 Ludvigsson J, Johannesson G, Heding L, Häger A, Larsson Y. Sensory nerve conduction velocity and vibratory sensibility in juvenile diabetics. *Acta Paediatr Scand* 1979; 68: 739–43.

26 Gamstorp I, Shelburn SA, Engleson G, Redondo D, Traisman HS. Peripheral neuropathy in juvenile diabetes. *Diabetes* 1966; 15: 411–18.

27 Young RJ, Ewing DJ, Clarke BF. Nerve function

and metabolic control in teenage diabetics. *Diabetes* 1983; 32: 142–7.

28 Heimans JJ, Bertelsmann FW, de Beaufort CE, de Beaufort AJ, Faber YA, Bruining GJ. Quantitative sensory examination in diabetic children: assessment of thermal discrimination. *Diabet Med* 1987; 4: 251–3.

29 Hoffman WH, Hart ZH, Frank RN. Correlates of delayed motor nerve conduction and retinopathy in juvenile onset diabetes mellitus. *J Paediatr* 1983; 102: 351–5.

30 Aubrey AV. A clinical investigation into the use of 40% urea cream for the medical avulsion of nails. *Chiropodist* 1986; 41: 381–2.

31 Formulary of Wound Management Products. David A. Morgan, Clwyd Health Authority.

9 Neurology

Robin Grant and Edwin J. Harris

Neural organisation and development

Neurons and neuroglia (nerve supporting cells) are all produced from embryonic neuro-ectoderm, which has become specialised on the dorsal surface of the embryo, during the third week of gestation (Fig. 9.1). The lateral margins of this neural plate invaginate and close dorsally into the central nervous system (CNS). At the same time neural crest cells proliferate and migrate through the mesoderm and later differentiate into the dorsal root, sensory and motor nerves, autonomic, ganglia and Schwann cells which make up the peripheral nervous system (PNS). The first point of fusion of the neural tube is in the medulla and fusion progresses rostrally and caudally until week 7. Differentiation at the rostral and caudal ends of the developing nervous system then commences. Disturbances around this time produce anencephaly or myelomeningoceles.

Between weeks 8 16 neural proliferation occurs. Chromosomal abnormalities, teratogens (irradiation, toxins, e.g. alcohol) or infections may prevent proliferation. Migration of cells to specific sites producing nerve tracts and nuclei occurs mainly between weeks 12 and 22. Incomplete migration of cells results in agenesis of the corpus callosum or severe abnormalities such as schizencephaly. Organisation of neurons occurs from week 20 onwards and continues for several years after birth. The major changes that occur are alignment and orientation of cortical neurons, sprouting of dendrites and axons, and development of synapses. Failure of complete organisation is usually the result of perinatal insults but also occurs in Down's syndrome and primary mental retardation. Myelination of axons starts around the second trimester, occurring first in the PNS, in motor then sensory roots, and next in the CNS in the major sensory and then motor tracts. Myelination in the cerebral and cerebellar hemispheres starts well after delivery, continues over the first two decades and is necessary for the development of fine motor and sensory control, refinement of balance and coordination, and for development of reasoning and intelligence.

The grey matter contains nerve cell bodies and the white matter contains myelinated axons. The neurons are supported by glial tissue (astrocytes and oligodendrocytes). Afferent (or sensory) neurons transmit action potentials from peripheral receptors, e.g. in the skin, to central neurons, e.g. in the sensory cortex. Efferent neurons send axons from central cell bodies, e.g. in the motor cortex, to peripheral effector organs, e.g. in muscle.

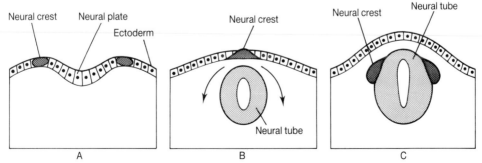

Figure 9.1 Transverse section through the dorsal structures of the embryo at 3 weeks (A) to 7 weeks (C) gestation demonstrating development of the neural tube and neural crest.

Control of posture and movement

Voluntary movement is initiated from the cerebral cortex, although there is some evidence that deeper structures such as the thalamus, cerebellum and basal ganglia aid in initiation of movement by their actions on the motor cortex.

Descending tracts

Corticospinal tracts

The upper motor neurons (UMNs) descend via the posterior limb of the internal capsule in the corticospinal tracts and corticobulbar tracts. At the level of the medulla most of the corticospinal fibres cross the midline and descend as the lateral corticospinal tracts. A smaller percentage do not decussate and they descend as the anterior corticospinal tracts and only cross at their segmental levels. Most corticospinal fibres end on interneurons in lamina VII of the spinal cord. These pathways are concerned with fine movements.

Reticulospinal and vestibulospinal tracts

The reticulospinal tracts start in the pons and medulla and partially decussate and synapse with interneurons in lamina VII. Reticulospinal tracts control movements that do not need conscious attention. Vestibulospinal tracts from the vestibular nuclei in the medulla descend uncrossed and end on interneurons in the spinal cord. These neurons mediate extensor tone and allow us to maintain an upright posture.

Basal ganglia and cerebellum

The basal ganglia and cerebellum do not have descending tracts, but they do modify movement and possibly store learned patterns of behaviour. The basal ganglia (caudate nucleus, putamen and globus palidus) are concerned with posture, truncal movements and gross limb movements. The role of the cerebellum is to smooth and to coordinate movement. The cerebellum has extensive afferent input from motor cortex (via the pontocerebellar tracts),

spinal afferent systems (spinocerebellar), and vestibular (vestibulocerebellar) receptors. The efferents from the cerebellum relay to the thalamus (and brain stem nuclei) which in turn influence the motor cortex (thalamofrontal projections). These supraspinal projections ultimately affect the rate and pattern of discharge from the lower motor neurons (LMN) in the brain stem (cranial motor nuclei) and spinal cord (anterior horn cells).

Peripheral nervous system

Axons from the anterior horn cells exit the spinal cord via the anterior (motor) nerve roots and then join with the sensory nerves to form a mixed nerve (Fig. 9.2). Mixed nerves contain

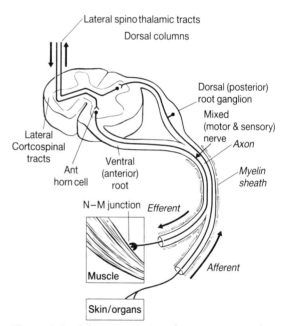

Figure 9.2 Afferent pathways from sensory and organs in the periphery to the spinal cord and efferent (motor) pathways from spinal cord to the neuromuscular junction.

large and small diameter fibres. The somatic motor nerves and sensory nerves subserving joint vibration and position sense are well myelinated and conduct action potentials quickly, while the smaller fibres subserving pain and temperature or to muscle spindles are poorly myelinated and have slower conduction velocities. At the distal end of the mixed peripheral nerve and motor and sensory elements once more part company, the former to muscle and the latter to specialised sensory nerve endings. The LMN terminates at the neuromuscular junction by forming the pre-synaptic terminal which lies over a specialised motor end plate. Motor control is finely controlled by a feedback loop in the PNS via gamma efferent neurons to muscle spindles and via Ia afferent fibres from muscle spindles which provide information about small changes in muscle stretch.

Neurotransmitters

Neurotransmitters are chemicals released at synaptic junctions and are present in the CNS and the PNS. These chemicals are different from hormones in that they produce their effect locally, i.e. at a synapse rather than at a distant site. There are many different types of neurotransmitter and many subsets of each type. The neurotransmitters that have most effect on movement and posture are acetylcholine (Ach), dopamine (DA) and gamma-amino-butyric acid (GABA).

Acetylcholine acts through two types of receptors: nicotinic or muscarinic. Cholinergic neurotransmission in the cortex and subcortical areas is mediated through both types of receptor whereas in the spinal cord and at the neuromuscular junction neurotransmission is through nicotinic receptors. In the CNS its action is still ill defined but it may be important in memory. Stimulation of the lower motor neuron causes release of acetylcholine from pre-synaptic vesicles and this binds to post-synaptic nicotinic receptors which results in the release of calcium from muscle sarcoplasmic reticulum which in turn causes muscle contraction. Acetylcholine is also the neurotransmitter present in all pre-ganglionic neurons, parasympathetic post-ganglionic neurons and sympathetic post-ganglionic neurons. Stimulation of these causes bradycardia, bronchoconstriction, small pupils, vasodilation and sweating.

Dopaminergic neurons in the basal ganglia are necessary to enable proper control of posture, tone and speed of movement. There is a relative balance of action of DA and Ach in basal ganglia and when there is a net reduction of dopamine a Parkinsonian state is produced with flexed posture, increased tone (rigidity), slowed movement (hypokinesia) and tremor. When there is relative excess of dopamine, movement disorders such as dyskinesia may predominate.

Gamma-aminobutyric acid (GABA) is an inhibitory transmitter within the brain, spinal cord and cerebellum. Activation of the GABAa receptor produces a post-synaptic inhibitory action potential. The GABAb receptor is inhibitory to noradrenaline, glutamate, dopamine and serotonin. Following any damage to the upper motor neurons in the brain or spinal cord, excitatory influences predominate. Benzodiazepines and valproate facilitate GABA binding and thus produce an anticonvulsant action. Baclofen is a GABAb agonist and therefore acts as a muscle relaxant.

History and examination

Neurological evaluation should start by obtaining a history of the presenting complaint, past medical history, the birth and the mother's obstetric history, family history, drug and social history. In neonates and young children, history should be obtained from the parents. Most neurological diagnoses can be made from history alone and examination and investigations only confirm what is usually apparent.

Neonatal examination

The most important aspect of neurological examination in neonates is observation. Level of alertness, ability to suck and to swallow, morphological features such as weight and length, head shape and circumference, symmetry and position of all limbs and digits and normal spinal and facial features should all be recorded. Level of alertness will vary with time of feed and examination is best performed prior to a feed when the baby is active and unlikely to vomit. When the baby is held upright, the hips are usually flexed and the head hangs limply forward. However, when the baby is supported under the abdomen it may momentarily lift the head up, and when it is laid supine the head will turn to one side. The hands are usually fisted at rest but when the baby is being fed the arms may partially extend and the baby will try to grasp at the breast. Eye contact with the mother occurs early during breast feeding. A healthy baby will startle at a loud noise and will have an active cry when hungry. Muscle tone may be slightly increased and various primitive reflexes such as the grasp, Moro, sucking, rooting and tonic neck reflex are present. The plantar reflexes are extensor.

By three months the baby produces vigorous movements at rest with the hands open or loosely fisted. When the baby is held upright its head will bob, when prone the head will be held up for a few seconds and when supine the head is in the midline. The baby will be able to hold a toy for a short time. The Moro, tonic neck reflex and grasp reflex may now be suppressed. The baby will smile, vocalise and follow an interesting object. At six months the baby, when supine, can lift his head up, roll from supine to prone and can maintain his head and chest up in this position. He can support his weight when in the standing position, transfer a toy from hand to hand with a rather coarse grasp and recognise familiar faces and voices. At 9–10 months the child can pull himself into an upright posture and by 12 months can usually stand for a moment unassisted and walk when led. By 15 months the child can walk with a broad based gait and by 18 months he can manage a rather stiff run with only occasional falls. At two years he can run without falling and he can usually walk up and down stairs without help. It is also valuable to observe simple motor tasks, e.g. rising from a squatted position, walking on the heels to test the ankle dorsiflexors and on the toes to test gastrocnemius. Balance may be assessed by asking the child to stand with feet together with eyes open, in order to test cerebellar function, and then with eyes closed, to test joint position (Romberg's test). By three years the child can balance momentarily on one foot, at four years he can run and jump, and by age five he can skip and balance on one foot, for a short time, with the eyes closed. Testing tandem gait will often identify subtle cerebellar signs. Hopping is a good, quick, non-discriminative test, which if accomplished, usually means that the lower limb motor, sensory and cerebellar functions are normal.

The upper limbs can be quickly screened by means of three tests:

1. Hold arms out (palms upward) – if the arm cannot be raised or drifts downwards, there is usually proximal weakness.
2. Touch nose with eyes open – may demonstrate cerebellar incoordination.
3. Touch nose with eyes closed – when this test is normal with eyes open and abnormal with eyes closed, there is a sensory problem.

A valuable reproducible test of dexterity or test for clumsiness is the timed nine hole peg test (timed at putting nine pegs in nine holes, using one hand at a time).

These simple quick screening tests usually identify children who require a more detailed neurological examination.

Formal neurological examination

Limb symmetry, muscle bulk, tone, strength and reflexes should be compared on each side, both proximally and distally. Muscle strength can be tested in groups. In the lower limbs L1, 2, 3 supply the hip flexors (iliopsoas), L4, 5, S1 innervate the hip extensors (glutei), L2, 3, 4 supply the knee extensors (quadriceps), L5, S1, 2 innervate the knee flexors (hamstrings), L4, 5 supplies ankle dorsiflexion (tibialis anterior) and S1, 2 plantar flexion (gastrocnemius). Ankle inversion is supplied by L4 nerve root and eversion by L5, S1 root.

The reflex levels may be remembered by:

ankle jerk S1, 2
knee jerk L3, 4
biceps jerk C5, 6
supinator jerk C6
triceps jerk C7

The plantar response should be tested last by drawing a moderately sharp object from behind the lateral malleolus along the lateral border of the foot and then across the metatarsal heads (Chaddock's test). This is as effective as Babinski's method and is less likely to produce a withdrawal response.

Testing sensation requires much cooperation from the patient. When there are no sensory complaints, there are usually no significant sensory abnormalities and a brief screening examination should suffice. When there are complaints of numbness or tingling, the patient should be asked to map it out and the distribution should be confirmed and localised (i.e. nerve root, single nerve or glove and stocking). With the increasing AIDS problem, pain sensation should be tested using a safety pin which is then disposed of after testing. The dermatomes can be quickly tested.[1]

In the lower limbs anterior thigh is supplied by L1, 2, 3, the lower leg by L4 anteromedially, L5 anterolaterally, S1 the outer border of the foot and sole, S2 up the back of the leg and S3, 4, 5 over the buttock.

Joint position sense is tested by moving the finger or toe and asking the patient to identify the direction of movement with eyes closed. Vibration sense is tested by placing a vibrating tuning fork over a bony prominence and asking the patient if he feels vibration.

Cerebellar function should be tested last, because in the presence of motor or sensory problems it is difficult to comment on coordination. Cerebellar function is tested by checking for slurred speech (dysarthria), jerky eye movements (nystagmus), finger–nose–finger test, smoothly running the heel up and down the shin (heel–shin test), rapid alternating movements and tandem gait.

Abnormal neurological patterns

There is a spectrum of normal clumsiness when walking and some paediatricians consider that as many as 10% of children may be clumsy to a degree. Abnormal clumsiness with delay in reaching the appropriate motor milestones is much less frequent and merits full neurological examination.

1. *Upper motor neuron (UMN) damage* characteristically produces weakness of extensor muscle groups in the upper limb and of flexor groups in the lower limb with spasticity, hyperreflexia and extensor plantar response. When spasticity is unilateral the arm is held flexed and the leg extended. There is circumduction at the hip and the toes and outer aspect of shoes are often scuffed. When there is bilateral UMN damage, the gait is characteristically scissored and adductor tone results in the knees rubbing when walking coupled with plantarflexion and inversion of the feet. There may also be lordo-sis and a rather festinant precarious gait as is seen in cerebral palsy.

2. *Damage to the basal ganglia* produces tremor, increased tone (rigidity), slowed movement (hypokinesia) and flexed posture.

3. *Cerebellar damage* will result in slurred speech, nystagmus, incoordination in the upper and lower limbs and a wide based ataxic gait.

4. *Lower motor neuron disorders* produce wasting, fasciculations (spontaneous contraction of motor units), hypotonia, weakness, arreflexia and flexor plantar responses without sensory changes, e.g. anterior horn cell or motor root diseases.

5. *Neuropathies* generally produce sensory and motor signs. Loss of vibration distally in the lower limbs with reduced ankle jerks is often an early sign of a peripheral neuropathy before numbness or weakness appear. In peripheral neuropathies there is weakness of ankle dorsiflexion and this produces foot drop and a high steppage gait.

6. *Disorders of the neuromuscular junction* produces fatigable weakness without wasting, fasciculation, reflex changes or sensory loss.

7. *Primary muscle disorders* (e.g. polymyositis or Duchenne dystrophy) produce weakness (± wasting) proximally in the lower ± upper limbs, with normal reflexes and no sensory signs. The gait is characteristically swaggering, with rolling at the hips. Some dystrophies (e.g. myotonic dystrophy) result in distal weakness and wasting, producing a gait similar to that in a peripheral neuropathy but without sensory signs.

Diseases affecting the nervous system

Cerebral palsy

Cerebral palsy (CP) is defined as 'aberrant control of movement or posture of a patient which appears early in life as a result of a central nervous system lesion, damage or dysfunction and not the result of a recognised progressive or degenerative disease'.[2] Cerebral palsy can be classified into spastic, ataxic and dyskinetic forms, and the spastic form may be subclassified into quadriplegia, diplegia and hemiplegia.[3]

In most cases the diagnosis of CP is established during the first two years of life. The most common cause is intraventricular haemorrhage (IVH) in preterm infants. IVH varies inversely with gestational age and is frequently seen in premature babies with respiratory distress syndrome or general cardiovascular difficulties. IVH is present in 40% of infants weighing less than 1500 grams and in 40% of admissions less than 35 weeks preterm. It is neurologicaly silent in up to 78% of these cases.[4] One-third of patients with significant intraventricular haemorrhage develop severe handicaps.

Intraparenchymal and intraventricular haemorrhages may be identified by cranial duplex ultrasound scanning through the anterior fontanelle. Ultrasound scans performed early are as good as late scanning for predicting cerebral palsy. Poor outcome is increased when there are bilateral intraparenchymal lesions. Cerebral infarctions also seen in preterm infants, often in watershed areas between arterial supplies.

About 75% of cases of CP have predominantly spastic forms. Diplegia (40%) is slightly more common than quadriplegia (35%) or hemilegia (25%). Ataxic and dyskinetic syndromes occur in about 18% and 7% respectively.[5] Patients may suffer from mental retardation (53%), epilepsy (50%), sensory deficits (hearing or visual), and emotional problems.

Passive movement and braces prevent contractures. Extensive braces do not help and they inhibit normal muscle function.[6] Bobath developed a neurodevelomental treatment programme which attempts to inhibit abnormal infantile reflexes and to facilitate more normal movement patterns such as the righting reflex.[7] This is popular in many rehabilitation centres but well designed trials demonstrating objective benefit over other methods are still lacking. This programme may stimulate the child and improve social integration into the family and for future life, although it may not significantly reduce the number of operations that the child will require. Physiotherapy, such as positioning of the patient to avoid contractures, and lightweight night splints may be useful to keep ankles in a neutral position but these are often ineffective or uncomfortable.

Surgical intervention for muscle contractures should be approached cautiously especially in patients with athetosis, dyskinesia or chorea, because there is often a tendency for overcorrecting especially in the dyskinetic patient. Surgery to improve ambulation should be delayed until after the gait has matured (age 6–10 years) and the patient should be mobilised early with minimal casting. Sixty-eight per cent of severely or profoundly retarded children survive for more than five years.

Friedreich's ataxia

The most common hereditary ataxia is Friedreich's ataxia.[8] This is an autosomal recessive condition with a high spontaneous mutation rate. Degenerative changes occur in the cerebellum, posterior columns and lateral corticospinal tracts.

The classical presentation is with a clumsy ataxic gait in a child who has been slow to achieve motor milestones. In the space of a few years the ataxia is more obvious and clumsiness in the upper limbs becomes apparent. The ataxia is initially due to a mixture of cerebellar and dorsal column damage but later it is also complicated by an upper motor neuron weakness. Tendon reflexes in the lower limbs are nearly always absent due to peripheral sensory involvement, but the plantar responses are extensor. Vibration sense is lost early in the lower limbs and joint position sense becomes impaired later in the disease. Truncal instability may occur late in the disease requiring spinal support. Skeletal abnormalities, such as pes cavus and talipes equinovarus, are seen in 75% of sufferers and kyphoscoliosis will develop in nearly all cases. Cardiac murmurs and hypertrophic cardiomyopathy are common.[9]

While classical Friedreich's ataxia is clinically easy to diagnose, there are many atypical cases where separation from other forms of hereditary ataxia such as Lévy–Roussy syndrome (wasting in lower limbs and no cerebellar signs), hereditary cerebellar ataxia (no skeletal or spinal cord signs), or olivopontocerebellar ataxia (later onset, no spinal cord signs) may be difficult. Magnetic resonance imaging may demonstrate atrophy of the cerebellum and spinal cord. Nerve conduction studies (NCS) reveal severely slowed or absent sensory conduction with normal motor conduction velocities. Cerebrospinal fluid (CSF) shows mild elevation of protein and the electrocardiograph (ECG) and echocardiography are frequently abnormal. There is usually a steady decline in function with death in 10–20 years, but some cases with an autosomal dominant form have been reported with normal life span. Cardiac abnormalities along with diabetes mellitus, kyphoscoliosis and recurrent chest infections significantly contribute to morbidity and mortality.

Spina bifida

Spina bifida is defined as failure of closure of the spinal column leading to a defect in the vertebral column. This may vary in severity from asymptomatic spina bifida occulta, which affects 5–10% of the population, to myelomeningocele, where the spinal cord and roots lie in a cystic defect protruding through the skin and this occurs in the lower spine (80%), or cervical area (20%). The incidence of myelomeningocele varies from 1 in 3000 in Japan to greater than 1 in 300 in parts of Wales. There is often associated hydrocephalus, Chiari 2 malformation, scoliosis and foot deformities. Antenatal diagnosis of severe dysraphic states is possible, either by maternal serum alphafetoprotein levels, which are elevated, or by ultrasound screening in the first trimester.

At birth, myelomeningocele is all too obvious, but with spina bifida occulta, cutaneous abnormalities are usually not evident although lumbosacral dimple, sinus or hair tuft may point to an underlying dysraphic state such as spina bifida occulta, diastematomyelia, lipoma or dermoid cyst.

Clinically the patient has a flaccid paraparesis or paraplegia with loss of lumbosacral sensation and bladder atonicity, leading to frequent infections and renal damage. Detailed neurological assessment is extremely important when considering management.[10]

Severe cases of myeomeningocele often die in the first year from recurrent infections. Thirty-three per cent of survivors are totally dependent and only 20% are independent. Management requires a multidisciplinary approach involving paediatric, neurology, orthopaedics, urology, rehabilitation and podiatric services.[11] The aims are to develop independence, to promote ambulation where possible and to prevent respiratory and urinary tract infections, pressure sores and flexion contractures.

Guillain–Barré syndrome

Guillain–Barré syndrome is an acute post-infectious demyelinating motor neuropathy which predominantly involves the anterior spinal roots. The segmental demyelination is probably due to a cell-mediated immune response against peripheral nervous system myelin but when severe it can result in some irreparable axonal damage. About 50% of patients describe a preceding upper respiratory tract infection or diarrhoeal illness that has occurred one to three weeks before the onset of the weakness. Back pain is often an early symptom and although there may be sensory symptoms, motor weakness predominates. Reflexes are lost early in the course of the disease. The onset of weakness commonly occurs distally initially and ascends, but often it is generalised and progresses over the next three to four weeks. It becomes life threatening when the respiratory or bulbar muscles are involved or when there are autonomic disturbances producing swings in blood pressure and tachycardia. The inflammation of the motor roots results in a marked increase in cerebrospinal fluid protein with little or no elevation in CSF white cells. Nerve conduction studies may be normal initially as most of the demyelination occurs proximally in the nerve roots rather than distally in the nerve. Virological tests sometimes demonstrate elevations in titres of Epstein–Barr virus or cytomegalovirus.

Recovery of strength in this condition takes place over some months as remyelination occurs slowly. There is a 10% mortality rate in even the best series. Treatment is supportive with ventilation when required, control of autonomic disturbances and physiotherapy. In severe cases plasmapheresis reduces the amount of time spent in an intensive treatment unit on a ventilator and improves the grade of weakness sooner than in those who do not require plasmapheresis.

Charcot–Marie–Tooth disease

Charcot–Marie–Tooth disease is an autosomal dominant condition. Type 1 presents in the teens or twenties with slowly progressive foot drop, due to wasting of the peronei, and the peripheral nerves may be palpably enlarged. In type 2, the onset of muscle weakness is not until adult life and nerves are not palpable. Pes cavus and hammer toes are frequent accompaniments which contribute to instability at the ankles and these may be evident prior to the development of obvious weakness. Distal weakness and wasting in the lower limbs is accompanied by tendon hyporeflexia and a glove and stocking distribution of impaired sensation. In type 1, nerve conduction velocities are slowed to less than 15 m/sec (normal 50–60 m/sec), CSF protein is elevated and sural nerve biopsy demonstrates segmental demyelination and remyelination. In type 2, nerve conduction velocities are slowed to between 65% of normal velocity. CSF is normal and biopsy reveals axonal regeneration. Progression is very slow in both these types of hereditary sensory and motor neuropathies and effective splinting may prolong ambulation for many years.[12] Long-term results of posterior tibial tendon transfer as part of a staged procedure, in general, have been poor.[13]

Myasthenia gravis

Myasthenia gravis (MG) is a relapsing and remitting autoimmune disease where autoantibodies (AchR ab) are directed against the patient's own post-synaptic acetylcholine receptors at the neuromuscular junction. There are also abnormalities in the thymus gland, most commonly hyperplasia but occasionally neoplasia (thymoma). Myasthenia gravis may be divided into neonatal (NMG), congenital (CMG), juvenile (JMG) and adult (AMG) forms.

NMG appears transiently in 10–20% of infants born to myasthenic mothers and is probably due to placental transfer of AchR ab from the mother. These babies present within 48 hours of birth, with a poor cry and a poor ability to suck as a result of fatigable bulbar weakness. Less commonly there is generalised weakness or respiratory failure. The condition may last several weeks and the spontaneous improvement is paralleled by a steady reduction in neonatal AchR antibody titres.

CMG is rare and never life threatening. It is usually present at birth but is so mild it may go unnoticed until adulthood. There is a high familial incidence, but mothers do not have AchR antibodies.

Juvenile myasthenia gravis is similar to the adult form and usually presents at about eight years of age. It affects females three to four times as often as males and generally affects the cranial nerves first, with ptosis, diplopia or facial weakness.

Diagnosis is based on the symptoms of fatigable muscle weakness, demonstration of acetylcholine receptor antibodies in the serum, electromyographic evidence of a decremental response in amplitude of action potentials to repetitive muscle stimulation and a response to edrophonium chloride – a short-acting anticholinesterase which prevents the destruction of acetylcholine by cholinesterase at the neuromuscular junction.

In life threatening situations where there is respiratory or bulbar involvement, removal of circulating AchR ab by plasmapheresis can produce a short-lived improvement in muscle strength. Longer-acting anticholinesterases and steroids which suppress the autoimmune response occurring at the neuromuscular junction are the mainstay of treatment and may lead to long-term remission. Removal of the thymus gland may also produce improvement or even long-term remission.

Duchenne muscular dystrophy (DMD)

Dystrophies are hereditary myopathies. The most common and most severe progressive dystrophy is Duchenne muscular dystrophy, an X-linked recessive dystrophy which is due to a mutation at position 21 on the short arm of the X chromosome resulting in a defective gene product (dystrophin).[14] It therefore almost exclusively affects males with a prevalence of 1 in 25000.

DMD usually manifests before the age of five years, with delay in walking, abnormal gait, frequent falling and difficulty in climbing stairs. The important signs on examination are a waddling gait with lordotic posture, abnormal run and hop, difficulty in rising from the floor due to weakness of pelvic girdle muscles (Gower's sign) and pseudohypertrophy of the calves. The patient may try to accommodate for proximal weakness by 'toe-walking'. There may be associated cardiomyopathy, low IQ, and musculoskeletal deformities such as equinovarus, scoliosis and eventually fixed flexion contractures, as the disease progresses. There are no sensory or reflex abnormalities until a very late stage of wasting, plantar responses are flexor and the sphincters are not involved. The clinical course is usually relentless with progressive loss of function and eventual wheelchair existence by 12 years of age. Respiratory infections are common and death generally occurs by the early twenties. A slower progression and continued ambulation after 12 years of age should suggest the milder X-linked recessive Becker's dystrophy.

Investigations demonstrate an elevation in serum creatine kinase levels, increased echogenicity on ultrasound of muscle, myopathic EMG and muscle biopsy revealing degeneration of muscle fibres with evidence of regeneration with variation in fibre size, internal nuclei and excessive fat and connective tissue.

There is no effective treatment but it is important to avoid excessive immobilisation and to encourage physiotherapy in order to prevent fixed deformities. Physiotherapy and rehabilitation must be individualised for the patient. Timely use of splints or callipers may prolong active gait for years. Occasionally surgery for tendon transfer[10] or flexion contractures may be necessary but the price to pay may be discomfort from several operations and frequent hospital admissions with only transitory benefit. Eventually the energy expended from walking and the risk of falls and injury make the need for a wheelchair inevitable. Spinal supports, chair moulds and chest physiotherapy may reduce the likelihood of respiratory infections.

Treatment

Treatment of orthopaedic complications of neuromuscular disease may seem to be a chaotic and complicated task. Therapy becomes simple and effective with the setting of short and long-term goals. However, it is important that therapeutic goals be kept realistic based on knowledge of the natural history of the individual neuromuscular diseases as well as an understanding of the pathophysiology which causes dysfunction.

Physiological aberrations

Loss of cerebral control modulating inhibition of the simple reflex arcs results in clinical spasticity, which is a common feature of many neurological diseases and which produces hypertonicity and hyperreflexia. Purposeful movement is affected, acquisition of motor landmarks is delayed and abnormal posturing leads to contractures.

Loss of anterior horn cells results in denervation of muscle. The severity of muscle weakness reflects the degree of denervation and eventually atrophy of muscle with flaccid paralysis develops. This weakness interferes with the ability to balance the centre of gravity and to maintain articular stability. Locomotor skills are adversely affected and contractures frequently occur.

Fatigable muscle weakness, worsening with activity, may reflect failure of neurotransmission at the neuromuscular junction, resulting in the classical clinical finding of myasthenia. Although this is a very dramatic finding, it is fortunately rare.

Myotonia is defined as the inability to relax muscle after a sustained contraction and it produces problems which range from minor annoyance to significant loss of function. Patients with myotonic dystrophy may become severely disabled as they age. Eventually orthopaedic treatment may become necessary in order to allow the individual to function.

Symptoms may be associated with ultrastructural abnormalities in muscle. Congenital myopathic disease is being diagnosed more frequently because of increased awareness of these conditions. Advancement in techniques to identify ultrastructural abnormalities in muscle has resulted in an apparent increase in the incidence of congenital myopathies. Similarly, recognition of metabolic myopathic disease is increasing with developments in muscle cytochemistry.

Motor and sensory dysfunction may occur as the result of degenerative peripheral and central nervous system pathology. There is usually an hereditary component to these syndromes. Sensory involvement is frequently minimal and since it does not produce marked impairment, patients are frequently unaware of sensory change. The motor component produces significant muscle weakness and imbalance and these result in functional and static orthopaedic pathology which can severely interfere with locomotion.

Within the scope of this text, it is impossible to deal with the therapeutic considerations of each of these individual diseases. A rational approach to the clinical problems is more important since these problems are shared by many different diseases. Although accurate diagnosis is necessary to predict prognosis it is quite appropriate to approach the subject from the standpoint of clinical management of the symptom. In order to illustrate the management of these therapeutic problems, four models have been selected: cerebral palsy, muscular dystrophy, the hereditary sensory-motor neuropathies and myelomeningocele.

Specific clinical problems

From the orthopaedic prospective, neuromuscular diseases have their greatest impact on motor skills and ambulation. Problems with maintaining head control, trunk stability, effective sitting postures and useful mobility make it impossible for the child to realise his intellectual potential and to lead a socially useful life. In keeping with the goal-oriented approach to therapy, a number of clinical problems are seen repetitively in the various neuromuscular diseases. These problems form the basis for clinical therapy.

Contracture

Permanent shortening of muscle is a common complication of many neuromuscular diseases.

During childhood muscle grows in length by adding sarcomeres to the myotendinous junction. The major stimulus for increasing muscle length under physiological conditions is repetitive stretching of the muscle to its maximal length. When this stretching does not occur, the muscle contracts. In the early stages of the development of contracture it is possible to regain some length. For this reason, occupational and physical therapy are important for maintenance of range of motion. However, once a contracture develops no amount of physical therapy will recapture the lost length. Repeated attempts to stretch in the presence of an unyielding myostatic contracture will result in muscle or tendon injury.

Because of the decreased excursion of the muscle, limited range of motion of the affected joints results. Eventually the capsule and peripheral soft tissue structures around these joints also become contracted. Thus there are two reasons for decreased range of motion: (i) the decrease in range of motion produced by the short muscle; (ii) decreased range of motion produced by para-articular soft tissue contractures.

The most important therapeutic goal in the management of contractures is prevention. Occupational and physical therapy can do much to prevent the development of these particularly deforming and disabling changes. Once these changes occur the only successful clinical management is surgical lengthening of the contracted soft tissues. In the case of the contracted joint structures, this requires wide surgical release. In the case of the myotendinous unit, lengthening of the tendon is the treatment of choice. It should be noted that lengthening of the tendon does not increase the length of the muscle. Lengthening of the tendon simply allows a greater excursion of joint motion because the distance between the origin and insertion of the muscle has effectively been increased. The distance that the muscle mass itself traverses during contraction remains unchanged. Increased range of motion occurs at the expense of some loss of strength.

Imbalance

Purposeful coordinated movement and quality activity require that the individual joints in the extremities be balanced. This balance allows smooth, efficient activity and prevents the development of contracted para-articular tissues which may result when joints are continually held in one position. Balance may be upset by two very specific sets of circumstances. Firstly balance may be compromised when the power in the agonists and antagonists becomes unequal, and secondly, balanced activity may be disturbed when selective muscles are continually firing out of phase.

Especially in the case of unbalanced strength between opposing muscle groups, static deformity of the parts may result. A good example of this principle occurs when the tendo Achillis is inadvertently overlengthened surgically. The gastrocsoleus complex becomes significantly weakened, the posterior and lateral compartments are forced to assume some of the load through flexor augmentation, and the hindfoot–midfoot complex takes on a cavoid configuration (Fig. 9.3). This problem is

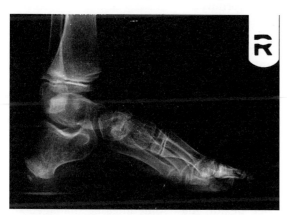

Figure 9.3 Cavus deformity resulting from overlengthening of the tendo Achillis. The ankle is maximally dorsiflexed in the ankle mortise and the forefoot is plantarflexed through the midtarsal joints.

best prevented by careful preoperative evaluation and attention to preoperative muscle strength assessment. Joint contractures can be prevented by well thought out bracing plans or by appropriate muscle transfer designed to support and to strengthen the activity of the weakened muscle.

Managing imbalance caused by out-of-phase muscle activity is an entirely different problem. This imbalance is the result of a strong muscle being activated or contracting at an inappropriate time. Transfer of a strong muscle to support out-of-phase activity usually fails even in the neurologically intact individual. In most cases these transferred muscles ultimately function as tenodeses.

Volitional control

One of the consequences of some central nervous diseases is loss of volitional control over muscle activity. This loss of control may be total or incomplete. The effect is that the child lacks the ability to perform controlled and coordinated movements and in addition he may have difficulty in locating body parts in space. The child may also have difficulty initiating a given motor response and at the same time, destructive patterned movements may take place. Occupational and physical therapy may help the child to suppress these patterned activities. These therapies may also assist the child to recruit new neuronal pathways in order to develop some purposeful activity.[15, 16] When this does not occur, carefully designed bracing is needed to overcome the loss of purposeful activity.

Persisting primitive reflexes

Primitive reflexes that persist into childhood may produce patterned activities which are evoked by an appropriate stimulus. In some cases (e.g. the symmetrical and asymmetrical tonic neck reflexes) mass activity is evoked by body part position. In almost all cases, these reflexes produce activities which are counterproductive to smooth efficient locomotion.

Seven of these reflexes are significant because they may be used to predict walking ability. Bleck[17] has designed a grading system which uses these seven primitive reflexes as predictors of independent ambulation (Table 9.1).

Specific foot and ankle problems in cerebral palsy

Equinus

The most common problem associated with cerebral palsy is ankle equinus. By definition,

Table 9.1   Predicting walking potential according to Bleck

Detrimental reflexes (score one point if present)	Favourable reflexes (score one point if absent)
Asymmetrical tonic neck reflex	Foot placement reaction
Neck righting reflex	Parachute reflex
Symmetrical tonic neck reflex	
Moro reflex	
Extensor thrust	

Prognosis	
0 points	= good prognosis
1 point	= guarded prognosis
2 or more points	= poor prognosis

equinus deformity exists when there is insufficient dorsiflexion of the ankle to allow for toe clearance during swing phase of the gait cycle and for heel contact at the initiation of stance phase. Equinus may produce excessive knee and ankle flexion as compensatory mechanisms to allow the toes to clear the ground during the swing phase (Fig. 9.4a, b, c, d). However, more commonly, equinus deformity of the ankle in cerebral palsy produces major gait alterations during stance phase. There are two patterns which are frequently seen. The first pattern is one in which the initial part of stance phase is initiated by toe contact. This is then followed by a modified full flat pattern which operates through the remaining one-half of stance phase. A second commonly produced gait pattern in stance phase is limited to toe contact with the heel never coming to the ground. The first pattern is frequently referred to as a toe–heel pattern and the second is referred to as toe-to-toe gait pattern.

Ankle equinus may be partially compensated for by subtalar joint pronation. Therefore there are two potential mechanisms for dorsiflexing the foot above neutral. The major excursion of motion (therefore the most physiologic) is at the level of the ankle. However, within certain defined limits, subtalar joint pronation can allow just enough dorsiflexion of the distal and lateral portions of the foot to clear the ground. When gastrocsoleus tone is high and body weight is comparatively small, the toe-to-toe pattern predominates. When increased body mass becomes great enough to

overcome the hypertonicity and the stretch reflex, then an equinovalgus deformity is produced.

When equinus operates for a sufficient period of time, the end result is the development of myostatic contracture of the triceps mechanism. This contracture becomes unyielding, and the altered gait pattern becomes fixed and permanent.

When tibialis posterior is spastic, a pattern of equinovarus may result. There may be some associated adduction of the forefoot and midfoot, and the whole picture may be complicated by a forefoot varus deformity when tibialis anterior is also involved.

The treatment of equinus and associated deformities should begin before the child begins to walk. Early physical therapy intervention maintains range of motion and prevents the development of contracture. This form of therapy should be started early without delay and the goal is to prevent fixation of the deformity.

The mainstay of therapy is bracing as long as the range of motion can be maintained. The equinus component of the deformity is controlled by designing an ankle–foot orthosis (AFO) with the heel in the same plane as the long axis of the tibia. The ankle is neutral in the sagittal plane. This may be accomplished as long as there are no hip and knee flexion contractures. Failure to take hip and knee flexion contractures into account will result in a persisting toe-walking gait when the child wears the AFO (Fig. 9.4d). In the absence of fixed hip flexion and knee flexion deformity, dynamic knee flexion may sometimes be managed by adding a ground reaction plate to the proximal portion of the ankle–foot orthosis. Occasionally knee flexion or hyperextension in gait may be controlled by bracing the ankle in slight plantar flexion or dorsiflexion respectively.

Equinovalgus patterns may be managed in much the same way as simple equinus. An AFO incorporating a well moulded heel seat and a well contoured medial longitudinal arch will control this deformity provided that the patient maintains a passive range of motion of the ankle which allows sufficient dorsiflexion above neutral that the patient is not required to pronate the subtalar joint to allow the ankle to be neutral.

Equinovarus patterns are almost impossible

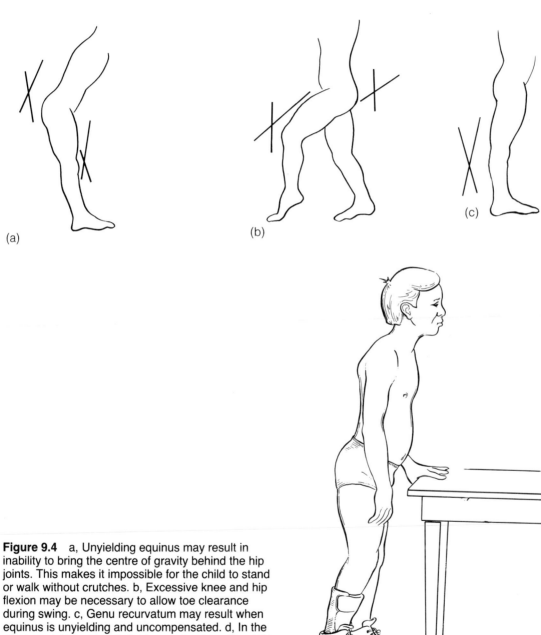

Figure 9.4   a, Unyielding equinus may result in inability to bring the centre of gravity behind the hip joints. This makes it impossible for the child to stand or walk without crutches. b, Excessive knee and hip flexion may be necessary to allow toe clearance during swing. c, Genu recurvatum may result when equinus is unyielding and uncompensated. d, In the presence of knee or hip flexion contracture, the child may 'stand or walk on his toes' – even in ankle–foot orthotics.

to brace. Although the equinus component is fairly straightforward, attempting to use orthotics to pronate the subtalar joint in the presence of spasticity almost always fails. Fractional lengthening of tibialis posterior (with lengthening of the tendo Achillis when a fixed contracture coexists) works well.[18-23] This surgery must be followed by the use of a carefully prescribed ankle–foot orthosis in order to maintain the correction.

When equinus becomes fixed by myostatic contracture physical therapy will not help. Since the foot and ankle cannot be placed in the desired position, bracing is contraindicated; it then becomes necessary to lengthen the tendo Achillis in order to bring the patient back to a functional state in which he can then be braced.

Before surgery is performed, careful attention must be paid in order to select the proper procedure. Although there are a number of procedures described, all may be classified into two categories. The first includes all procedures designed to lengthen the Achilles tendon. This goal may be accomplished by sectioning the tendon longitudinally and then by making proximal and lateral cuts in different directions so that when the tendon is subjected to stretch, the ends separate and slide along each other. The Z-plasty is the best example of this procedure (Fig. 9.5). Multiple hemi-sections of the tendon may also be made according to the technique of Hoke. When the tendon is then subjected to longitudinal stretch, these hemi-sections separate, and thus the tendon will separate longitudinally. The sliding component of the repair allows the tendon to remain in continuity (Fig. 9.6). This latter procedure can be performed percutaneously. It has been found in many cases that the Hoke type procedure is more satisfactory than the Z-plasty technique in children who have cerebral palsy because such children tend to have less postoperative muscle spasm. However, the disadvantage of the Hoke type procedure is that only a comparatively small lengthening can be achieved by this technique. When the surgeon underestimates the amount of lengthening required, tendon continuity may be lost and this will result in excessive scarring in the tendo Achillis and also convalescence will be delayed significantly.

When tibialis anterior is involved, it some-

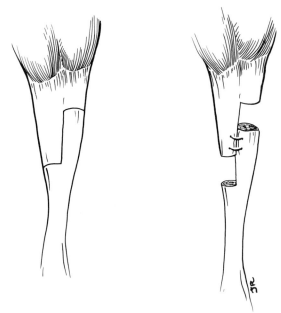

Figure 9.5 The Z-plasty of the tendo Achillis. The slide is constructed by creating a longitudinal splint in the tendon along its long axis. Peripheral cuts are then made as indicated. The separated segments of the tendon are allowed to slide. Integrity is maintained by suture of the arms of the cut tendon.

times becomes necessary to balance its effect on the forefoot. This may be accomplished in one of two ways: (i) The tendon can be moved laterally. It is important to move the tendon only as far in a lateral direction that it no longer inverts (supinates) the forefoot. When it is moved too far laterally a deformity in the opposite direction will result. (ii) Tibialis anterior may be split, with the lateral half being transferred to the area of the cuboid.[24] When performed properly, this procedure will balance the forefoot satisfactorily (Fig. 9.7a, b).

Hallux varus

Adduction deformity of the hallux may occur in cerebral palsy and most frequently, the pathology rests in the abductor hallucis, with early contracture of this muscle occurring. Generally, non-operative techniques (such as physical therapy, straight and outflare last shoes) fail. The problem is a surgical one. Thompson described a procedure in which he excised the entire abductor hallucis.[25] This procedure is rarely performed because of

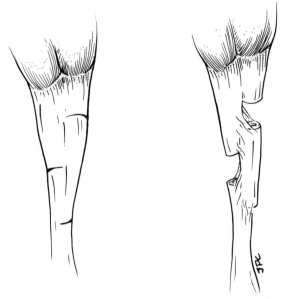

Figure 9.6 Tendon lengthening by the technique of Hoke. The transverse incisions are made in the tendon from the periphery to midline as indicated. The tendon is stressed longitudinally and the cut ends are allowed to slide. No sutures are used and the procedure can be performed through percutaneous stab incisions.

injury to the plantar neurovascular bundles, iatrogenic hallux valgus and because cosmetically unacceptable appearances have resulted. Tenotomy at the level of the first metatarsal base has also been described,[26, 27] although the possibility of contracture through the cut section of the muscle needs to be taken into consideration. Either lengthening or transfer of the distal abductor tendon with release of the muscle from the plantomedial skin and the medial first metatarsal has been very successful.

Hallux abductovalgus

Hallux abductovalgus occurs frequently in patients with cerebral palsy with the majority of cases beginning in the pre-teen years and with the deformity tending to progress rapidly. Since the condition is caused by muscle imbalance, soft tissue procedures (which are usually successful in the neurologically normal population) almost always fail. Surgery for this deformity needs to be extremely aggressive in patients with cerebral

palsy. In order to prevent progression or recurrence, it is frequently necessary to perform an arthrodesis of the first metatarsophalangeal joint. When there is an associated metatarsus primus elevatus, a 'reverse Jones' procedure is indicated, i.e. the tendon of flexor hallucis longus is transferred to the first metatarsal head.

Hammer toe deformities

Hammer toes are most likely to develop when there is augmentative action of the long toe flexors in an attempt to overcome weakened ankle plantar flexors. This deformity may be complicated by spasticity or weakness of the intrinsic muscles which should normally stabilise the proximal phalanges of the lesser toes. The development of painful keratotic lesions on the toes is a natural consequence and may progress to ulceration. Severe flexion deformity is incompatible with footwear.

Interphalangeal joint fusion coupled with appropriate tenotomy and capsulotomy frequently proves successful. When patients have no ambulatory potential the digits may be maintained in an acceptable alignment by performing tenotomies of the long and short flexor tendons. This latter procedure is purely palliative and should be reserved only for those patients who do not bear weight, but who have subjective symptoms from the digital deformities.

Calcaneus deformity

By definition, calcaneus occurs when the heel is on the ground, but the toes are not. This is rarely seen as a primary deformity in cerebral palsy, but it may occur as an iatrogenic complication following overlengthening of the tendo Achillis. When this happens, the foot adopts a calcaneocavus appearance. The ankle remains in calcaneus but the forefoot and midfoot plantarflex in global fashion in order that the metatarsal heads may reach the ground. Because of the calcaneus change which occurs in the ankle the patient actually has significant limitation of dorsiflexion since the dorsum of the talar neck abuts against the anterior lip of the tibia (Fig. 9.3).

Calcaneocavus deformity is best managed by preventing its occurrence in the first place. Careful preoperative assessment and strict

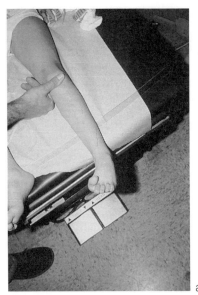
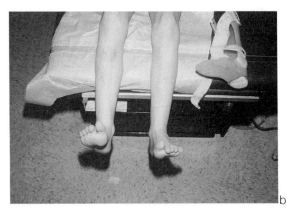

a

b

Figure 9.7   a, The left equinus with hindfoot and forefoot varus deformity in a child with spastic diplegia. b, Following tendo Achillis lengthening, fractional lengthening of tibialis posterior at the myotendinous junction and split tibialis anterior transfer.

adherence to technique are therefore mandatory for all cases in which tendo Achillis lengthening is contemplated.

Attempts to shorten an overlengthened tendo Achillis rarely succeed. Radical plantar release and transfer of functioning tendons to the posterior calcaneus may be of some benefit but the advantages and disadvantages must be weighed carefully in individual cases. It must be remembered that muscles which may be transferred are actually out-of-phase in function.[28–30]

Foot and ankle deformities in patients with muscular dystrophy

Equinus

The progressive form of muscular dystrophy described in boys by Duchenne is extremely well documented and studied and motor deterioration and subsequent deformities may be predicted. It is important to remember that certain static changes seen in patients with Duchenne's muscular dystrophy may actually be necessary for continued function:[31, 32] e.g.

equinus contractures of the ankle occur almost invariably as a compensatory mechanism for more proximal weakness. Without equinus, the patient would have extreme difficulty in balancing the centre of gravity posterior to the hip joint and anterior to the knee axis.

Initial functional losses begin proximally. Hip extensors are involved early on in the course of the disease and changes in gait are the first manifestation. The progressive weakness of hip extensors results in an inability to maintain the hip in extension by muscle power alone. In order to keep upright, the boy must extend the hips by posterior displacement of the centre of gravity behind the axis of hip motion. This requires increasing the lumbar lordosis so that the centre of gravity (which is located relatively high in the thorax) now comes to lie behind the hip joint axis. Additionally the hip abductors are also involved early. The end result is a gait pattern which is characterised by waddling from side to side as well as forward thrusting of the pelvis caused by hyperlordosis of the lumbar spine and decreased thoracic kyphosis.

As the disease worsens the knee extensors become involved. In order to continue functioning, the boy preferentially develops a toe-to-toe gait pattern. As this postural activity persists, over time the gastrocsoleus complex develops myostatic contractures and a fixed ankle equinus results which eventually becomes complicated by heel varus as the child becomes wheelchair-bound.

Once the child becomes chair-bound, equinus becomes a major problem. The child can no longer position his feet flat on the wheelchair platforms and this tends to destabilise the pelvis. This destabilisation results in pelvic obliquity, progressive knee and hip flexion contractures, hip abduction contractures and it may also play a role in the rapid progression of scoliosis in these children.

An additional disadvantage of the development of equinovarus contractures is that it becomes impossible to fit shoes on such malpositioned feet. It is important to remember that even the child with advanced muscular dystrophy must occasionally go outdoors in inclement weather.

The major therapeutic goal in those children with Duchenne muscular dystrophy is to keep them ambulating for as long as possible. This requires early aggressive physical therapy to maintain useful ranges of motion and to prevent the development of disabling contractures.

As long as the gait remains efficient, the child can remain walking in hyperlordosis, knee flexion and ankle equinus thus allowing him to participate in a relatively wide variety of physical activities.

Well designed and carefully made ankle foot orthoses are used at night in order to prevent the development of early and severe ankle contractures. For boys who have existing contractures bracing slows down the process.[33] Bracing the ankle at neutral during ambulation causes problems when the knee extensors become weak. Once this happens it becomes necessary to design knee–ankle–foot orthoses which will allow the child to function in some equinus, the knee slightly flexed but stabilised by the orthotic and weightbearing on the ischial tuberosity. Such devices must be kept light in order to allow the weakened boy to function.

Weakness

Eventually weakness becomes so profound that the child ceases to have any functional ambulation. When the child becomes wheelchair-bound it becomes necessary to design a trunk and pelvic support system to maintain the child upright. Careful attention to the set of the wheelchair is important in order to prevent the development of early pelvic obliquity. Support for the foot and ankle should be designed to keep the foot on the wheelchair platform as close to neutral in the sagittal plane as possible. Motorised wheelchairs eventually become the method of transportation.

Even though function becomes extremely limited, it is still necessary to continue active physical therapy in order to prevent the development of contractures which will interfere with normal sitting and sleeping. Marked knee and hip flexion contractures make it impossible for the child to sleep on his back. Hip flexion and adduction contractures make sitting difficult and they also interfere with perineal care.

Osteopenia

In certain cases osteoporosis caused by disuse is a significant problem. Weakened bone becomes liable to fracture from what otherwise would be trivial trauma. Even before the child ceases ambulating altogether, significant osteoporosis has already developed. Osteoporosis and progressive muscle weakness are both accelerated by immobilisation. Injury and limb surgery are major setback events in the child's motor function. It becomes necessary to start ambulation as soon as possible after trauma and surgery in order to maintain the previous level of activity. When function is lost, it is possible through therapy and careful bracing to recover some of the previous skills.

The hereditary sensory-motor neuropathies

In 1968 Dyck and Lambert classified the combined sensory and motor neuropathies with heritable characteristics. Although this classification has been revised by several different authors it is still very useful today.[34, 35]

These diseases are characterised pathophysiologically by degenerative changes in the peripheral nerves which result from loss of myelin and from fragmentation of the axons. It is quite probable that these conditions represent a spectrum of degenerating conditions affecting the peripheral and central nervous systems. The classification of these varying syndromes is outlined in Table 9.2.

Table 9.2   The hereditary motor-sensory neuropathies (HMSN types)

HMSN type I	Hypertrophic neuropathy (peroneal muscle atrophy)
HMSN type II	Neuronal type of peroneal muscle atrophy
HMSN type III	Hypertrophic neuropathy of infancy (Dejerine–Sottas)
HMSN type IV	Hypertrophic neuropathy with excess phytanic acid (Refsum's disease)
HMSN type V	Peripheral neuropathy with spastic paraplegia

The most familiar and best studied of these is Charcot–Marie–Tooth syndrome. Affected patients may either fully express this disease or they may present with formes frustes with varying degrees of neurological expression. Certain patients have early and severe disabling symptoms, while others run a much more benign course.

The initial presentation almost always affects the feet. Frequently abnormality in gait is the initial complaint and occasionally the gait is described as clumsy. Instability in walking may actually be the common factor in most disturbances. This is especially noted in the invertor–evertor muscle pairs. Although uncommon, equinus may be a presenting gait disturbance. When this occurs, posterior contractures are usually well established.

Cavus deformity

With progression, hindfoot varus becomes a major clinical finding. Since the anterior and lateral compartment muscles of the leg are affected early, the peroneals and tibialis anterior show early weakness but tibialis posterior is fairly well preserved. This muscle then becomes the deforming force which produces varus deformity. As further progression occurs, a cavoadductovarus pattern presents.

Two patterns of cavovarus may occur. In the first pattern subtalar joint motion becomes re-

stricted. However, supinatory motion is usually unaffected. Subtalar joint pronation becomes limited and a primary hindfoot varus deformity results. In certain patients this hindfoot varus deformity is compensated for, while in others the hindfoot varus becomes totally uncompensated.

In the second variation, pronatory excursion of the subtalar joint is preserved. However, the forefoot takes on a cavoadductus configuration which produces a rigid forefoot valgus. These patients then function with the subtalar joint abnormally supinated.

It is important to make the distinction between these two since the therapeutic approach to each of these is radically different. The Coleman Block Test helps to distinguish the two types (Fig.9.8a, b).

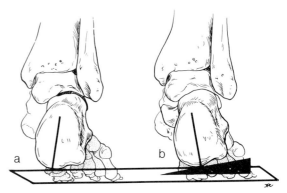

Figure 9.8   The Coleman Block Test is designed to separate fixed rearfoot varus deformity from the flexible type. a, In stance, the heel is in varus. b, A wedge or block is placed under the lateral heel and lateral forefoot. If the hindfoot varus is flexible (sufficient range of motion of the subtalar joint complex), the heel will move into valgus when the foot is placed on the wedge as shown. If there is no subtalar range of motion, the heel will stay locked in varus.

The intrinsic muscles of the feet and the hands are involved early and the loss of stability normally provided by these intrinsic muscles results in flexion deformity of the digits. This is complicated by the fact that flexor substitution is an important compensation for muscle weakness and early hammer and mallet toe deformities result. As the disease progresses, myostatic contractures develop. These contractures further the static deformity of cavoadductovarus.

Although there is definitely sensory involvement in many of these syndromes, patients do retain protective sensation and they do not seem to develop ulcers or neuropathic joint changes. Therapy centres around the prevention of contractures and the management of static deformities. Early involvement in physical therapy is important since major contractions can be delayed.

Gait disturbances

The gait disturbances are somewhat more difficult to manage and there are two components which need to be addressed here: (i) mediolateral instability is usually a major problem. Such patients feel unstable, frequently develop supinatory ankle injuries, and additionally wear shoes markedly. (ii) In more advanced cases, anterior compartment weakness results in foot drop and such patients then have difficulty clearing the floor during swing phase. Posterior contractures result in fixed ankle equinus.

Effective management of both problems may be achieved by the use of an ankle–foot orthotic which allows both frontal and sagittal stability of the foot and the ankle. Although it is possible to hinge the ankle in such a way that plantar flexion is limited while relatively unrestricted dorsiflexion is allowed, most patients do better when the ankle is fixed at or near neutral in the sagittal plane. Although an ankle–foot orthotic provides stability, it does not affect the overall relentless progression of the cavus deformity.

The role of in-shoe orthoses is somewhat controversial. Frequently Schaffer plates are used and although they do not modify the progression of the cavus deformity, they do provide some symptomatic relief for pain and fatigue which occurs in the plantar musculature. The role of in-shoe orthotics which are designed to evert the heel by posting the forefoot in valgus is even more controversial. Since these children have relatively plastic skeletal structures as a consequence of their skeletal immaturity, there has been some concern that devices of this type might actually worsen any deformity in the long term. Although this has never been satisfactorily proved, the possibility must be kept in mind.

Eventually the cavus deformity becomes so advanced that surgical intervention is necessary. Conceptually there are two approaches to the surgical management of the cavoid component in the hereditary sensory motor neuropathies. The first consideration is intimately concerned with the age of the patient. Even in childhood the rapid development of the cavus deformity becomes intolerable and even in those patients who are very skeletally immature steps must be taken to arrest the advancement of this deformity. Frequently it is impossible to achieve full correction and as an interim measure the approach is one of slowing or stopping the progression at the expense of incomplete reduction. Since tibialis posterior is relatively spared during the course of Charcot–Marie–Tooth syndrome, this muscle may be regarded as the principal deforming force. Transfer of tibialis posterior through the interosseous membrane into the dorsolateral aspect of the foot in the area of the third cuneiform is a logical approach to the problem.[36,37] It also becomes necessary to release the contracted plantar fascia. In certain cases too it becomes necessary to enhance dorsiflexion of the forefoot by transferring the digital extensors into the metatarsals according to the techniques outlined by Hibbs[38] and Jones.[39]

In adolescence and early adulthood osteotomy of the midfoot becomes the therapy of choice. The Cole procedure[40] involves resection of a wedge of bone from the lesser tarsus and when combined with a plantar release the cavus component will effectively be reduced. This procedure has one significant drawback in that it produces overall shortening of the foot and this may be intolerable because of the already small size of the involved foot. The Japas procedure,[41] when combined with a plantar release, reduces the cavoid architecture without producing the additional shortening of the foot that is undesirably produced by the Cole procedure. This method has been proven to be satisfactory.

Digital deformities are a major problem with respect to patient comfort. The proximal and distal interphalangeal articulations become contracted early in the course of the disease. These joint contractures interfere with shoe fitting and produce subjective discomfort when the dorsa of the interphalangeal joints rub on the shoe, although this does not occur usually until adolescence. Since such children are older it is appropriate to manage the digital deformities by appropriate joint resection, tendon transfer and interdigital joint arthrodeses.

Myelomeningocele

Patients with myelomeningocele present an unusual orthopaedic challenge. By virtue of the pathology, function of the spinal cord cephalad to the lesion itself remains intact but function at and below the level of the lesion is lost.

Functional levels may be asymmetric when comparing one side to the other. Segments of the cord below the level of the defect may remain intact. The simple reflex arcs governed by the cord at this level may also remain intact. However, these are not under modulation by higher areas of the central nervous system. Although there is no volitional control, there may be spontaneous activity. This spontaneous activity may make functional level determination more difficult for the inexperienced and it may raise false hope among the family. More importantly these intact reflex arcs may result in imbalance of muscle with consequent deformity.

Functional level may actually deteriorate.[42] Most frequently this is caused by progressive tethering of the spinal cord which produces symptoms with growth. Additionally hydromyelia, syringomyelia, progressing hydrocephalus and shunt failure may present with deteriorating peripheral control and loss of trunk stability and milestone regression.

Once the spine lesion is closed, rehabilitation of the child begins. This involves the efforts of orthopaedic specialists, neurosurgeons, urologists, paediatricians, physical therapists, occupational therapists and orthotists. Since most patients with myelomeningocele have caudal lesions, much of the rehabilitation is directed towards the spine, hips, knees and feet. The lower the level, the better the overall prognosis for function and independent ambulation. In order to fully appreciate the complexities of these problems, it is important to review the muscle activities in the lower extremities as they relate to the functional neurological levels.[43] It must be borne in mind that there is some disagreement about the relationship between levels and function.

Although innervation of an individual muscle may come from several levels, there is a certain innervational threshold which is required for meaningful function. This threshold is usually more caudal than the level required to produce deformity.

Levels

The iliopsoas muscle is the major hip flexor. It derives its innervation from L1, 2, 3. Some significant function of the iliopsoas is present when the child has functional activity down to the level of L1.

The quadriceps and the adductors may be considered together since they derive their innervations from L2, 3, 4. Although the quadriceps is considered to be an L4 muscle from the standpoint of deep tendon reflexes, considerable quadriceps function is present when L3 is intact.

Tibialis anterior derives its innervation from L4, 5. When L4 is intact, tibialis anterior is capable of producing a major foot deformity since the remaining anterior compartment muscles are not functioning.

Extensor hallucis longus, extensor digitorum longus and brevis, gluteus medialis and the medial hamstrings all derive their major innervation from L5.

Tibialis posterior and flexor digitorum longus derive their major innervations from L5 and S1. Flexor hallucis longus completes the posterior compartment, and derives its innervation from L5, S1, 2.

Peroneus longus and brevis, gastrocnemius, soleus, gluteus maximus and the lateral hamstrings are all considered to be fundamentally S1 muscles.

The foot intrinsics are S2, 3, 4 muscles. Additionally, at this level, bladder control and anal sphincter control are acquired.

Armed with this information, it is possible to consider the functional level as a predictor of useful activity as well as a predictor of static deformity when muscles remain unbalanced. It is important to remember that both motor deficits and sensory loss occur together. The patient has not only paralysis but also loss of protective sensation for the skin and joints. Additionally vasomotor stability below the functioning level is frequently involved.

When L1 is the lowest functional level there

is usually no volitional activity at the hip, knee and ankle. There may be a degree of flexion deformity at the hip due to some activity at the iliopsoas, but the knees and ankles predictably are flail.

When L2 is the lowest functioning level there is volitional flexion and adduction activity at the hips and also there is some degree of partial extension at the level of the knees, but the ankles are flail. Since iliopsoas and the adductors are unopposed, predictably there will be flexion and adduction deformity at the level of the hip. Generally there is no deformity at the knee and the foot is usually flail.

When L3 is the lowest functioning level there is active hip flexion and adduction as well as extension activity of the knee. There is no ankle activity. Flexion, adduction and external rotation deformity at the hip are observed. The knee is fixed in extension and the ankle is flail.

When L4 is the lowest functioning level, the child has active flexion and adduction at the hip. The knees will extend and the foot will dorsiflex and invert. The hip is fixed in flexion, adduction and lateral rotation but the potential for dislocation of the hips is high. The knees demonstrate extension deformity and the feet demonstrate dorsiflexion and inversion deformity.

When L5 is the lowest functioning level the hips have active flexion, adduction and abduction. The knees show active extension as well as partial flexion which is produced by activity of the medial hamstrings. The feet will dorsiflex and invert. Generally the hips show flexion deformity but they are balanced in the frontal plane. The knees are partially balanced by active extension from the quadriceps along with some flexion from the medial hamstrings. The feet show typical calcaneus deformity since the entire anterior compartment is now functional. The posterior compartment is still paralysed. On occasion the feet will show severe pronation deformity because of partially innervated but unopposed peroneals.

When S1 is the lowest functioning level, the hips have full activity. The hips are almost completely balanced by the addition of most of the gluteal maximus. The knees are fully balanced because of the addition of the lateral hamstrings. The feet show full dorsiflexion,

inversion and eversion but there is only partial plantar flexion. The hips and knees are both balanced without resulting deformity. The incidence of toe deformities, calcaneovalgus and vertical talus is common with function at this level.

When S2 is the lowest functioning level, the hips, knees and feet are almost totally functional except for certain of the foot intrinsic muscles. The hips and knees are balanced and so also are the ankles. The absence of certain of the intrinsic foot muscles results in late onset cavovarus and also flexion deformities of the toes.

The therapeutic intervention for myelomeningocele may be divided into four periods: the immediate postnatal period; the period between birth and the onset of ambulation; the period of functional walking; and the period of late adolescence and adulthood.

It is important to evaluate the infant shortly after birth. Before closure of the defect it may be difficult to assess realistically the true functional level. Some additional functional loss may occur during operative closure. The effects of hydrocephalus may make it difficult to determine function. Attention should be directed toward evaluating deformities of the extremities. Three factors are operative: (i) muscle imbalance produced by a loss of volitional control will produce predictable deformity; (ii) in the absence of volitional control a deformity may result when spasticity from persisting reflex arcs below the level of the defect occurs; (iii) intrauterine malpositioning may result in deformity caused by contractures from undesirable prenatal postures.

Deformities such as equinus, equinovarus and calcaneus of the feet require to be treated early. Flexion and hyperextension deformities of the knees may occur and these may be very disabling when left untreated. Hip instability and dislocation require to be recognised early and treated appropriately if long-lasting stability is possible. This is particularly important when dislocation is unilateral. The early management of foot and ankle deformities is complicated by the fact that the infant's medical condition may make it difficult to manage these problems effectively. For a period of time following closure the infant must remain prone. It becomes somewhat impractical to have both feet unavailable for intravenous access and heel sticks for haematological test-ing. During this critical period therapy is largely confined to manipulation. Once the infant is stable, taping and plaster of Paris splinting may be applied as indicated.

Presuming the functional levels are appro-priate, a variable period of time will elapse before any useful independent ambulation is possible. During this period continued splint-ing and physical therapy are in order. Since sensation is impaired, meticulous care of the skin is necessary to prevent breakdown. Orth-otics must fit well. Additionally growth makes continued orthotic monitoring mandatory.

When the child can maintain hip extension and knee extension some independent ambu-lation is expected. Even when the child cannot manage hip and knee extension by himself, appropriate orthotics may perform this move-ment for him. Orthotic management and physical therapy will allow the child to max-imise his potential for independent ambula-tion.

Children who have no potential for indepen-dent ambulation need to be placed in the upright position in order for them to ad-equately interact with the environment and achieve their maximal possible mental poten-tial.

For those patients who have high functional levels, the physiological burden of ambulation becomes so great that they choose wheelchair transportation for its ease and speed. In these groups too it is important to try to maintain periodic upright posturing in order for them to develop some bone mass. Osteopenia of disuse is a major problem for these patients and fractures become a part of life.

Specific treatment for the feet and ankles depends on the lowest level of function. Indi-vidual muscles derive innervation over several levels but overall function demands complete or almost complete innervation. Incompletely innervated muscles lack sufficient strength and their antagonists will produce deformity.

Ambulation requires hip and knee exten-sion. This extension may come from balanced musculature or it may come from extrinsic bracing. The amount of ambulation becomes level dependent.

Children who have function at S2 and below have no major orthopaedic problems. Sen-sation is intact and the child has protection for the entire foot. The only predictable ortho-paedic problem that may result is instability of the toes as the result of incomplete innervation of the intrinsic muscles. Claw toes may de-velop later in childhood but no immediate therapy is necessary in the majority of cases.

Treatment considerations

Children who function at S1 almost always have balanced knees and hips. All extrinsic muscles to the feet have sufficient strength in order to produce a normal heel-to-toe gait. There may be some weakness of the gastroc-soleus complex. A degree of cavus deformity may result in later childhood. An additional possible complication is flexion deformity of the toes which is produced when the long toe flexors augment a weakened gastrocsoleus group. Observation for progressing cavus de-formity is in order. There is no specific bracing for this possible complication and significant cavus deformity ultimately becomes a surgical problem.

In the grey area between functioning L5 and S1 levels, pes planus is frequently found and this is usually a significant deformity. The ma-jority of these patients do well when UCBL-type orthoses are prescribed provided that the peroneals are not too strong. These devices maintain the heel vertical and prevent the secondary development of an independent forefoot varus.

When the lowest functioning level is L5, the anterior compartment muscles are generally intact. Predictably the resulting deformity is one of calcaneus. For several reasons calcaneus is a very difficult deformity to manage clini-cally, e.g. (i) when the foot is dorsiflexed the only way the child can obtain the upright pos-ition is to assume a crouch position with the hips and the knees flexed; (ii) calcaneus de-formity is very difficult to brace but an AFO with an anterior clamshell will maintain the foot at right angles. The posterior component of such an orthosis then serves to keep the knee extended although occasionally it may be necessary to add a ground reactive component to the anterior of the AFO. In selected cases, transfers from very strong anterior compart-ment muscles to the tendo Achillis will balance the ankle near neutral.[44] This makes it easier to functionally brace these children. Naturally the feet are partially insensate and special attention must be paid toward good brace fitting as well as periodic inspection to prevent the development of trophic ulcers. In spite of such problems many of these children achieve a high degree of independent ambulation throughout adolescence.

Patients whose lowest functioning level is L4 have problems with frontal plane as well as sagittal plane balance. Usually there is function of tibialis anterior which results in a varus position of the forefoot. Frequently there is also a calcaneus component and together the combination of forefoot varus and calcaneus deformity is extremely difficult to brace. A further complication is the fact that much of the foot is insensate. AFOs with carefully designed anterior clamshell components will help to prevent secondary deformity as well as allowing the child a degree of upright posture.

Additional complications in neuromuscular disease

There are a number of additional orthopaedic problems which are common to many of the neuromuscular diseases. Such problems include (a) osteopenia, (b) fractures, (c) antetorsion and (d) internal and external tibial torsion.

Osteopenia

Disuse produces osteopenia and both appendicular and axial skeleton are involved. The problem is partially managed by producing stress loading of the extremities. When functional ambulation is not anticipated, placing the child in the upright position is critical towards developing reasonably strong bone in the extremities and in the spine. Consequently, considerable effort is made both in physical therapy and in orthotic management to ensure that the child will spend some time in the upright position.

Fracture

Frequently fractures occur in children with neuromuscular disease. These may occur as a consequence of therapy, or they may be intrinsic to the disease process itself. Even although the likelihood of fractures is well known, classical presenting patterns are frequently overlooked.

Trauma, which might be insignificant under other circumstances, may result in complete or incomplete fracture patterns and additionally fatigue fractures occur. Sudden onset of pain without associated trauma or pain following what should have been insignificant trauma frequently means fracture. Occasionally the fracture patterns are occult. Such fractures resemble stress fractures in other areas of the body and they may not show positive X-ray changes for 5–15 days following the actual insult. Occasionally the fracture pattern may be purely cancellous. The cortex is not involved and the true nature of the problem becomes evident only when cancellous bone condenses in the repair process.

Equinus deformity is a frequent cause of fracture of the calcaneus in children with neuromuscular disease. This may occur at any time but frequently follows immobilisation for medical or surgical procedures. Body weight directed from above through the tibia into the talus is countered by the ground reactive force against the forefoot as well as the upward vector produced by activity of the tendo Achillis. When the ankle will not allow sufficient dorsiflexion for neutral position to be reached, fracture of the posterior body of the calcaneus may result. This may happen spontaneously or it may follow minimal trauma. The initial radiographs are often negative. The physical examination shows oedema in the retrotibial triangle behind the ankle. Generally there is moderate to severe pain when the medial and lateral sides of the posterior calcaneus are compressed. These injuries are best treated by immobilisation. It is imperative that the period of immobilisation be as short as possible to allow both for relief of pain as well as for consolidation of the fracture. Prolonged immobilisation actually worsens the osteoporosis and predisposes the patient to the additional risk of fracture.

Patients with myelomeningocele frequently fracture. This disease is characterised by lack of sensation in all or the major portion of the limb distally. Fractures may occur following immobilisation for medical and surgical procedures.[45–47] A particular risk for fracture occurs when orthoses become too short, e.g. an ankle–foot orthosis may become so small that the proximal portion of the orthosis approaches mid-calf. This produces a significant stress riser and fracture of the tibia can result.

Salter–Harris type I fractures occur at a disproportionately higher incidence in children with myelomeningocele[47] and such fractures may or may not displace. These fractures heal but they do so with very exuberant callus formation. The periosteum may be stripped for some distance away from the cortex and large sub-periosteal haemorrhages result. Since the patient is usually insensate at the level of the fracture, the physical findings draw attention to the fracture. The child may develop swelling in the area with increase in temperature and he may become irritable. Hyperpyrexia frequently occurs and the child may develop a leucocytosis. These clinical findings tend to complicate the picture as it may be difficult to distinguish early infection from fracture. Due to ongoing urological problems, the risk of osteomyelitis and septic joints in such patients is higher than in normal children.

Antetorsion

It is important to recognise the persistence of femoral antetorsion in children with neuromuscular disease. In cerebral palsy, particularly, the incidence of abnormal antetorsion is especially high. It is beyond the scope of this chapter to discuss antetorsion in great detail except to say that angles well above the upper norm for the age produce clinical intoeing. Frequently associated with antetorsion is coxa valga although it is unclear how these two problems are related. Coxa valga does not influence the position of the limb in the sagittal or transverse plane. However, it does influence the amount of femoral head coverage by the acetabulum.

Femoral antetorsion produces clinical intoeing. It cannot be managed by non-operative techniques such as physical therapy and bracing. Unlike the normal child population, antetorsion occurring in neuromuscular disease does not reduce with age. When the problem produces significant gait disturbance in a child who would otherwise ambulate well, it may be necessary to perform a proximal

femoral derotational osteotomy in order to surgically reduce the angle of antetorsion.

Internal and external tibial torsion

Internal and external tibial torsion are frequently seen in patients who have cerebral palsy as well as in patients who have myelomeningocele.[48] These problems generally tend to spare children with muscular dystrophy. The most likely explanation for both internal and external tibial torsion is hamstring imbalance. This may be complicated by modification of toe-off in patients who have fixed internal or external tibial torsion. As a result of this abnormal gait pattern, the problem tends to worsen. Unlike in the normal child, spontaneous change in tibial torsion for the better is unlikely to occur. Provided the problem is static, derotational osteotomy of the tibia will usually provide sufficient correction to justify its performance.

References

1 *Aids to the Examination of the Peripheral Nervous System*. London, Baillière Tindall, 1988.
2 Nelson KB, Ellenberg JH. Epidemiology of cerebral palsy. In *Advances in Neurology* (Ed. BS Schoenberg). New York, Raven Press, 1978, p. 421.
3 Hagberg B, Hagberg G, Olow I. The changing panorama of cerebral palsy in Sweden. 1954–70. II Analysis of the various syndromes. *Acta Paediatr Scand* 1975; 64: 193–200.
4 Papile L, Burstein J, Burstein R *et al*. Incidence and evolution of subependymal hemorrhage: A study of infants with birth weights less than 1500 grams. *J Paediatr* 1978; 92: 529–43.
5 Kudrjavcev T, Schoenberg BS, Kurland LT, Groover RV. Cerebral palsy: survival rates, associated handicaps and distribution of clinical subtype. *Neurology* 1985; 35(6): 900–3.
6 Sparrow S, Zigler F. Evaluation of a patterning treatment for retarded children. *Paediatrics* 1978; 62: 137.
7 Bobath B. The very early treatment of cerebral palsy. *Dev Ment Child Neurol* 1967; 9: 373.
8 Harding A. The inherited ataxias. *Adv Neurol* 1988; 48: 37–46.
9 Ackroyd RS, Finnegan JA, Green SH. Friedreich's ataxia: a clinical review with neurophysiological and echocardiographic findings. *Arch Dis Child* 1984; 59(3): 217–21.
10 Carroll NC. Assessment and management of the

lower extremity in myelodysplasia. *Orthop Clin North Am* 1987; 18(4): 709–24.

11 Liptak GS, Bloss JW, Brisken H, Campbell JE, Herbert EB, Revell GM. The management of children with spinal dysraphism. *J Child Neurol* 1988; 3(1): 3–20.

12 Bird TD. Hereditary motor sensory neuropathies. Charcot Marie Tooth syndrome. *Neurol Clin* 1989; 7(1): 9–23.

13 Miller GM, Hsu JD, Hoffer MM, Rentfro R. Posterior tibial tendon transfer: a review of the literature and analysis of 74 procedures. *J Paediatr Orthop* 1982; 2(4): 363–70.

14 Mandell JL. Dystrophin. The gene and its product. *Nature* 1989; 339(6226): 584–6.

15 Bobath K. The neuropathology of cerebral palsy and its importance in treatment and diagnosis. *Cerebral Palsy Bulletin* 1959; 1(8): 13.

16 Bobath K, Finney N. Re-education of movement patterns in everyday life in the treatment of cerebral palsy. *Occupational Therapy* 1958; 21(6): 23.

17 Bleck EE. Locomotor prognosis in cerebral palsy. *Dev Med Child Neurol* 1975; 17: 18–25.

18 Banks HH. The foot and ankle in cerebral palsy. In *Orthopaedic Aspects of Cerebral Palsy* (Ed. RL Samilson). Philadelphia, JB Lippincott, 1975, p. 213.

19 Baker LD. Triceps surae syndrome in cerebral palsy. *Surgery* 1954; 68: 216.

20 Silfverskiold N. Reduction of the uncrossed two-joint muscles of the leg to one-joint muscles in spastic conditions. *Acta Chir Scand* 1923–1924; 56: 315.

21 Strayer LM. Recession of the gastrocnemius, an operation to relieve spastic contracture of the calf muscles. *J Bone Joint Surg* 1950; 32-A: 671.

22 Vulpius D, Stoffel A. *Orthopaedisch Operationslebre*, 2nd edn. Stuttgard, Ferdinand Enke, 1920.

23 White JW. Torsion of the achilles tendon: its surgical significance. *Arch Surg* 1943; 46: 784.

24 Hoffer MM, Reiswig JA, Garrett AM, Perry J. The split anterior tibial tendon transfer in the treatment of spastic varus hindfoot of childhood. *Orthop Clin North Am* 1974; 5: 31.

25 Thomson SA. Hallux varus and metatarsus varus. *Clin Orthop* 1960; 16: 109.

26 Jones CA, McCrea JD. Tenotomy of the abductor hallucis for correction of residual metatarsus adductus. *J Am Podiatr Med Assoc* 1980; 70(1).

27 McCrea JD. *Paediatric Orthopaedics of the Lower Extremity*. Mount Kisco, Futura Publishing, 1985, p. 313.

28 Banta JV, Sutherland DH, Wyatt M. Anterior tibial transfer to the os calcis with achilles tenodesis for calcaneal deformity in myelomeningocele. *J Paediatr Orthop* 1981; 1: 125.

29 Herndon CH, Strong JM, Heyman CH. Trans-

position of the tibialis anterior in the treatment of paralytic talipes calcaneus. *J Bone Joint Surg* 1956; 38A: 751.

30 Turner JW, Cooper RR. Posterior transposition of the tibialis anterior through the interosseous membrane. *Clin Orthop Rel Res* 1971; 79: 71.

31 Kelly CR, Redford JB, Zilber S, Madden PA. Standing balance in healthy boys and in children with Duchenne muscular dystrophy. *Arch Phys Med Rehabil* 1981; 62: 324.

32 Williams EA, Read L, Ellis A, Morris P, Galasko CSB. The management of equinus deformity in Duchenne muscular dystrophy. *J Bone Joint Surg* 1984; 66B: 546.

33 Seeger BR, Caudrey DJ, Little JD. Progression of equinus deformity in Duchenne muscular dystrophy. *Arch Phys Med Rehabil* 1985; 66: 286.

34 Dyck PJ, Lambert EH. Lower motor and sensory neuron disease with peroneal muscle atrophy. I. Neurologic, genetic and electrophysiologic findings in hereditary polyneuropathies. *Arch Neurol* 1968; 18: 603.

35 Dyck PJ, Lambert EH. Lower motor and primary sensory neuron disease with peroneal muscle atrophy. II. Neurologic, genetic and electrophysiologic findings in various neuronal degenerations. *Arch Neurol* 1968; 18: 619.

36 Williams PE. Restoration of muscle balance of the foot by transfer of the tibialis posterior. *J Bone Joint Surg* 1976; 58B: 217.

37 Tachdjian MO. *Paediatric Orthopaedics*, 2nd edn, Vol. III. Philadelphia, WB Saunders, 1990, p 1680.

38 Hibbs R. An operation for 'claw-foot'. *JAMA* 1919; 73: 1583.

39 Jones R. The soldier's foot and the treatment of common deformities of the foot. *Br Med J* 1916; 1: 749.

40 Cole WH. The treatment of claw-foot. *J Bone Joint Surg* 1940; 22: 895–908.

41 Japas LM. Surgical treatment of pes cavus by tarsal V-osteotomy. Preliminary report. *J Bone Joint Surg* 1968; 50A: 927.

42 Bunch WH, Scarff TB, Dvonch VM. Progressive neurological loss in myelomeningocele patients. *Orthop Trans* 1981; 5: 32.

43 Hoppenfield S. *Orthopedic Neurology: A Diagnostic Guide to Neurologic Levels*. Philadelphia, JB Lippincott, 1977.

44 Sharrard WJW, Grosfield I. The management of deformity and paralysis of the foot in myelomeningocele. *J Bone Joint Surg* 1968; 50B: 457.

45 Anshuetz RH, Freehafer AA, Shaffer JW, Dixon MS. Severe fracture complications in myelodysplasia. *J Paediatr Orthop* 1984; 4: 22.

46 Drennan JC, Freehafer AA. Fractures of the lower extremities in paralytic children. *Clin Orthop Rel Res* 1971; 77: 211.

47 Kumar SJ, Cowell HR, Townsend P. Physeal, metaphyseal and diaphyseal injuries of the lower extemity in children with myelomeningocele. *J Paediatr Orthop* 1984; 4: 25.

48 Diaz LS, Murali JJ, Collins P. Rotational deformities of the lower limb in myelomeningocele. *J Bone Joint Surg* 1984; 66A: 215.

Further reading

Asher M, Olson J. Factors affecting the ambulatory status of patients with spina bifida cystica. *J Bone Joint Surg* 1983; 65A: 350.

Bach J, Alba A, Pilkington LA. Long-term rehabilitation in advanced stage of childhood onset, rapidly progressive muscular dystrophy. *Arch Phys Med Rehabil* 1981; 62: 328.

Bennet GC, Rang M, Jones D. Varus and valgus deformities of the foot in cerebral palsy. *Dev Med Child Neurol* 1982; 24: 499.

Diaz LS. Ankle valgus in children with myelomeningocele. *Dev Med Child Neurol* 1978; 20: 627.

Drennan JC. *Orthopaedic Management of Neuromuscular Diseases*. Philadelphia, JB Lippincott, 1983.

Dubowitz V. *Muscle Disorders in Childhood*. Vol. XVI in the series Major Problems in Clinical Pediatrics. London, WB Saunders, 1978.

Dubowitz V. *Color Atlas of Muscular Disorders in Childhood*. Chicago, Yearbook Medical Publications, 1989.

Fulford GE, Cairns TP. The problems associated with flail feet in children and their treatment with orthoses. *J Bone Joint Surg* 1978; 60B: 93.

Kling TF, Kaufer H, Hensinger RN. Split posterior tibial tendon transfer in children with cerebral spastic paralysis and equinovarus deformity. *J Bone Joint Surg* 1985; 67A: 186.

Levitt R, Canale ST, Gartland JJ. Surgical correction of foot deformity in the older patient with myelomeningocele. *Orthop Clin North Am* 1974; 5: 19.

Lindseth RE, Glancy J. Polypropylene lower-extremity braces for paraplegia due to myelomeningocele. *J Bone Joint Surg* 1974; 56A(3): 556.

McCall RE, Lillich JS, Harris JR, Johnston FA. The Grice extra-articular subtalar arthrodesis: A clinical review. *J Paediatr Orthop* 1985; 5: 442.

McCall RE, Schmidt WT. Clinical experience with reciprocating gait orthoses in myelomeningocele. *J Paediatr Orthop* 1986; 6: 157.

Spencer GE, Vignes PJ. Bracing for ambulation in childhood progressive muscular dystrophy. *J Bone Joint Surg* 1962; 44A(2): 234.

Stillwell A, Menelaus MB. Walking ability in mature patients with spina bifida. *J Paediatr Orthop* 1983; 3: 184.

10 Orthopaedics

George Rendall, Paul R. Stuart and Sean P. F. Hughes

Orthopaedics is that branch of medicine concerned with the maintenance of the skeletal system and its related structures. This is very much the concern of both the orthopaedist and the podiatrist and this chapter attempts to accommodate the views and therapeutic approaches of both disciplines.

Flatfoot

Flatfoot is a useful lay term to describe a group of conditions with the common feature of a flattened medial longitudinal arch, a tendency to medial bulging in the hindfoot and midtarsus and eversion of the calcaneus.

The incidence and significance of flatfoot in children changes from infancy, where almost all early walkers present with flatfoot, to adolescence, where those with persistent flatfoot are likely to produce symptoms, deformity and dysfunction in later years. Reliable prediction of which children will retain their flatfoot into adulthood is therefore a major aim of the practitioner.

Flatfoot in children may be loosely subdivided into two major groups: those with structural origins and those with functional origins (Table 10.1).

Structural flatfoot consists of those types, mainly congenital, which are incapable of attaining an arch, even in non-weightbearing situations, without therapy. Functional flatfeet are those which only flatten on weightbearing. In infants the vast majority of flatfeet have a functional origin which is generally either treatable conservatively or will resolve spontaneously. The initial diagnostic approach is therefore to differentiate between structural and functional flatfoot.

Although no single mechanism has proved entirely reliable in diagnosis, two useful clinical indicators are the tiptoe test (Fig. 10.1) and the big toe dorsiflexion (Jack) test (Fig. 10.2). Such tests utilise Hicks' windlass effect where first toe dorsiflexion tightens the plantar fascia and compresses the first ray, simultaneously fixing the calcaneus and dorsiflexing the talus. The ultimate effect is subtalar supination which, in the tiptoe test, is assisted by contraction of the tendon Achillis group. This demonstrates that the subtalar joint and talonavicular joints are capable of a degree of normal function and motion which is unlikely to be the case where the major sources of structural flatfoot are present, i.e. tarsal coalitions and vertical talus. Both conditions are comparatively rare but are potentially very damaging and often require surgical therapy. The dangle test, where the child is picked up and the feet allowed to dangle, is also useful in young children. When suspended in such a way the child's foot will normally dangle in the supinated position. Eversion or abduction may indicate structural abnormality.

Table 10.1   Types of flatfoot

Structural flatfoot*	Functional flatfoot‡
Tarsal coalition	Ligamentous laxity
Congenital vertical talus	Accessory tarsal navicular
	Os tibiale externum
Arthritides	Compensation for plantar
Trauma	abnormalities in the lower
Iatrogenic	limb and foot
	Neuropathy
	Myopathy
	Muscle spasm
	Congenital pes calcaneo-valgus

* By far the most important types in children are congenital vertical talus (CVT) and the various forms of tarsal coalition.
‡ Foot types which function with a flattened medial longitudinal arch but have sufficient form to retain an arch when non-weightbearing are extremely common in children.

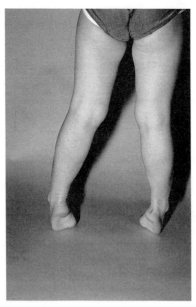

Figure 10.1   The tiptoe test.

Structural (rigid) flatfoot

Tarsal coalitions

Tarsal coalitions are rare, congenital deformities which, when untreated, tend to lead in early adolescence to painful, rigid everted feet and spastic peronei. In infancy only the stiffness and flatfoot are likely to be present as although the coalition or bar is intact, it will not ossify for another decade or so. The cartilaginous nature makes diagnosis by X-ray difficult, particularly where there is navicular involvement, until late childhood. Recent literature describes the use of computer aided axial tomography (CAT scans) in order to ease identification problems.[1]

Almost any of the bones in the midfoot may coalesce and a number of rare types have been described in the literature. The effect is usually similar. As the coalition ossifies it becomes rigid and possibly painful. Foot movement which produces pain is limited by spasm of peroneous brevis everting and immobilising the foot.

Treatment of subtalar coalitions and the determining criteria have been described in some detail and are outlined briefly as follows. Where symptomatic, surgical removal of the bar is usually recommended unless such a move would, due to the extent of the bar, leave a non-viable articular surface. In such cases triple arthrodesis may be performed in order to produce painless but immobile stability. Surgical treatment is usually effective and, combined with orthotic therapy in the immediate postoperative period, should leave a relatively functional foot.[2]

Results for conservative management are more variable and, on balance, surgery appears to be the treatment of choice and will remain so unless criteria are identified which indicate conservative management.

Vertical talus

Vertical talus is a congenital anteroplantar dislocation of the talus which is thought to result from an abnormality of fetal tarsal derotation. Typical features include:

1. Increased talonavicular angle with the talus more plantarflexed relative to the navicular and the calcaneus.
2. Disarticulation of the calcaneocuboid joint.
3. Hypo-plasticity of the head and neck of the talus.
4. Abnormal and incomplete calcaneal subtalar facet (so that attempts at surgical reduction are frequently doomed to failure unless wired).
5. Markedly flat or convex plantar surface due to the vertical attitude of the talus and dorsiflexion of the forefoot relative to hindfoot (i.e. congenital convex pes valgus or 'rockerbottom' foot).
6. Relatively normal forefoot and navicular/first ray relationship.
7. Rigidity of the ankle and subtalar joints.
8. Contraction of the tendo Achillis with resultant equinus of the calcaneus.
9. Limited soft tissue mobility, although the forefoot may be mobile across the modified midtarsal joint.

The condition is often associated with other syndromes or abnormalities. Hamanishi's[3] (1984) classification by aetiology includes association with neural tube defects, neuromuscular disorders, malformation syndromes and chromosomal aberrations but suggests that around two-thirds are idiopathic, including in this latter group, inherited and familial incidences. Hamanishi also classifies by severity

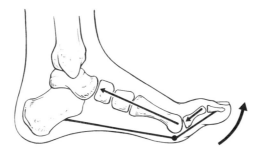

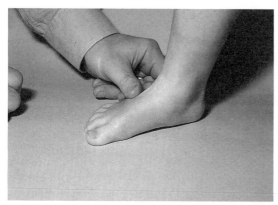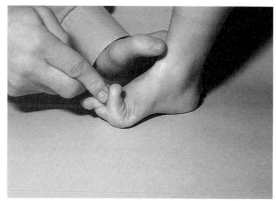

Figure 10.2   The Jack test. Dorsiflexion of the big toe creates tension in the plantar fascia which pulls on the calcaneus. The reaction to this tension is compression through the line of the first ray. In the structurally normal foot, these forces effect a rise in medial longitudinal arch because of plantarflexion of the first ray and supination of the subtalar joint. Absence of calcaneal supination may be due to abnormal subtalar joint structure.

using the angles of talar and calcaneal dislocation from the forefoot as the criteria. He measured the angles formed at the base of the first metatarsal with the talus (TAMBA) and the calcaneus (CAMBA). In his classification the critical point dividing rigid and flexible congenital vertical talus is 60° of TAMBA and 20° of CAMBA. (This compares with a normal TAMBA of 3.3 ± 6.4° and a CAMBA of −9 ± 4.5°.) He describes those below 60/20° as oblique talus and believes these resolve conservatively. For all other cases open reduction is recommended at three months and all authors recommend surgical intervention in early infancy for true vertical talus.

The aim of treatment is to provide a stable platform for walking. Due to the types of surgical procedure required and the common

aplasty of the talus, the prospect of achieving normal foot function is very limited.

Prospects of producing foot function consistent with normal life are, however, very good where appropriate surgery is used and when concurrent general problems are not preclusive.

Talipes calcaneovalgus

Talipes calcaneovalgus must be differentiated early from vertical talus. This common deformity is probably a result of fetal malposition and is characterised by excessive dorsiflexion and possibly limited plantarflexion of the ankle joint.

There is little evidence relating to therapeutic results and most mild cases appear to resolve spontaneously. Moderate degrees respond to maternal manipulation against the direction of the deformity (see Chapter 11, p. 246). These measures will usually produce normality within a few weeks and are of value in reasurring a concerned mother.

Retention of calcaneovalgus tends to produce a specific pattern of problems in adulthood. The foot frequently functions with comparatively few symptoms but gait is apropulsive, heel weightbearing excessive and the heel is broad and large compared to a comparatively under-developed forefoot. Therefore treatment with manipulation and observation is recommended.

Calcaneovarus

A similar but rarer condition is calcaneovarus. The general pattern is similar as is the approach to therapy (i.e. manipulating out of the deformity) but the forefoot is markedly inverted. This may predispose to a rigid adult forefoot varus which is likely to function with marked arch flattening and propulsive pronation as well as the heel symptoms previously described (see forefoot varus).

Functional mobile flatfoot

Flatfoot associated with functional or postural instability is very common in the infant and the early walker. All normal early walkers have to some extent a flattened medial longitudinal arch. There has long been a debate about the normality of functional flatfeet, the source of the debate being not so much the normality of the finding, as its implications for future dysfunction in certain cases. Therefore there is a need to focus on criteria for predicting which abnormality is likely to persist into later childhood, and also the biomechanics which justify the concern about pronated feet.

Perceptions of normality are highly variable and this situation is compounded by a paucity of literature describing reliable predictors for persistent flatfoot and the disagreement which exists in the opinion based literature makes determination of reliable good practice guidelines difficult.

Diagnostic considerations

1. Calcaneal eversion in relaxed stance. This is normally around 7° at one year old and it decreases by approximately 1° per year, so that by the age of seven years the relaxed calcaneal stance position should be within 1–2° of vertical.

On examination, a useful rough guide would be to subtract the child's age from seven and calcaneal eversion which deviates markedly from the result may be considered abnormal and a possible predictor of future problems.

2. Malleolar/tibial torsion. This measurement is typically 0° at birth. However, the tibia externally rotates at around 2° per year for the first 7–8 years and malleolar torsion should reach adult norms of 13–18° by 8–10 years. Malleolar deviation in the transverse plane reflects, but is approximately 5° less than, true tibial torsion which is difficult to assess clinically without resort to X-ray. Findings of low external tibial torsion in the child should be monitored and may require in-shoe orthoses. Internal, as opposed to low external, torsion is unlikely to resolve without treatment.

3. Tibial varum/valgum. Tibial varum may be due to intrauterine compression. Persistent pronounced tibial varum (Fig. 10.3) in school-

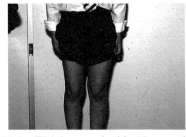

Figure 10.3 Tibial varum in this 10 year old girl has produced significant subtalar joint pronation and associated marked internal rotation.

children and adolescents leads to pronation and medial foot instability and should be treated with functional orthotics.

4. Ankle joint dorsiflexion. From a position of virtually unrestricted movement at birth, ankle joint dorsiflexion will normally reduce gradually as structural stability and calf muscle tone increase. A child of three years should have approximately 25° of motion and a child of 10 years 15° of motion. Low ranges of dorsiflexion should prompt a long-term programme of monitoring and when appropriate the practitioner may instigate a calf muscle stretching programme and the use of in-shoe orthoses. Complete lack of, or negative, dorsiflexion accompanied by hyper-reflexia necessitates further investigation and is unlikely to respond to conservative treatment.

5. *Gait analysis.* Gait and stance analysis provide useful indicators of the effects of underlying abnormalities on walking. In the hands of the experienced practitioner gait analysis should direct further investigations. Early heel lift or toe walking may indicate equinus. Pronatory movement in gait should be observed and related to the underlying features. Marked internal position of the patellae in stance or gait necessitates further investigation in order to determine the level and source of the abnormality. (Normally the patellae are slightly externally rotated in infancy and gradually move into the frontal plane by age 10.) Asymmetry, slouching, scoliosis, hyperactivity, unsteadiness and thumping may all be indicative of underlying pathology.

6. *Intoeing.* Excessive intoeing may be indicative of torsional or postural abnormalities in the hip, femur, knee or tibia and where the foot is structurally normal, is usually frequently accompanied by excessive subtalar pronation. Such features will tend to persist when untreated but, particularly where the problem is primarily postural, may be helped by stretching and strengthening programmes for the internal and external rotators of the hip. There is no evidence to support the notion that internal femoral rotation protects the foot from pronatory forces or is an attempt to do so.

7. *Toe walking.* Toe walking may be an indication of equinus and demands further investigation as persistent equinus is likely to alter the forefoot/hindfoot relationship.

8. *Abducted gait patterns.* Abducted gait patterns may produce excessive stress on the medial border during propulsion and may, where excessive, lead to persistent ligamentous flatfoot and possibly to the development of supinatus.

9. *Asymmetry.* Asymmetry of rotation, step length, or limb length may be indicative of abnormal development and demands further investigation and vigilant monitoring.

10. *Plantar weightbearing patterns.* Plantar weightbearing patterns are a useful guide as they may produce evidence of gross deformity. Whilst all normal infants and toddlers would have weightbearing patterns which would show a degree of weightbearing in the medial longitudinal arch, actual convexity of the medial border would indicate medial instability and possibly subluxation of the talonavicular joint. A mirrored stance-imager is useful in assessing plantar weightbearing patterns (Fig. 10.4).

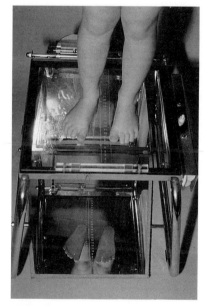

Figure 10.4 The mirrored stance imager enables observation of plantar weightbearing patterns.

The biomechanics of functional flatfoot

Functional flatfoot is almost invariably associated with abnormal pronation of the subtalar joint. In the new walker, this is most likely to be due to general hindfoot instability and to the very high ranges of subtalar motion which are to be found in the infant foot (45–50°).

Excessive pronation of the subtalar joint

(STJ) may also be due to minor functional aberrations which force the STJ into pronation in order for the foot to become plantigrade in stance. The main causes of abnormal STJ pronation are hindfoot and forefoot varus in the frontal plane, ankle equinus in the sagittal plane and internal tibial or femoral torsion or rotation in the transverse plane.

Causes of abnormal STJ pronation

Hindfoot varus

Hindfoot varus is a condition where, when referenced to subtalar joint neutral in stance, the calcaneus is inverted relative to the transverse plane (i.e. the supporting surface). Its source may be calcaneal or talar or may be due to tibial varum and in the mobile STJ hindfoot varus will cause pronation. Pronation occurs until the foot becomes plantigrade and in the stable foot with a normal forefoot/hindfoot relationship this should coincide with the calcaneal vertical position. Here the foot may be slightly hypermobile in the propulsive phase and some degree of lowering of the medial longitudinal arch will occur in stance but, in general, mild hindfoot varus in the normal child is not a major cause for concern with regard to future development. However, a high hindfoot varus combined with ligamentous laxity may produce more damaging forces in gait.

Hindfoot varus responds well to conservative therapy combined with functional orthoses.

Forefoot varus

Forefoot varus is a fixed frontal plane deformity where, with the STJ referenced to neutral and the forefoot maximally everted, the forefoot is inverted relative to the hindfoot (Fig. 10.5). Pronation occurs until the foot becomes plantigrade but this does not occur until the hindfoot is everted to the extent of the forefoot deformity. This means that in stance the calcaneus will be everted, the talus adducted and plantarflexed and the leg internally rotated. The pronation occurs in the middle to late part

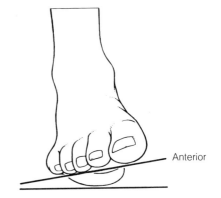

Figure 10.5   Forefoot varus.

of the gait cycle when the foot requires to be a rigid lever. Therefore the forefoot is at its most mobile in propulsion when reaction forces are at a peak.

Forefoot varus is a major cause for concern in the growing foot and should be treated and monitored with great care in order to ensure that the foot is protected from abnormal stresses and is allowed to develop to its full potential. A mild degree of forefoot varus in the infant is probably an acceptable finding, particularly as the general hypermobility makes certain diagnosis of such a problem difficult. However, persistent deformity in the early schoolchild is less likely to resolve and is highly damaging to the developing foot so that even at this young age it may necessitate intervention with functional orthotic therapy. Where practitioners cannot reconcile themselves to this approach in young children an interim measure is to use the California Triplane wedge (Fig. 10.6).

Ankle equinus

Ankle equinus is a restriction of ankle dorsiflexion to less than 10°. This level is used as a guideline for the amount of dorsiflexion required to permit the heel to remain in ground contact as the centre of mass passes over the body in mid-stance and prior to heel contact of the opposite foot. Lack of dorsiflexion at this phase imposes high stresses on the forefoot and may well lead to 'buckling' across the calcaneocuboid/talonavicular joints in the mobile foot. This buckling is achieved by pronating the STJ, thereby lowering the axis of motion of the MTJ oblique axis and increasing

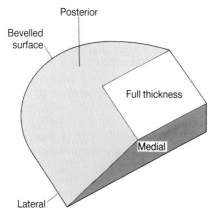

Figure 10.6 Tri-plane wedge.

the parallelism of the calcaneocuboid and talonavicular axes. The effect is to both increase the overall range of motion and to increase the sagittal component available at the oblique axis of the MTJ.

This compensation occurs after mid-stance, from a position approximating calcaneal vertical, so that pronation leads to calcaneal eversion and forefoot hypermobility during propulsion. This is potentially very damaging to the growing foot and necessitates early intervention.

Equinus may also indicate underlying neuromuscular problems so that a finding of equinus in young children, particularly when accompanied by abnormally brisk reflexes, should always stimulate further investigation.

Mobile equinus may respond well to a combination of stretching exercises and to orthotic therapy providing the child can be persuaded to adhere to the set programme. This invariably demands both parental and patient compliance and may involve frequent changes of programme in order to maintain interest as well as regular review to assess progress and reinforce the message. Where equinus has a neuromuscular origin and where there is a lack of heel weightbearing, conservative therapy is unlikely to produce improvement and a resort to surgery may be indicated. However, the validity of surgical approaches has been questioned since there is a tendency for the spastic foot to rapidly resume its pre-surgical malposition after tendo Achillis lengthening.

Orthoses are not helpful in cases of equinus unless there is good heel function. Even then

functional orthoses may be considered a risk since sagittal plane forces absorbed in the pronating foot may, in the absence of pronation, be transferred to the extended knee and may possibly lead to hyperextension and instability. Such factors combine to make ankle equinus one of the most destructive and most difficult functional problems to treat.

Ankle calcaneus

Ankle calcaneus is a common congenital disorder in which an abnormally high range of dorsiflexion of the ankle joint is the main feature. It is frequently associated with frontal plane abnormalities of the forefoot (see calcaneovarus and calcaneovalgus), and will normally resolve spontaneously by, or shortly after, early walking, probably as a result of increased tone and strength of the tendo Achillis muscle group. Absence of early resolution need give little cause for concern unless there is persistent forefoot varus.

The foot frequently functions with few symptoms but gait is apropulsive, heel weightbearing excessive and the heel broad and large with a comparatively underdeveloped forefoot. The lack of tone in the triceps surae group leads to retarded plantarflexion and to prolonged heel weightbearing. Associated pronation may lead to failure to prepare for contact and therefore subjects the heel to excessive stress at contact.

The heel hypertrophies as a result of overuse and the subtalar and ankle joints may develop osteoarthrosis in such cases. Therefore treatment with manipulation and orthoses, and observation is recommended.

Hindfoot valgus

Hindfoot valgus may originate in the STJ but it is more commonly associated with genu valgum. The line of action of the centre of mass is considerably more medial to the feet than is normally the case. This is due to the splayed tibia and the calcaneus tends to retain a position of eversion relative to the ground. The forefoot becomes plantigrade by inverting/supinating at the longitudinal axis of the midtarsal joint. This may lead to development of a supinatus deformity in the long term. Knee pain and medial instability are common sequelae and there may be a problem with late pronation, particularly in the presence of supinatus.

Mild genu valgum in young children will usually resolve spontaneously by the age of 10. Persistent genu valgum, particularly when associated with obesity and ligamentous laxity, can produce significant instability of the knees. Treatment of hindfoot valgus is also difficult but functional orthoses may help to restore foot function thereby reducing associated lower limb trauma.

Forefoot valgus

Forefoot valgus is a fixed frontal plane deformity where, with the STJ referenced to neutral and the forefoot maximally everted, the forefoot is everted relative to the hindfoot. Supination of the longitudinal axis commonly occurs as compensation and late pronation may occur but this is not considered a serious source of foot problems in children.

Treatment of forefoot valgus is difficult and orthoses with lateral forefoot and medial hindfoot posts have both been tried with mixed success. Fortunately the effects of non-intervention are minimal so that in children forefoot valgus should be monitored for improvement and otherwise left to develop.

Internal rotation

Torsion of the lower limbs may produce major pronatory disturbance. Far from protecting the growing foot from pronation, internal rotation (as opposed to torsion) is often a result of abnormal subtalar pronation and puts excessive transverse plane torque on the forefoot. Foot loading, in the internally rotated/torqued limb, tends to be more lateral than normal, particularly after mid-stance. This foot loading increases ground reaction on the lateral border of the forefoot. Due to the rotation, the lateral border is required to function as a pivotal point for the sagittal as well as for the frontal plane movement and is not stabilised by the medial border.

Evertory ground reaction forces acting through the midtarsal joint may cause medial displacement of the head of the talus thus producing the characteristic medial bulge. This occurs because eversion of the forefoot will normally only allow it to become parallel to the hindfoot. Therefore the foot must pronate at the subtalar joint. Furthermore internal torsion decreases the obliquity of the axes of the subtalar and oblique mid tarsal joints relative to the frontal plane and increases the sagittal plane motion available at these joints and also their susceptibility to distortion by sagittal ground reaction forces.

Pronation associated with torsional problems is resistant to therapy with functional orthoses and may require a high cant in order to produce an antipronatory effect. This would not be used in young children. Certain practitioners recommend the use of gait plates. High levels of torsion in the infant may be treated by the use of derotational splints or by serial casting. Derotational surgery may be considered in the older child with persistent high torsion.

Congenital talipes equinovarus

Congenital talipes equinovarus (CTEV) (Latin talus – ankle; pes – foot; equinus – horselike; varus – grown awry), or clubfoot is a structural deformity of the foot, ankle and calf which is present at birth and which varies considerably in severity. The calf muscle atrophy is a constant feature and is present even after successful treatment. No definitive cause has been identified but many theories have been proposed. When treatment is not instituted at birth the abnormality progresses to a fixed bony deformity of increasing severity as the foot grows. When the deformity is part of a systemic skeletal dysplasia or neurological anomaly, as it often is, the deformity is more resistant to treatment and the ultimate prognosis less favourable (Fig. 10.7).

Congenital talipes equinovarus is the most common orthopaedic congenital anomaly. In Western populations the incidence is 1–2 per 1000 live births. A racial and geographical variation in incidence exists, i.e. low in Oriental peoples and higher in Caucasians and Polynesians. Most studies show a sex ratio in incidence of 70:30, male:female with slightly more than 50% being bilateral and an equal laterality amongst unilateral cases.

The cause of the idiopathic clubfoot deform-

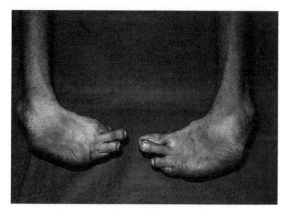

Figure 10.7 Untreated talipes equinovarus.

ity remains unknown but theories abound. The most widely accepted theories are:

1. Hereditary: family and twin studies have shown a marked increase in incidence in siblings and offspring of index cases and a 33% concordance in monozygous twins. No simple hereditary pattern exists but it has been shown that it is a polygenic multifactorial trait possibly sensitising to environmental factors.
2. Extrinsic pressure in utero: the earliest theory, but still proposed as a contributing factor. It is proposed that oligohydramnios causes decreased fetal movement and abnormal intrauterine position. Against this theory is the fact that the fetus is free float ing at the 20–60 mm stage when the foot is being formed and that there is no increased incidence in twins or primipara where there is increased intrauterine pressure.
3. Arrested fetal development: it has been shown that during the formation of the foot and ankle a growth 'spurt' occurs first in the fibula (21–30 mm stage), and then in the tibia (31–50 mm stage). It has been suggested that a local growth arrest at different stages of this process may cause the various grades of clubfoot deformity.
4. Primary germ plasm defect: extensive dissections have shown that the only consistent abnormality is in the cartilaginous anlage of the talus where deficiency is found in the region of the talar neck.
5. Neurological defect: CTEV is always associated with smaller calf musculature on the affected side together with a smaller foot

size and sometimes a slightly short leg. Certain studies have shown histochemical evidence in the calf muscles of a neurogenic factor in the causation of the deformity.
6. Vascular aetiology: injection studies of aborted fetuses and stillborn babies have suggested an ischaemic area at the level of the sinus tarsi and these studies have also shown that the vascular nucleus of the forming talus is abnormal.

The clubfoot deformity has been classified by the ease of correction into type I – postural and easily correctable, and type II – rigid and incompletely correctable. The type II deformity, associated with spina bifida, other neurological anomalies and arthrogryposis congenita multiplex is termed the teratological or type III clubfoot.

The precise anatomy of the type III deformity is highly variable and depends greatly on the underlying pathology. The type I and II deformities have the same underlying pathological anatomy. There is an abnormal relationship between the tarsal bones. A rotational deformity exists between the talus and the navicular and calcaneus, i.e. a congenital subluxation of the talocalcaneonavicular (TCN) joint. A secondary abnormality occurs in the anatomy of the talus during growth and development. The subluxation of the TCN joint may be considered as an exaggeration of the extreme of equinovarus movement of the normal joint. Alongside this hindfoot deformity is an adduction deformity of the forefoot, an anterior displacement of the talus in the ankle mortise and a posterior displacement of the lateral malleolus. A cavus deformity of the foot may or may not be present.

Extensive soft tissue contractures are present on the posteromedial aspect of the ankle and foot. The medial displacement of both the anterior and of the calcaneus and the navicular around the talus leads to the talonavicular capsule, deltoid and spring ligaments, and the tibialis posterior tendon being represented by a dense fibrous tissue mass which obscures the TCN joint. The posterior ligaments are shortened, viz. talocalcaneal, calcaneofibular, peroneal tendons and retinaculum, and the tendo Achillis is shortened and attached more medially than is usual to the calcaneus.

Radiographs provide a useful baseline not only for assessment of the deformity in clubfoot but also for monitoring progress of treatment and for determining recurrence following treatment. Anteroposterior (AP) and lateral films are taken using a standardised technique. The AP film is taken with the foot flat on the plate and with the ankle in 30° of plantarflexion and a tube-plate angle of 30°. The lateral film is produced with the child lying on the affected side and with the lateral border of the foot flat on the plate (Fig. 10.8a, b).

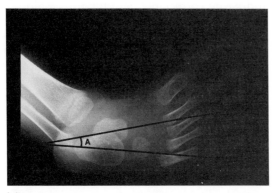

(a)

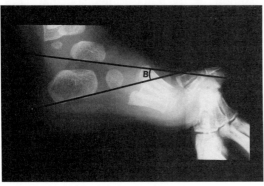

(b)

Figure 10.8 AP (a) and lateral (b) radiographs of clubfoot. A = talocalcaneal angle. B = lateral talocalcaneal angle. For normal ranges see text.

By using these standard exposures certain lines can be drawn on the film in order to assess the deformity. In the AP film the intersection of the long axes of the talus and calcaneus forms the talocalcaneal angle (normal range 20–40°), which will be less than 20° with the hindfoot varus of clubfoot. Similar lines drawn through the long axes of the talus and

calcaneus on the lateral film form the lateral talocalcaneal angle (normal range 35–50°). The equinus deformity of the clubfoot reduces this angle to −10 to 35°.

In the normal foot the anterior ends of both the talus and calcaneus overlap in the lateral view, whereas in clubfoot no such overlap exists, and this is a useful guide to completeness of correction.

The aim of treatment of clubfoot is to achieve a plantigrade, flexible and cosmetically acceptable foot. Relapse of the deformity may occur up to the age of 10 to 15 years and therefore long-term follow-up is necessary.

Treatment must start as soon as possible after birth of the affected infant. An attempt at conservative treatment is warranted in all cases – failed conservative management may have given sufficient improvement to allow a less extensive operative approach at a later date.

The conservative methods available involve manipulation and serial casting or stretching and strapping with or without the aid of a splint (see Chapter 11, p. 244). Both methods are demanding and time consuming, especially in the first few weeks of life. The gentle stretching of the soft tissues allows a gradual resumption of the normal interrelation of the tarsal bones and maintaining this position allows remodelling and stabilisation to occur.

Regardless of the method of treatment, the result must be critically evaluated at two to three months by clinical and radiological examination. Approximately 35% of clubfeet will be corrected by these methods, viz. all cases of type I and certain cases of type II. However, incomplete correction with no further improvement occurring at this stage is an indication for surgical management.

Surgery for clubfoot may be divided into soft tissue release procedures and bony surgery. The former is generally used at an early age in order to correct the initial deformity; the latter as salvage procedures for neglected cases and also to correct persistent deformity or to alleviate degenerative changes in the older child.

Soft tissue releases consist of lengthening and releasing in order to allow correction of the four elements of the deformity: posteriorly for equinus, medially for the varus and adductus elements and occasionally a plantar release for cavus deformity.

No specific operation is applicable in all instances as each patient requires a specific degree of release which will be dictated by the rigidity and the extent of the deformity. A move has occurred over recent years towards earlier surgery; i.e. as soon as the failure of conservative measures to improve the deformity becomes evident.

Surgery at the 6–8 week stage is very demanding; structures are difficult to identify and great care is required in order to prevent damage to the neuromuscular bundle.

A posteromedial release is the most commonly required procedure. This procedure may be performed through a curved incision running along the medial border of the Achilles tendon and around on to the medial side of the foot or through the increasingly popular Cincinnati or 'shoe-top' incision which has no vertical element and is more easily extended when extensive releases are required. It is also less likely to produce skin healing problems and leaves a cosmetically more acceptable scar.

The release commences posteriorly with a Z-lengthening of the Achilles tendon and, where necessary, release of the posterior ankle and subtalar joint capsules. The medial element involves the release of the abductor hallucis from its origin on the calcaneus, protecting the neurovascular bundle and lengthening the tibialis posterior tendon. The capsule of the talonavicular joint is incised and the subluxation reduced. The thickened mass of tissue which comprises the deltoid ligament, the spring ligament, the talonavicular capsule and the insertion of the tibialis posterior tendon is carefully excised and the medial subtalar joint capsule thus exposed is released.

Such releases allow correction of the deformity in most cases but occasionally a more complete release will be required. Stability may need to be established with Kirschner wires after extensive release. Postoperatively the leg is held in a cast in the corrected position.

Bony surgery

Bony surgery is not appropriate until the child is six to eight years of age or older, when the foot has undergone most of its growth. The indications have already been discussed and the operations most commonly used are as follows:

1. Calcaneocuboid wedge resection and fusion (Evans procedure), which achieves shortening of the lateral column.
2. Metatarsal osteotomy for persistent adduction deformity after six years of age.
3. Wedge osteotomy of the calcaneus (Dwyer's procedure), in order to correct persistent heel varus. This operation may be performed as a medial opening wedge or as a lateral closing wedge; the former when the heel is small and high riding.
4. Triple arthrodesis, as a salvage procedure in order to produce a plantigrade foot in severe late deformity.

Most series have shown overall good or excellent results (i.e. complete correction) in approximately 70% of cases. Such series have also shown that 60% of cases will recur after initial conservative management. Up to 85% of good results have been reported following one stage posteromedial release. It must be remembered that even after excellent correction the child is still left with hypotrophic musculature, a foot that is often smaller than the normal side and in certain cases shortening of the affected leg.

Pes cavus

Pes cavus is a fixed deformity of the forefoot on the hindfoot.[4] The clinical presentation of the foot is that of a high medial arch, producing an equinus deformity with the heel in varus, resulting in an overall equinovarus deformity. In association with this deformity are clawing of all toes including the hallux.

Such changes present as clinical problems which range from abnormality in gait from the equinovarus deformity to pain in association with plantar callosities as a consequence of the clawing of the toes.

In 1963 Brewerton et al.[5] demonstrated that pes cavus may be the sign of another condition. These authors reviewed a group of patients with pes cavus and noted that two-thirds of them had a distinct neuromuscular condition.

These conditions included:

- Peroneal muscular atrophy
- Poliomyelitis
- Spinal dysraphism
- Spina bifida
- Duchenne muscular dystrophy
- Friedreich's ataxia
- Cerebral palsy
- Polymyelitis

With more sophisticated techniques for investigating neuromuscular problems now available, the proportion of patients presenting with pes cavus caused by a neurological origin would clearly be much higher. Hence any child who presents with a pes cavus deformity requires to be examined carefully to detect a neurological condition.

The question as to how the cavovarus deformity and clawing of the toes occurs has unfortunately not yet been answered. There are several theories which partly explain the abnormality, but none explain the total deformity.

Muscle imbalance between a weak anterior tibial muscle and a strong peroneus longus tendon

Benton (1933)[6] proposed this idea as the cause of the problem. The weak tibialis anterior, which is inserted into the medial cuneiform, is overcome by strong peroneous longus inserted into the first metatarsal bone. The result is pronation of the forefoot and a decrease in dorsiflexion and inversion. Hence there is a *dynamic* imbalance which would account for some of the clinical presentation.

The main criticism of this theory is the fact that tibialis anterior functions well in many patients with pes cavus.

Isolated weakness of peroneus brevis muscle

In this theory, the paralysed peroneal brevis is compensated by hypertrophy of peroneus longus thus producing an effectively pronated foot coupled with plantar flexion of the arch of the foot. This pulls the toes into hyperextension and in turn results in clawing of the toes.

The hindfoot varus would also be an act of compensation to the forefoot eversion.

Paralysis of intrinsic muscles of the foot

Loss of the intrinsic muscles of the foot, similar to that seen in an ulnar nerve lesion of the hand, will produce clawing of the foot. This intrinsic contracture would explain many of the forefoot deformities that are seen but not the varus heel.

Electrophysiological studies have been used with some success to study this intrinsic muscle contracture.

Muscle fibrosis and contractures

This certainly occurs but it is not clear whether this is a secondary phenomenon.

Therefore it seems that whilst everything points to pes cavovarus being caused by a neurological abnormality, the actual muscles involved have not been completely identified.

The intrinsic contracture theory is popular but it does not explain the whole presentation. The most attractive theory is that of weakness of peroneus brevis[4] and further study of this theory seems to be the way forward.

The child with a pes cavovarus deformity presents with: (a) high plantar arch, (b) varus heel, (c) clawing of the toes, with or without (d) callosities.

The heel is in varus and this is obvious with the child standing. The high arch is fixed and is not correctable in established cases. However, the toes may still be mobile and correctable. This suggests that the contracture of the intrinsic muscles is secondary to the primary deformity in the hindfoot.

Callosities may be a major problem in early adult life, producing significant pain and deformity.

Investigations

1. Electrophysiological studies are required in patients who present with pes cavovarus. Such studies should include consideration of nerve conduction, electromyography and somatosensory evoked potentials.

Muscle biopsies may be necessary in

patients with, for example, Duchenne muscular dystrophy.

2. Radiographs. Standing lateral radiographs are of value in defining the extent of the cavus and also the structure of the midtarsal bones. Hibbs' (1919) angle[7] was introduced to measure the angle between the first metatarsal and the axis of the varus. Anything less than 60° is considered a true cavus (Fig. 10.9).

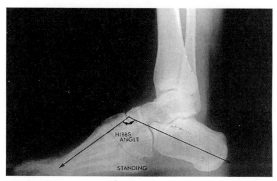

Figure 10.9 Hibbs' angle.

3. Other investigations include photographing the weightbearing foot through a glass plate in order to demonstrate the state of the medial arch.

New techniques such as dynamic pedobarographs[8] and gait analysis have a place in identifying the extent of the problem.[9]

Treatment

Early

Passive stretching and medial supports have a place in the early management of these conditions, particularly when the foot is still supple.

Late

This is when this deformity has developed into a fixed condition. Treatment can be addressed to each of the underlying problems.

1. Cavus. This deformity needs to be corrected as it is possibly the whole cause of the con-

dition. The treatment is therefore surgical. The effect of whatever is the deforming force, is a high arch and before bony changes occur, consequent to the muscle imbalance, the normal plantar arch requires to be restored.

Steindler[10] described the operation of plantar release. The plantar fascia and flexor accessories are reflected from the os calcis, and in the relatively supple foot the deformity is corrected (Fig. 10.10).

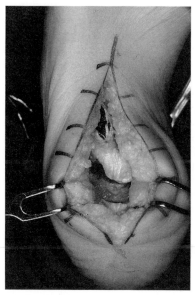

Figure 10.10 Steindler plantar release.

2. Varus heel. Whilst a Steindler release may correct the varus deformity, usually it is fixed. Thus a bony operation is necessary and is performed either by introducing an opening wedge or by a sliding osteotomy to the os calcis.[11]

3. The toes. The toe hyperflexion may be corrected by removing the extensor tendon from its insertion into the proximal phalanx and then rerouteing it through the head of the first metatarsal, in order to elevate that bone by means of a dynamic splint. The floppy toe then needs to be stabilised by an arthrodesis of the interphalangeal joint. This is the Robert Jones procedure.[12]

The clawing of the other four toes may be corrected by taking the flexor tendon of each toe and inserting it into the extensor tendon. Once again this produces a dynamic splint which controls the deformity.[13]

4. Bony procedures. Ultimately, when soft tissue correction can no longer be achieved, bony resection and arthrodesis is necessary. This requires resection of part of the bones that are involved in midtarsal movement: the talus, navicular, calcaneus and cuboid.

Wedge resection described by Lambrunidi[14] allows for correction of the cavus deformity of the foot but the varus heel may need to be addressed separately.

Sufficient bone is resected in order to correct the deformity, which is then held in situ by staple fixation and fused with cancellous graft when necessary.

Pes cavovarus is a fascinating clinical problem. Caused mainly by neuromuscular conditions its effect is demonstrated with time and unfortunately produces significantly painful and deformed feet. In adults the result may be troublesome and can be so severe as to warrant amputation on occasion.

Metatarsus varus

This is a common condition, in which there is a forefoot varus deformity. The incidence is about 1:1000 live births[15] and it is observed more commonly in females than males.

The condition may present as either *Metatarsus adductus* in which the forefoot is adducted but not inverted, or *skewfoot*[16] in which there is a complex varus deformity of the forefoot (Fig. 10.11).

In both conditions the hindfoot is essentially normal and is in valgus, not in varus, thus differentiating the deformity from congenital talipes equinovarus.

Although metatarsus varus is a congenital deformity present at birth it is usual for the child to present to the medical practitioner after one year when the child is walking. The mother notices that the child's feet tend to turn inwards and that the child has a tendency to fall over. Hence metatarsus varus is one of the causes of intoeing to be differentiated from: (a) femoral anteversion; (b) tibial torsion.

Another problem is that as the child be-

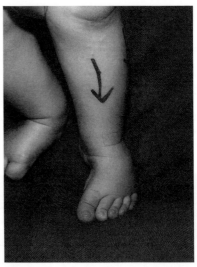

Figure 10.11   Skewfoot.

comes older and because of the shape of the forefoot, fitting of shoes may be difficult or troublesome.

A standing plane radiograph is helpful in order to demonstrate the normal configuration of the hindfoot (Fig. 10.12a), thus showing the difference from congenital talipes equinovarus, although in the skewfoot there is much more rotation of the forefoot (Fig. 10.12b).

Rushforth[17] demonstrated that in the UK, most children i.e. 87% of a large retrospectively collected series, corrected their deformity by the age of three years, without or irrespective of any treatment. This certainly seems true of metatarsus adductus.

The conflict in management is the uncorrected 13% and the true skewfoot. Treatment options in the early stages of diagnosis are numerous and include:

1. Exercises.
2. Reversing shoes, i.e. right shoe on left foot and vice versa.
3. Pronation shoes.
4. Denis Browne boots and splints.
5. Serial casting.

Probably the only really effective way of correcting metatarsus varus in the early stages is serial casting. There is no evidence that any of the other methods of treatment influence the outcome in any way.

In the UK those patients who by the age of three have not corrected by masterly neglect

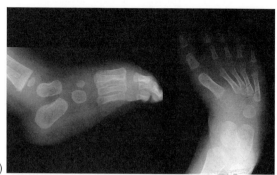

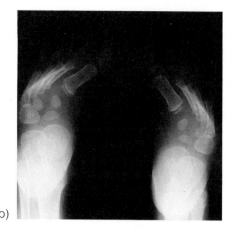

Figure 10.12 a, Metatarsus adductus. b, Skewfoot.

combined with hawk-like observation are selected for surgical release of the adductor hallucis muscle or tendon. The site of the release depends upon the extent of the deformity.

Patients who have a skewfoot which has not corrected after serial casting require a more aggressive approach.

The Heyman, Herndon, Strong procedure[18] is an extensive mobilisation of the intermetatarsal joints coupled with ligamentous release. This procedure may be combined with osteotomies of the base of the metatarsus in order to correct the forefoot deformity.

Skeletal abnormalities of the foot

Such relatively rare conditions may be classified according to Frantz and O'Rahilly as follows.[19]

Terminal transverse
1. Amelia of the lower limb.
2. Hemimelia of the lower limb.
3. Apodia.
4. Complete adactylia.
5. Complete aphalangia.

Terminal longitudinal
1. Complete paraxial hemimelia – absence of part of the leg and foot.
2. Incomplete paraxial hemimelia – as above with part of the tibia or fibula present.

3. Partial adactylia – absence of one or four digits of the foot.
4. Partial aphalangia – absence of one or four phalanges of the foot.

Intercalary transverse
1. Complete phocomelia – in which the foot is attached to the trunk.
2. Proximal phocomelia – in which the foot and lower leg is attached to the trunk.
3. Distal phocomelia – in which the foot is attached directly to the thigh.

Intercalary longitudinal
1. Complete paraxial hemimelia – as in terminal longitudinal, but the foot is more or less complete.
2. Incomplete paraxial hemimelia – similar also to terminal longitudinal but the foot is also more or less complete.
3. Partial adactylia – absence of proximal or middle digits.
4. Partial aphalangia – absence of proximal or middle phalanges.

These skeletal abnormalities manifest themselves in the foot as described below.

Lobster clawfoot

This is a rare congenital deformity in which there is absence of two or three central metatarsals and digital bone, i.e. a *partial adactylia*. Lobster hindfoot is invariably associated with other abnormalities such as cleft palate, syndactyl triphalangeal thumb and deafness.[20] Surgical correction by osteotomies of the metatarsus may be required, usually early on in the child's life.

Polydactylism

Supernumerary digits are common in the foot and usually require to be removed for cosmetic reasons alone. It is extremely rare for a complete functional unit to form. Such digits will usually actually consist of an extra digit attached to the main one or possibly no more than two conjoined distal phalanges which would go unnoticed but for the appearance of a second nail plate.

Macrodactylism

Fortunately gigantism of one or more toes is rare and may well be associated with neurofibromatosis. Surgery is required for cosmetic reasons.

Microdactylism

Rarely do small toes require surgical treatment.

Syndactylism

Congenital webbing of the toes does not cause disability nor does it interfere with function. The cosmetic appearance is not unreasonable and surgical treatment may not be necessary.

Fortunately skeletal abnormalities of the lower limb are not common and when they occur they need to be considered along with the whole limb and not in isolation.

When a part is missing it may not be possible to reconstruct the limb as the growing part may be absent. On the other hand, many of the four abnormalities lend themselves to surgical correction in order to improve function and also for cosmetic reasons.

Injuries of the bone and growth plate in children

Introduction to fractures and their management

A fracture is a loss in continuity of the substance of a bone.

Fractures are common in children and are more common than dislocations. This reflects the relative strengths of bone and ligamentous structures. As bone mass and strength increase in adulthood the relative frequency of dislocations increases.

The treatment of bony injury in children is gratifying as their bones heal quickly, possess great facility for remodelling, and post-immobilisation joint stiffness is generally not a problem.

Against such benefits the possibility of injuries to the growth plates and also the potentially devastating sequelae of growth arrest must be monitored. Non-accidental injury is an all too frequent occurrence, and a constant high index of suspicion, and early referral to an expert in the field is of paramount importance.

There are many complex classifications of individual fractures, but any professional who manages fractures must be able to describe such an injury in 'language' and conventions which are accepted in the field.

Fractures may be classified by their aetiology, configuration and displacement, or whether they are simple or complicated, i.e. by injury to surrounding soft tissue structures as well as to the skin.

Aetiology

1. Traumatic. Most fractures are traumatic in nature and are caused by falls or by externally applied trauma. They may be subdivided into low velocity injuries such as minor falls, kicks and blows, and high velocity injuries such as motor vehicle accidents, falls from a great height or by penetrating missile injuries. High velocity injuries impart more kinetic energy to the bone and are therefore prone to comminute the bone and to create greater soft tissue damage around the fracture – an important factor to be considered in fracture healing.

2. Pathological. A pathological fracture is a fracture through abnormal bone of any type. In children this is often through a simple bone cyst and indeed such lesions frequently present as pathological fractures. The bone may be dysplastic rather than a space occupying lesion and this predisposes a child to fracture, e.g. osteogenesis imperfecta.

Configuration of fractures

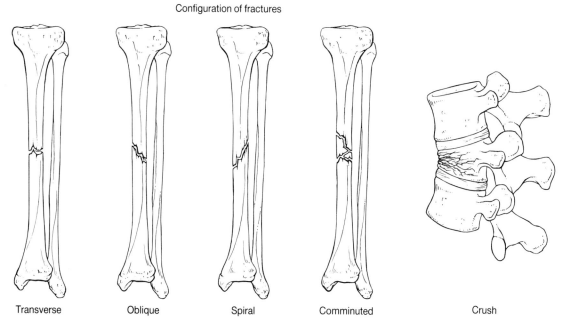

| Transverse | Oblique | Spiral | Comminuted | Crush |

Figure 10.13   Configuration of fractures.

3. Fatigue (stress). Unaccustomed, repetitive activity may place repeated stresses on a bone below the yield point (the point at which it would fracture). Eventually such stresses will cause a fatigue fracture, unless the stress is applied over a sufficiently long period in order to allow remodelling of the bony architecture. A stress fracture may be caused by several applications of a load just below its yield point. This type of fracture is most frequently seen as the 'march' fracture of the second metatarsal shaft.

Types of fracture

A standard terminology has been adopted to describe the configuration and displacement of fractures. It is important that radiographs of fractures include two views taken at right angles to each other, and that the joints above and below the fracture are visualised. The shape of the fracture fragments – the configuration of the fracture – imparts information about the nature of the causative force. The displacement of the fragments may provide information about the muscle forces which are acting upon the fragments. When studying radiographs of fractures it is not only the 'visible' bony fragments that should be con-

sidered. The 'invisible' muscle and ligamentous attachments must also be visualised in the mind's eye (Fig. 10.13).

Fractures through shafts of bones occur through cortical bone. Bones of a mainly cancellous structure (calcaneus, vertebral body) tend to undergo crush type fractures when loaded beyond their yield point.

The fracture pattern confers a stability or otherwise upon a fracture. Transverse fractures are inherently stable once they have been reduced. Oblique and spiral fractures tend to shorten by sliding or rotating respectively. Comminuted fractures tend to lack any inherent stability.

The position of the distal fragment is always described in relation to the proximal. The distal fragment may be displaced in the coronal (frontal) plane or sagittal plane, or it may be angulated, or shortened (or occasionally distracted) and finally it may be rotated.

Any combination of such displacements may occur in the same fracture. Coronal and sagittal displacements are readily observed on radiographs of a fracture as is shortening. However, a high index of suspicion must be maintained in order to detect rotational deformity which is less obvious because of the near circular cross-section of many bone shafts. Rotational deformity is important not only because of the functional problems of a foot in permanent internal or external rotation, but also because even children, with their great ability to remodel malunited fractures, have little or no capacity to remodel rotational deformities.

A fracture may be said to be complicated when nerve or vessel damage occurs at the fracture site. Damage to the overlying skin and muscle is also of great importance.

Open fractures are those in which the bone ends are exposed or are potentially exposed by an overlying breach in the skin and soft tissues. These constitute orthopaedic emergencies and their management is now discussed.

Arterial occlusion requires immediate investigation and treatment as distal limb viability may be compromised. Vessels may be compressed or kinked by severely displaced fractures, reduction of which will restore the circulation. When flow is not restored by reduction an intimal tear, or transection, may have occurred and angiography and exploration is indicated.

Injury to nerves may take the form of 'incontinuity' traction lesions with a reasonably good prognosis for recovery, or divisions of the nerve that require repair and therefore carry a far worse prognosis.

Bone is a vascular tissue and a fracture brings about the formation of a haematoma between the bone ends. It is from this haematoma that fracture healing starts. Necrosis of the bone ends occurs as the local blood supply is traumatised and empty lacunae are observed on microscopy. An inflammatory response is mounted with migration of macrophages and polymorphs to the fracture site in order to remove debris and dead tissue. Capillary loops and fibroblasts invade the haematoma in order to organise it into granulation tissue which forms the initial fibrous (soft) callus. Osteoblasts form by transformation of osteoprogenitor cells, stimulated by inductive factors, and migrate from the endosteum, periosteum and surrounding tissues in order to lay down a matrix of woven bone in the fibrous callus. Cartilage is produced in peripheral callus and this ossifies by the process of endochondral ossification.

Providing that there are no intervening soft tissues and that the gap is not too large callus grows from both sides of the fracture in order to form a bridge. The greater the movement occurring at the fracture, the larger the diameter of the callus; this maximises the mass of tissue as far as possible from the axis of rotation and provides the greatest strength to the fracture–callus unit.

Once a fracture is stabilised by external bridging callus, endosteal new bone formation occurs. Osteoblasts and blood vessels migrate from osteons of the bone ends and replace the woven bone of the callus with new osteons in order to re-establish cortical continuity. This process is followed by a period of remodelling which is governed by the principles of Wolff's law – bone being laid down along the lines of maximal stress. This usually leads to a complete return to pre-fracture bone architecture in children.

Principles of fracture treatment

Blood loss from isolated pelvic or femoral injuries or from multiple fractures may be sufficient to cause cardiovascular decompensation and shock. A patient's general condition and general resuscitation must take the highest priority in any trauma case – life must be saved before limb. However, fractures must not be ignored in the multiply injured patient.

Simple splinting of fractures will reduce blood loss and control pain. Early rigid fixation of long bone and pelvic fractures significantly decreases the incidence of fat embolism and adult respiratory distress syndrome which is a severe pulmonary condition found in trauma patients.

Certain general principles may be applied to fracture management in isolated fractures or once the general condition is stable in multiply injured.

The three components in managing any fracture are reduction, maintenance of reduction, and rehabilitation.

Reduction

A fracture must be reduced into an acceptable position and in most fractures this equates to the anatomical position. The methods available for reduction include manipulation, open reduction and traction.

Manipulation under anaesthesia involves

manually manoeuvring the fragments back into place and is the most commonly used method of reduction in children's fractures.

Open reduction at operation is usually undertaken in conjunction with internal fixation and confers the advantages of anatomical reduction under direct vision.

Traction is occasionally used to reduce fractures as well as to hold them reduced. The unstable supracondylar humeral fracture is the commonest fracture to be treated in this way.

Maintenance of reduction

A fracture must be held in its reduced position until it has sufficient inherent stability to maintain this position. Union is said to have occurred on clinical grounds when there is no local tenderness on stressing the fracture site. Full radiological union usually lags a little behind clinical union. This period of fracture treatment is a balancing act between achieving union and preventing the so-called 'fracture disease' – joint stiffness, muscle wasting and osteoporosis.

The most widely employed method of holding reduction in children's fractures remains splinting with a plaster of Paris cast. Plaster casts do not supply rigid immobilisation of fractures, but a well applied cast will prevent significant displacement of a fracture whilst allowing a jog of movement at the fracture site which stimulates callus formation.

Pulling on the limb or traction may be applied through the skeleton by means of a percussion pin passed through the bone, or by skin traction using adhesive tape. Traction exerts its effect by supplying a tense 'tube' of muscle in order to hold the fracture ends approximated. Traction has the advantage of not immobilising the joints adjacent to the fracture but its main disadvantage is that of keeping the patient in bed until union occurs.

Operative fixation of fractures may be achieved by means of an external fixator frame (Fig. 10.14), or internal fixation with wires, screws, screws and plates, or intramedullary nails. The latter are rarely used in children because of potential damage to growth plates.

The advantages of internal fixation include those of open reduction and of providing an immediate rigid fixation of fractures which

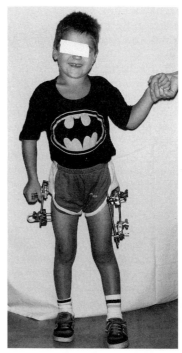

Figure 10.14 External fixation of bilateral femoral fractures. © University of Newcastle upon Tyne.

allows early mobilisation of adjacent joints in most instances.

However, internal fixation has the disadvantage of requiring an open operation with its attendant possible complications, the most important of which must be conversion of a closed fracture to an open fracture.

The use of an external fixator is generally restricted to open fractures where it has the advantages of stable fixation without the possible introduction of foreign material into the fracture site and it also allows the wound to be inspected and dressed with ease. As can be imagined from Fig. 10.14, patient acceptability may be a problem.

Rehabilitation

This is the most important part of fracture management and it is the only part in which the patient is really interested, i.e. 'When am I going to be back to normal?'

Early joint motion will allow an early return to function and physiotherapy may have a part to play in maintaining muscle bulk and joint function. Generally children pass through the phase of rehabilitation very quickly and in part this is due to reflection of their shorter bone healing times and thus a decreased immobilisation time.

All open fractures are potentially infected and must be treated accordingly. Immediate treatment consists of the application of an antiseptic dressing to the wound, anti-tetanus prophylaxis, and parenteral antibiotic administration. Definitive treatment must proceed as soon as the patient's general condition allows. A delay in excess of six hours risks severe infective complications. Once in theatre the soft tissue wound is excised and all devitalised, crushed and heavily contaminated tissue, including bone, is removed. The wound is then lavaged with up to 10 litres of saline. Rigid fixation may be appropriate and this instils greater host resistance to infection of the fracture. Open fracture wounds must never be primarily closed and wounds are reinspected at 48 hours. Further excision may be required or delayed primary closure or skin grafting may be appropriate.

Complications of fracture management

General complications

Blood loss, shock and visceral injury have already been discussed but such problems are so important that they must always be borne in mind when treating injured patients. The fat embolism syndrome is a complex alteration of homeostasis which occurs as a complication of fractures and causes respiratory insufficiency, petechial haemorrhages, psychological symptoms and fever. Two theories are currently postulated to account for the presence of the circulating fat globules that produce such signs and symptoms. One theory postulates that fat from the medullary cavity of the fractured bone is forced into the venous sinuses at the time of injury and the other is that trauma upsets lipid metabolism which consequently interferes with chylomicron formation and leads to intravascular fat globule formation.

Local complications

Delayed union is said to have occurred when a fracture has not healed in the expected time. This is a rather arbitrary diagnosis that is arrived at in the knowledge of average healing times for particular fractures at particular ages. Delayed union may progress either to healing or to non-union in which there is permanent failure of a fracture to unite. Two types of non-union occur: the atrophic form with narrow, porotic, avascular bone ends, and the hypertrophic type with sclerotic flared bone ends, i.e. where the fracture is 'trying' to heal.

Predisposing factors to non-union include increasing age of the patient, avascularity of bone fragments, excessive mobility at the fracture site and separation of the bone fragments commonly by soft tissue interposition.

Malunion of a fracture is a state of healing in a non-anatomical position and this will be discussed later with respect to remodelling of fractures.

Joint stiffness frequently complicates fractures and this may be due to mild soft tissue contracture secondary to immobilisation as previously discussed. More seriously it may be due to muscle tethering at the fracture site, intra-articular:articular fracture leading to joint surface incongruity and degeneration or myositis ossificans. This latter is a post-traumatic condition with ossification of muscle around the damaged joint and it is seen frequently around the elbow in children.

In certain sites avascular necrosis of fragments of bone may occur due to the anatomy of the blood supply. The proximal pole of the carpal scaphoid, the body of the talus and the femoral head are particularly prone to devascularisation by fracture. Nerve and vessel injury may occur at the time of fracture but their diagnosis and treatment are beyond the scope of this chapter.

When a high index of suspicion is maintained and distal neurovascular function is assessed in all fractures such potentially devastating injuries will not be overlooked.

Muscle viability as well as distal neurovascular function may be compromised by increased pressure in the tight fascial compartments of the limbs which is caused by trauma. The diagnosis of such compartment syndromes is

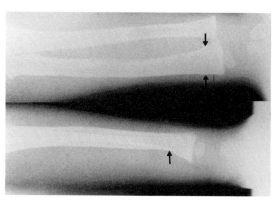

a

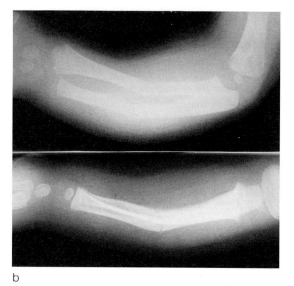

b

Figure 10.15 a, Buckle fracture. b, Greenstick fracture.

important and rapid treatment by surgical decompression is mandatory.

Distinctive characteristics of children's fractures

The general principles of fractures and their management apply to children and to adults but there are certain important differences in children which must be borne in mind.

Children's bones are growing and the physeal plates and injuries thereof present special problems. The bones of children are less brittle than those of adults and this feature leads to some unique fracture patterns. The continual growth of bones in children permits a far greater degree of remodelling of malunited fractures.

Fractures are more common than dislocations in children since the ligaments are relatively very strong. Growing bone is more porous and elastic than in the adult thus allowing incomplete fractures to occur under tension. The periosteum is strong and thick in children and rapidly produces abundant callus. The periosteum remains intact in paediatric fractures and forms a bridge which may help in their reduction.

Fractures unique to children include the buckle and greenstick fractures. Children's bones may also bend and may reach a point beyond its elastic limit but short of its yield point thus producing a gentle curve or bowed appearance to the bone.

A buckle fracture (Fig. 10.15a) represents the buckling of the cortex on the compression side of a metaphyseal segment of bone. Typically this is seen in the distal radius after a fall on the outstretched hand.

Greenstick fractures as their name implies are incomplete fractures of the tension side of a bone (Fig. 10.15b).

The principles of treatment are generally as for any fracture. The strong and usually intact periosteal bridge aids manipulative reduction.

Buckle fractures require to be protected only until pain free. This usually takes two weeks or less and they have no propensity to displace.

Greenstick fractures tend to spring open on the intact cortical/periosteal bridge. This fact is taken into account by certain authors' preference of overcorrecting the deformity in order to intentionally snap the opposite cortex. A well moulded plaster cast will usually allow satisfactory management without this rather drastic measure, which decreases the stability of the fracture. Careful follow-up with repeated radiographic examinations will allow any loss of reduction to be detected early and to be corrected.

A simple guide to possible healing times of children's fractures is given in Table 10.2. This guide is purely an outline since all fracture healing must be assessed clinically and radiologically. Clinical union may be said to exist when there is no pain on stressing the fracture. Radiological union, which frequently lags behind clinical union, exists when there is bony continuity of callus across the fracture site.

As noted from Table 10.2 the location of the

Table 10.2   Approximate healing times (weeks)

Age (years)	Physeal	Diaphyseal
0–3	3	6
4–10	4	8
11–15	5	10

fracture is of some relevance to healing times. Fractures closer to the epiphyseal plate heal faster with less callus and with a greater ability to remodel than those in midshaft. Head injury, especially when accompanied by brain injury, increases the speed of healing of limb fractures.

Remodelling of all fractures occurs under the influence of Wolff's law to a greater or lesser extent regardless of age. Children's bones have a far greater capacity for remodelling in certain circumstances. Large amounts of callus especially in the diaphyseal region are formed by children's fractures. Remodelling occurs over an 18 month to 2 year period with the callus disappearing completely in the prepubertal child and smoothing off and decreasing in size in the older child. Overgrowth occurs in shaft fractures of long bones in growing children. This is due to the hyperaemia associated with fracture healing stimulating the growth plate and it only occurs to a functionally significant amount in femoral shaft fractures. This length discrepancy does not remodel and thus the ideal position in which to hold a healing fracture of this type is with about 1–1.5 cm of overlap.

Up to 20–30° of angular malunion may correct itself with growth and will occur more in the plane of movement of the adjacent joint than in a plane at right angles to this. This ability is not an excuse for not reducing a dis-

placed fracture, as an obvious deformity may cause much anxiety to child and parents alike over the year or two which remodelling takes to occur.

Little or no correction occurs to rotational deformities with growth. Translational displacement and persistent apposition will remodel very well and is desirable in femoral fractures.

Growth plate injuries

Bone grows in length by endochondral ossification in the growth plates or epiphyseal cartilages.

Two types of epiphysis occur: (i) the pressure epiphysis at the ends of long bones from which longitudinal growth occurs, and (ii) the traction epiphysis at major tendonous insertions.

The weakest area of the epiphyseal plate is the zone of calcifying cartilage and fractures tend to occur through this layer. Thus the epiphyseal plate always stays attached to the epiphysis. The physis itself is cartilaginous and thus is not visible on radiographs.

The classification of epiphyseal fractures most commonly referred to is that proposed by Salter and Harris in 1963 (Fig. 10.16).

Such injuries have the potential to cause temporary or permanent growth disturbance. Bony bars may form across the physis, causing growth arrest or angulatory deformity. Incongruity of the joint surface may also occur and this predisposes to degenerative changes. When growth arrest or deformity do occur as sequelae to these injuries, the younger the child is the worse will be the resultant deformity and the more complex the treatment.

Type III and IV injuries are most commonly associated with growth disturbance and must be treated with early anatomical reduction and usually internal fixation (type IV always). If at all possible the internal fixation is not placed across the physis. Screws and wires are restricted to the metaphyseal fragment (types II and IV) and to the epiphysis in type III. If fixation must be used across the plate (unstable type I), unthreaded wires are used, and these are removed as soon as possible. The type V injury is rare and can only really be diagnosed in retrospect when growth disturbance is noted.

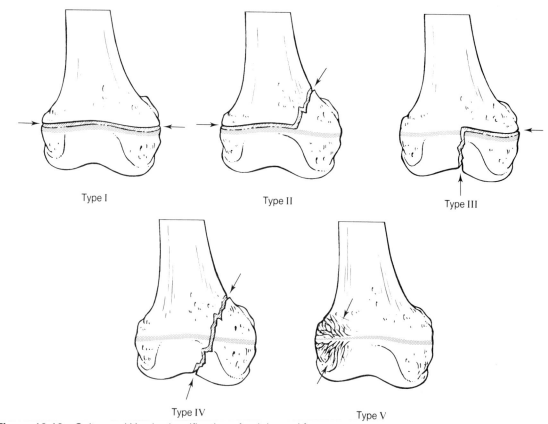

Figure 10.16   Salter and Harris classification of epiphyseal fractures.

Very careful follow-up of all physeal injuries is indicated in order to ensure that normal growth is proceeding. When arrest of a physis occurs the anatomy must be carefully defined in order to outline the position of the bar across the plate. This is usually carried out by the use of tomography or CT scanning. Surgery may be performed in order to attempt to resect a bony bridge across the physis and to hold it open with a fatty plug. However, this is technically very difficult and results are variable.

Angular deformities from physeal injuries may require to be corrected by periarticular osteotomy, which may have to be repeated as the child grows. Complete growth arrest near the end of the growth period may be treated by surgically closing (epiphysiodesis) the contra-lateral epiphysis.

A discussion of leg length discrepancy is beyond the scope of this chapter. However, various lengthening and shortening procedures do exist.

Specific fractures of the foot and ankle

Ankle fractures

Distal tibial and fibular epiphyseal fractures are common and are frequently caused by indirect trauma, with the foot being fixed and the body rotating around it. Ten per cent of all physeal injuries occur to the distal tibial epiphysis and are more common in boys in the 11–15 year age group. Towards the end of this period the growth plate is beginning to close and certain specific fracture patterns occur. The most distal tibial injury is the type II fracture.

The metaphyseal fragment may be medial, lateral or posterior depending on the direction of the injuring force. It usually reduces easily and may be held in a plaster of Paris cast. Severely displaced fractures may pull a flap of periosteum from the metaphysis and this flap may slip into the fracture preventing its reduction and therefore surgical treatment may be required. These fractures are usually associated with greenstick fractures of the distal fibula.

Type III and IV fractures of the medial malleolus occur which bring about a far greater incidence of growth arrest and which always require accurate open reduction and internal fixation. The type I distal fibula fracture is common and is frequently difficult to diagnose as it often slips back to its anatomical position after injury and thus it is not apparent on X-ray. This fracture is diagnosed on clinical suspicion and is treated by rest in plaster until comfortable.

The Tillaux and triplane fractures are complex distal epiphyseal injuries that occur during the period of physiological epiphyseal closure. The Tillaux fracture is a type III injury of the anterolateral part of the distal tibial epiphysis. This is caused by lateral rotation of the foot on the leg and produces a compression torque effect of the talar dome on the distal tibial epiphysis thus causing shearing. Accurate reduction is essential in order to reconstruct the tibial joint surface. Growth arrest is not a problem as physiological closure is already occurring.

The triplane fracture appears as a type III injury in the AP plane and as a type II fracture in the lateral plane. It is again an external rotation injury but occurs in a slightly older age group than the Tillaux fracture (average 13 years). The fracture may be two or three part.

Reduction may be by manipulation but it is important to restore the joint surface accurately. A proportion of such fractures will require open reduction.

Fractures of the foot

Accessory bones have been reported in many positions in the foot and ankle. They are frequently misdiagnosed as fractures, particularly during their ossification and may have a fragmentary appearance on X-ray.

Talar fractures are uncommon. Vertical talar neck fractures are the commonest and are usually undisplaced and may be treated in a non-weightbearing cast. When displacement has occurred they can usually be reduced by plantarflexion and can be held either in a plaster

or with percutaneous wires. Open reduction risks devascularisation of the talar body. Inversion and eversion injuries may cause ligamentous 'pull-off' fractures of the medial or lateral side of the talar body. Such fragments are osteochondral in nature and usually heal with rest in plaster, but non-union may occur and late excision of the fragment may be necessary. Osteochondral fractures of the talar dome occur with lateral ligament rupture thus allowing varus impingement on the tibial plafond. Here open reduction and internal fixation or excision may be required. Severe fractures and fracture–dislocations occur rarely and all may progress to avascular necrosis of the talar body with possible late collapse and osteoarthrosis.

Calcaneal fractures are still relatively rare but are the commonest tarsal fractures in children. These fractures are caused by falls from a height on to the heels and are always accompanied by extensive soft tissue swelling. Fracture blisters may occur. Initially treatment is by elevation in order to reduce the swelling and early active range of movement exercises. Most children's fractures are extra-articular and occur through the anterior or posterior processes and cause few long-term sequelae. The intra-articular fractures disrupt the subtalar joint and the crushing of the cancellous bone of the calcaneus causes decreased height and increased width of the heel which frequently lead to degenerative changes in the subtalar joint.

'Pull-off' fractures of the posterior process by the tendo Achillis occur and require either casting in plantarflexion or open reduction and internal fixation.

Injuries to the other tarsal bones are rare but may be associated with major crushing injuries or Lisfranc (tarsometatarsal) fracture dislocations. Soft tissue swelling and possible compartment syndromes must be considered with all major foot injuries. Elevation of the foot and possibly surgical decompression of the interosseous compartments may be required. Such fractures and dislocations are usually easy to reduce and may be held with percutaneous K-wires and plaster casts.

Avulsion fractures of the base of the fifth metatarsal by the peroneus brevis tendon are the commonest fractures of the foot. The secondary ossification centre at the base of the fifth metatarsal is frequently misdiagnosed as a fracture but this secondary centre lies longitudinally at 90° to the plane of most fractures. These fractures may be treated for two to three weeks in a short leg walking plaster for comfort.

Isolated metatarsal fractures most commonly occur in the shaft of the first or fifth. Direct trauma, such as dropping a heavy weight on to the foot, is the commonest cause. Isolated second metatarsal fractures suggest fatigue fractures.

Most metatarsal fractures are undisplaced because of the presence of strong interosseous membranes. Markedly displaced fractures should be reduced and should be held with wires as the capacity for remodelling, especially of plantarflexion deformities, is limited. Damage to the growth plate of the metatarsals may interfere with the proper formation of the arches of the foot. There is no association between trauma and Freiberg's infarction.

Fractures through the proximal phalangeal growth plate are more common than metatarsophalangeal dislocations which are commonly found in adults. Type III injuries occur here in older children and require accurate reduction and fixation when significantly displaced. Fractures of the lateral toes seldom require much treatment other than symptomatic, but a fracture of a hallux must be well aligned in order to prevent a varus or a valgus deformity. Crush injuries and puncture wounds of the toes must be treated according to the general principles for compound fractures already discussed.

Juvenile osteochondroses

Sever's disease

Sever's disease, a traction apophysitis of the calcaneus, is a problem of early adolescents and it most commonly affects boys between 10 and 12. The condition is characterised by posterior and postero-plantar heel pain. Initially the pain is a low grade dull ache which typically occurs on activity after rest (post-static dyskinesia) or after prolonged exercise. The pain may be produced by palpation or by contraction of the tendo Achillis (TA) group against resistance. In many instances the low grade pain persists for weeks or months before gradually fading. However, in certain patients it may become severe and disabling and can have a consider-

able effect on mobility, particularly on high stress activity such as games, climbing stairs or walking uphill. Here the gait is limping on tiptoe and marked supination is a frequent accompaniment. Limping may often be absent in periods between pain and its absence may lead to accusations of hypochondria from teachers, peers and family. Therefore its diagnosis may prove a relief.

Radiologically the apophysis may appear fragmented and of irregular density but findings in symptomatic and asymptomatic feet may be very similar.

Frequent microtrauma, due to compression and/or to traction by a tight tendo Achillis, and which are frequently associated with excessive subtalar joint pronation, may damage the ossifying, and the increasingly brittle, adolescent calcaneal apophysis. High activity levels in adolescent boys may be a contributing factor. Infection, trauma and avascular necrosis have also been suggested as causes.

Treatment is to relieve TA tension and is usually carried out by the use of a soft (closed-cell rubber or felt) heel raise. Where pronation is a likely cause antipronatory orthoses should be used. The use of corticosteroids, short wave diathermy or ultrasound is discouraged as these may influence growth.

Complete immobilisation with plaster casting is rarely necessary but may be used as a last resort where symptoms are severe.

Osteochondrosis of the navicular

Kohler's disease is a rare compression osteochondrosis in which the navicular becomes flattened and irregular. Radiological investigation with X-ray may detect patches of sclerosis and rarefaction.

The peak incidence is among four year old girls and five year old boys. Four out of five cases are found in boys. The problem is symptomatic in approximately one-third of cases.

Symptoms include tenderness and possible swelling over the navicular. Inflammation may be noted at the insertion of the posterior tibial tendon. There may be a marked limp but normally there is no loss of motion and passive movement may cause little or no discomfort.

The cause is probably compression due to repeated microtrauma. This compression traumatises the ossification centre of the navicular and creates tension or compression of the vascular supply thus producing a crushing aseptic necrosis in affected areas.

Usually pain is functional so that a supportive in-shoe orthosis is a useful and effective therapy. When the condition is more painful it may be necessary to immobilise with a walking plaster and to discourage all weightbearing for two to three weeks. During the healing period (six to eight weeks), strenuous activity should be discouraged although this may not prove easy in an active four to five year old.

Treatment appears to have little bearing on prognosis which is excellent and should therefore be aimed at providing maximum comfort.

Freiberg's infraction

This condition is a relatively common crushing osteochondrosis which is observed mainly in adolescents (peak incidence 12–14 years). Occasionally, active adults may be affected and here the condition is related to trauma. The second metatarsal head is most frequently affected, but the third and fourth may also be affected. Seventy-five per cent of cases are female.

Classicially described as an avascular necrosis, recent work using bone scintigraphy[21] supports the idea of an infarction occurring in the early stages of the disease process. The origin of such an infarction is often related to identifiable trauma, but in certain cases it is likely that focal ischaemia could result from repeated microtrauma such as stubbing.

Symptoms are of pain in the affected area on walking, on tip-toeing and on palpation. This pain will frequently fade without treatment, but when there is flattening of the articular surface it may persist into adulthood when osteoarthrosis may develop. Radiographs may show thickening, patchy rarefaction and the presence of loose bodies.

Treatment is by means of rest and the provision of a metatarsal bar. Where there is a functional problem orthoses may help. Prognosis is uncertain since many cases of apparently resolved juvenile Freiberg's develop osteoarthrosis in adulthood. Adults with traumatic Freiberg's tend to develop osteoarthrosis as part of the disease process.

Osteochondritis of the talus

Osteochondritis of the talus accounts for around 4% of all cases of osteochondritis. Causation is generally traumatic and is brought about by compression of the talar dome associated with plantarflexion/inversion. Frequently detection is difficult although modern radiographic techniques may help to overcome this. The investigating practitioner should ensure that the talar dome is not overlooked in traumatic disruption of the ankle while searching for a more common/obvious fracture.

Classification is by severity in four stages:[22]

Stage I involves chondral and subchondral damage as the lateral side of the talar dome is compressed against the fibula.

Stage II involves rupture of the lateral ligamenture of the ankle joint, a small degree of subluxation of the ankle and displacement of the osteochondral fragment.

Stage III involves complete detachment of the fragment.

Stage IV may see the rotation of the fragment within the joint.

Prognosis is good when the condition is treated early but relatively poor when types II, III and IV are subject to delayed therapy. Arthroscopy makes removal of fragments reasonably straightforward although its long-term effectiveness has yet to be established.[23,24] Such fragments should be removed early, particularly when displacement or complete fracture has occurred. Failure to remove fragments may cause damage and may lead to degeneration of the ankle joint. Generally, treated areas heal well.

Osteochondritis dissecans

This is a common condition in adolescents which may affect any mobile articular surface and which is usually associated with trauma. In the foot, trauma may be brought about by a single major episode, e.g. osteochondritis dissecans of the talus after a fall or bad inversion sprain, or from a series of microtraumata such as may result from a functional disorder or from a change in activity.

Typically the articular surface or a small area of it becomes avascular. Overlying cartilage becomes softened and there is usually a small fragment of bone which may become either fully detached or displaced but remains attached by soft tissue. Where complete separation has occurred this fragment may float around in the joint capsule thus acting as an irritant. Incomplete separation may result in readhesion/resolution or in detachment. Detachment leaves a roughened, pitted articular surface which is obviously unsuited to its smooth articulation and therefore remodelling and infilling occurs. Frequently the result is a smooth but flattened articular surface with a loss of articular cartilage which often leads to a loss of joint function. Even when this is not apparent in the short term, osteoarthritic changes are common in the long-term. Common sites are the superior surface of the body of the talus and the first metatarsophalangeal joint where hallux rigidus is classically the long-term end result.

Pain on pressure is the main clinical feature. This pain, which is relieved by rest, often occurs following trauma although it may only be reported once other symptoms have subsided, e.g. bruising, swelling. X-ray through the joint shows detached fragments.

Where a fragment is attached, compression and rest will encourage resolution and complete recovery with excellent long-term prognosis. Where detachment has occurred, rest will help to reduce inflammation but there is a high incidence of loss of function. Certain authorities advocate surgical excision and excoriation of the pit in order to encourage healing.

The rare forms of osteochondritis which have been reported are so varied that it must be accepted that any joint in the foot may be affected. A few are described briefly here.

Osteochondritis of the cuneiforms (Buschke's)

Osteochondritis of the cuneiforms (Buschke's) is similar to Kohler's disease. Features include irregular outline and an occasional limp. Duration is around three to four months.

Osteochondritis of the os tibiale externum

This condition is associated with pain and possibly with dysfunction in tibialis posterior.

Osteochondritis of the fifth metatarsal base (Iselin's disease)

This condition is a traction apophysitis brought about by repeated trauma and is observed in active children and adolescents, with a higher incidence in boys. The condition should be differentiated from fracture (see dancer's fracture) by X-ray. Treatment is by the use of orthoses in order to reduce stress.

Accessory bones

Accessory bones are small 'extra' bones which are commonly found in many sites all over the body and a large number have been described in the foot. They may be categorised either as post-fractional fragments, sesamoids, unossified secondary centres of ossification or as vestigeal evolutionary remnants. When congenital and hereditary these bones are usually symmetrical. Where an ossicle is found in one limb only a traumatic origin may be found. Whilst a large number have been described in the literature they are nearly always asymptomatic and therefore usually remain undetected. Only those which are seen commonly or are likely to produce symptoms or concern to the patient are described here.

Os tibiale externum (syn. accessory navicular)

Os tibiale externum is a relatively common accessory bone. Incidence has been suggested at between 10 and 20% in children and all but 2% of these bones have fused with the navicular by adulthood. The bone is sited on the posteromedial side of the navicular and may be seen as a sesamoid in the substance of the tibialis posterior tendon (type I), as an extra ossicle or bump on the navicular (type II), or as an extension of the posteromedial edge, i.e. the cornuated navicular (type III). The bone may be fixed or moveable and is frequently bilateral and it may be bifid. It is thought to originate as a secondary centre of ossification for the tuberosity of the navicular.

Although the problem is usually asymptomatic, in cases of painful flatfoot the area around the os tibiale externum may be inflamed and tender. It is often suggested that either due to the associated pain or due to anterior displacement of the tendon and its insertion, the accessory bone in some way reduces the effect of the tibialis posterior muscle. Alternatively it may be that mobile flatfoot instigates hyperactivity of the muscle, thereby increasing the tensile and shear stress on the accessory bone attached to the tendon, or simply that pronation associated with flatfoot results in compression and shear over the ossicle and that the muscle involvement is coincidental.

Lawson *et al.*[25] suggest that the pain is due to a combination of shear and compression (against footwear and/or the supporting surface) and traction (created by the pull of tibialis posterior). Such factors suggest that the pain is secondary to pronation and to flattening of the medial longitudinal arch. Whatever the cause this condition may be painful and disabling and should always be excluded in cases of medial navicular pain.

Treatment may be difficult in the early stages as the medial edge of orthoses may irritate the tender area. Identification by X-ray may be difficult and inconclusive. Surgical excision and reattachment of the tibialis posterior tendon relieves persistent pain but any restoration of foot function is unlikely.

Os trigonum

Os trigonum is a common accessory bone which is located at the postero/medial aspect of the talus. Wood Jones[26] suggests an incidence of around 8% in the adult population. In pre-adolescents the os trigonum is a secondary centre of ossification for the talus but normally it fuses to become part of the posterior edge of the groove for flexor hallucis longus at the posteromedial aspect of the talus. Trauma may play a significant role in the separation or non-fusion of these small bones.

The majority of os trigonum accessory bones produce no symptoms. In a minority of cases, limitation of plantarflexion of the ankle joint may be present but rarely is there any discomfort.

Os vesalii

Os vesalii is a common accessory ossicle which is positioned at the base of the styloid process of

the fifth metatarsal. Where bilateral, it is usually seen as a true accessory bone although there is some debate as to whether it is an unattached tubercle, an unfused secondary centre of ossification, or a sesamoid in the peroneus longus tendon. Where unilateral, a history of inversion sprain of the ankle may often be found. Here, in the so-called 'dancer's fracture', the posterior tubercle of the styloid process is either (i) pulled off by traction as peroneus brevis contracts strongly in protective reflex, or (ii) fractured by compression as the foot inverts, or (iii) a combination of these factors.

Toe deformities

Perhaps the most common clinical presentation of paediatric foot problems is one of the worried parent and of the child with 'curly toes'. Almost invariably asymptomatic, curly toes cause parental concern, and in some certain cases may lead to symptomatic toe deformities in later life. Therefore toe deformities merit a sympathetic approach and sometimes treatment.

Classification may be by structure, site or aetiology.

Common acquired deformities of lesser toes have been well classified by structure as follows:

1. Hammer toe – dorsiflexion of the metatarsophalangeal joint (MPJ) with fixed plantarflexion of the proximal interphalangeal joint (IPJ). It is very rare in children although the condition may develop in certain adolescents.
2. Claw toe – dorsiflexion of MPJ, plantarflexion of both IPJs, without fixation and with apical loading in stance. It is common in children of all ages.
3. Retracted toe – dorsiflexion of MPJ, plantarflexion of both IPJs, without fixation or apical loading in stance. Most typically the condition occurs in association with neurological disturbance.
4. Mallet toe – neutral MPJ and proximal IPJ but plantarflexed distal IPJ. Fixation may or may not be present. The condition is common in children.
5. Burrowing 5th toe – here the adducted underlying fifth toe may produce problems

by dorsally displacing the fourth toe and thereby bringing about plantarflexion and overloading of the fourth metatarsal.

Deformities of the first MPJ

1. Cock-up or trigger toe – hyperextension of the first toe at the MPJ which is almost invariably due to overpull of extensor hallucis longus. The condition is commonly associated with retracted or clawed toes and highly arched foot types.
2. Hallux limitus/rigidus is associated with functional disorders or trauma and may be seen in adolescence. More common in children is functional hallux limitus. Here limitation exists due to the hyperextension of the first ray and is seen in closed chain subtalar pronation. Intervention is important in such cases prior to the development of osteoarthritic changes.
3. Hallux abductovalgus (HAV) is rare in young children but may develop in early adolescence particularly where function is impaired due to pronation, forefoot hypermobility or forefoot adductus. The prevalence of juvenile HAV may vary according to footwear trends. The current predilection for broad sporty footwear is probably beneficial both in terms of removal of a major exciting cause and of providing footwear which is conducive to accommodating therapy where it is found to be necessary.

Congenital toe deformities

Congenital toe deformities are fairly common and a family history may frequently be present. Common inherited abnormalities include digiti quinti varus, syndactyly and less frequently polydactyly (see above). Factors which predispose to neuromuscular or functional abnormalities may also be inherited.

Digiti quinti varus (DQV) is an adduction deformity of the fifth toe which may be congenital. When left untreated the over-riding fifth will become floppy, flattened and hypoplastic.

Functional causes of toe deformities

Forefoot or metatarsus adductus may predispose the foot to toe deformities due to the cre-

ation of intrinsic muscle imbalance. With the metatarsals adducted relative to the calcaneus, the long flexors and extensors are straightened by flexor accessorius. The toes tend to run in line with the hindfoot and therefore they are abducted relative to the metatarsals. Abduction of the metatarsophalangeal joints provides a mechanical advantage to the lateral intrinsic digital stabilisers. Lumbrical imbalance leads to sagittal plane instability whilst imbalance of the interossei exaggerates the transverse plane deviation. The end result is frequently clawed/retracted and abducted digits. In children hallux abductovalgus is frequently a result of forefoot adductus.

Neuromuscular causes

Neuromuscular disorders which produce imbalance or hypertonicity are likely to produce clawed or retracted toes even in the youngest of children.

Paralytic and spastic disorders, which weaken muscle power or which lessen control, tend to disadvantage the already weaker anterior group. Typically this leads to pes cavus type disorders and to retracted or clawed toes.

References

1 Scranton PE. Treatment of symptomatic talocalcaneal coalition. *J Bone Joint Surg* 1987; 69A: 533–8.
2 Sartoris DJ, Resnick DL. Tarsal coalition. *Arth Rheum* 1985; 28: 331–8.
3 Hamanishi C. Congenital vertical talus: Classification with 69 cases and a new measurement system. *J Paediatr Orthopaed* 1984; 4: 318–26.
4 Tachdjian MO. *Pediatric Orthopaedics. Vol. 2. C. 7. The Foot and Ankle*. Philadelphia, Saunders, 1972, pp. 1263–442.
5 Brewerton DA, Sandifer PH, Sweetnam DR. The aetiology of pes cavus. *Br Med J* 1963; ii: 659.
6 Benton PGK. Pes cavus and the metatarso peroneus longus. *Acta Orthop Scand* 1933; 4: 50.
7 Hibbs RA. An operation for claw foot. *JAMA* 1919; 73: 1583.
8 Hughes J, Klenermann L. The Dynamic Pedobarograph. Vol. 4 (2): 99–110, 1989.
9 Gaga JR, Ounpuu S. Gait analysis. *Clinical Practice Sem Orthopaed* 1989; 4 (2): 72–87.
10 Steindler A. Stripping of the os calcis. *J Orthop Surg* 1921; 2: 8.
11 Dwyer FC. Osteotomy of the calcaneum for pes cavus. *J Bone Joint Surg* 1959; 41B: 80.

12 Jones R. The soldiers foot and the treatment of common deformity of the foot. Part II, Claw foot. *Br Med J* 1916; i: 749.

13 Taylor RL. The treatment of claw toes by multiple transfers of flexors into extensor tendons. *J Bone Joint Surg* 1951; 33B: 539.

14 Lambrunidi C. An operation for claw toes. *Proc Roy Soc Med* 1927; 21: 239.

15 Wynne-Davies R. Family studies and the cause of congenital club foot – talipes equinovarus, talipes calcaneovarus and metatarsus varus. *J Bone Joint Surg* 1964; 46B: 445.

16 McCormick DW, Blount WP. Metatarsus adduced-varus 'skewfoot'. *JAMA* 1949; 141: 449.

17 Rushforth GF. The natural history of hooked forefeet. *J Bone Joint Surg* 1978; 60B: 523–30.

18 Heyman CH, Herndon CH, Strong JM. Mobilisation of the tarso-metatarsal and intermetatarsal joints in the correction of resistant adduction of the fore part of the foot in congenital club foot in congenital metatarsus varus. *J Bone Joint Surg* 1958; 40A: 229.

19 Frantz CH, O'Rahilly R. Congenital skeletal club deficiencies. *J Bone Joint Surg* 1961; 43A: 1202.

20 Phillips RS. Congenital split foot (lobster claw) and triphalangeal thumb. *J Bone Joint Surg* 1971; 53B: 247.

21 Mandell GH, Harcke HT. Scintigraphic manifestations of infraction of the second metatarsal (Freiberg's disease). *J Nucl Med* 1987; 28: 249–51.

22 Berndt AL, Harty M. Transchondral fractures (osteochondritis dissecans) of the talus. *J Bone Joint Surg* 1959; 41A: 988–1020.

23 Pritsh M, Horoshovski H, Favine I. Arthroscopic treatment of osteochondral lesions of the talus. *J Bone Joint Surg* 1986; 68A: 802–65.

24 Parisien JS. Arthroscopic treatment of osteochondral lesions of the talus. *Am J Sports Med* 1986; 14: 211–17.

25 Lawson JP, Ogden JA, Sella E. Barwick KW. The painful accessory navicular. *Skeletal Radiol* 1984; 12: 250–62.

26 Wood Jones F. *The Foot*. Baillière, Tindall and Cox, 1943, pp. 83–92.

Further reading

Charnley J. *The Closed Treatment of Common Fractures*, 3rd edn. Edinburgh, Churchill Livingstone, 1961.

Cummings RJ, Lovell WW. Current concepts review – operative treatment of congenital idiopathic club foot. *J Bone Joint Surg* 1988; 70: 1108–12.

Rang, M. *Children's Fractures*, 2nd edn. Philadelphia, Lippincott, 1983.

Tachdjian MO. *The Child's Foot*. WB Saunders, 1985.

Tax H. *Podopaediatrics*, 2nd edn. Wiliams and Wilkins, 1985.

Turco VJ. *Clubfoot*. Edinburgh, Churchill Livingstone, 1981.

Valmassy RL. Biomechanical evaluation of the child; Symposium on Podopaediatrics. *Clin Podiatry* 1984; 1 (3): December.

Yablon IG, Segal D. Leach RE. *Ankle Injuries*. Churchill Livingstone, 1983.

11 Physical Therapy

Jill Pickard

Physical therapy may be defined as 'A systematic method of assessing musculoskeletal and neurological disorders of function including pain and those of psychosomatic origin and of dealing with or preventing those problems by natural methods based essentially on movement, manual therapies and physical agencies.'

Following the initial assessment of the child's problems, methods of treatment employed by the physiotherapist may include the use of massage, exercise mobilisation techniques or electrotherapeutic modalities.

The paediatric physiotherapist will work within the multidisciplinary team, either in the hospital setting or in the community. Other members of a health care team may include the podiatrist, the nurse, the social worker, the occupational therapist and the school teacher. The wide variety of specialisms in which the paediatric physiotherapist will be involved often necessitates close liaison with orthopaedic and neurosurgeons, obstetricians, paediatricians and rheumatologists. A suitable treatment programme which takes into account the child's age and problems and their severity is devised. The child should be fully involved in his own management when old enough, as well as the child's carers who are vitally important in continually reinforcing the therapeutic measures and advice that has been given. It is essential that parents are always able to contact the therapist and to discuss any worries or difficulties that they may have.

The objectives of physiotherapy for any paediatric foot condition may be broadly stated as:

1. To relieve pain and muscle spasm.
2. To increase range of movement at affected joints.
3. To increase the extensibility of shortened soft tissues.
4. To strengthen weakened muscles.
5. To re-educate balance and coordination.
6. To re-educate a normal gait pattern.
7. To restore normal movement and to allow the individual to be as functionally independent as possible.

Not all of these objectives will be relevant in each particular case and careful assessment of the child's condition will determine the identification of relevant problems and also their priority leading to more effective physiotherapy management. Careful assessment is the corner-stone of good physiotherapy intervention.

The therapeutic modalities used by the physiotherapist may be divided into the following categories:

1. Movement and exercise therapies.
2. Hydrotherapy.
3. Provision of orthoses.

Electrotherapy modalities are rarely used with paediatric foot disorders and therefore are not covered here.

Psychomotor development

The physiotherapist requires a thorough knowledge of the sequence of psychomotor development as a basic foundation for any effective treatment including foot disorders. The term 'psychomotor development' describes the maturation of both motor skills and intellectual complexity. The principles of maturation are especially important when dealing with children below the age of five. It would be inappropriate to employ hopping activities in the treatment of the child who is not physically capable of weightbearing. Conversely, a child will soon tire of an activity which is neither physically demanding nor intellectually stimulating. The newborn child is governed by a series of primitive reflexes and movements which are superseded by more complex movement patterns as the child grows older. The pattern of development is a continuous one with all children passing through the sequence in the same order although not necessarily at the same rate. All children, for example, can raise their heads in prone before they can crawl with the former being essential for the latter to occur.[1] The myelination process begins at the head and trunk and moves distally along the limbs. This explains why head and trunk control is gained before limb control. At birth the brain volume is about 25% of the adult and this rises to 75% by the age of one due to the increase in myelin present. As the maturation is dependent upon physiological events, practice alone will not hasten the child's ability to perform a task until the sensorimotor system is sufficiently developed to produce controlled actions of the relevant muscles. Children who are born prematurely or with neurological impairment, e.g. in cerebral palsy, will be delayed in their passage through this developmental progression and in severe impairment there may be no progress at all.

From the point of view of locomotion the most important development milestones are listed in Appendix VI.

Movement and exercise therapies

This aspect of physical therapy is undoubtedly the most commonly used when managing paediatric foot disorders. All congenital foot abnormalities that may be helped by physiotherapy should be treated as soon after birth as possible. When they are not treated, secondary bony or joint changes may occur and these may lead to further deformity and loss of function.

In the neonatal stage treatment must be entirely passive but, as the child becomes older, more emphasis should be placed on play in order to reinforce favourable muscle action and appropriate joint positioning. Therefore the objectives of treatment will depend upon the chronological age and the level of psychomotor development of the child.

Exercises cannot be prescriptive and great skill and ingenuity are required on the part of the therapist to make a movement regime stimulating and fun. The attainment of small measurable goals will help to motivate the child and keep his interest.

Techniques to increase range of movement and soft tissue extensibility

Movement at joints in the foot may be limited for several reasons including the following:

1. Damage to the articular surfaces and periarticular structures which may occur in children with juvenile chronic polyarthritis where there may be loss of movements such as inversion and eversion.
2. Adaptive shortening of soft tissues as might occur in the tendo Achillis in some congenital foot deformities, prolonged immobilisation and rheumatological conditions. When a muscle is immobilised for a short period of time it will adopt a shortened position and will form a contracture. If the contracted muscle is not treated there will be a long-term faulty positioning of the joint which that muscle passes over and this will produce pain and loss of function. Similarly, when ligaments are immobilised especially in a shortened position they too will shorten and become fibrosed.
3. Increased muscle tone (i.e. hypertonia or spasticity) may lead to loss of range of movement because affected muscles resist lengthening in order to allow normal joint positioning. When such tonal abnormalities are not treated permanent joint changes may occur. This may be seen in the plantarflexed inverted foot of a child with spasticity. The following physiotherapeutic techniques are most commonly employed to increase joint range of movement and soft tissue extensibility:

   (a) Passive stretching.
   (b) Active stretching.
   (c) Mobilising exercises.
   (d) Mobilisation techniques.
   (e) Soft tissue massage.

Passive stretching

A passive stretch may be defined as a manual or mechanical stretch applied to the shortened tissues whilst the patient is relaxed or, in the case of small infants, well supported. Most commonly this is used to stretch contracted tissue in the infant with talipes equinovarus, but may be used for any contracted muscle.

Two physiological mechanisms must be borne in mind when passively stretching soft tissue.

1. The stretch reflex. Within a muscle there is a specialised group of muscle fibres which lie parallel to the rest of the muscle fibres. These respond to the degree of stretch placed upon them by sending sensory impulses via the spinal cord to the motor fibres that return to the muscle. Impulses also travel to the cerebellum in order to produce smooth muscle function. When the muscle is stretched quickly, the intrafusal fibres send impulses to the spinal cord where stimulation of the motor fibres causes the muscle to contract and the tension on it to be removed. This series of events occurs very quickly and is called a stretch reflex. It prevents a muscle from being overstretched.

When a muscle is passively stretched it is important that the stretch is applied smoothly and slowly in order to decrease the likelihood of the stretch reflex mechanism being initiated. It is suggested that when the muscle is stretched for 30–60 seconds there is minimal activity of the stretch reflex.[2] When stretch is applied quickly to the muscle, the stretch reflex will be initiated and the muscle may be torn as it contracts against the stretching force.

2. The tendon reflex. There are specialised sensory nerve endings found wrapped around the fibres that comprise the muscle tendon as it attaches into bone. These fibres, known as 'Golgi tendon organ', are sensitive to tension in the tendon and thus the muscle. When a tendon is stretched very strongly, either by an active muscle contraction or by the muscle being stretched, the Golgi tendon organ sends impulses to the spinal cord. This causes the anterior horn cells of that muscle to be inhibited and leads to muscle relaxation and removal of the tension. Therefore, as tension develops in the muscle as it is stretched, so the tendon reflex is initiated and the muscle relaxes. This principle underlies the technique of passive stretching.

Technique for passive stretching. Passive stretching may only be used when there are muscle contractures. For this reason careful assessment should precede treatment to ensure that this is the case. The child, usually newborn, should have all lower garments except a nappy removed, and he should be positioned so that the stretch may be performed in the opposite direction to the tightness; which usually means supine.

The procedure should be explained to parents or guardians as it is usually necessary for them to perform the technique regularly at home.

When a muscle passes over more than one joint, e.g. gastrocnemius, flexor hallucis longus or flexor digitorum longus, each component of the movement that it performs must be stretched individually, before the whole muscle can be stretched over its entire length (Fig. 11.1).

The joint involved should be moved to the point of restriction and the therapist should then grasp either side of the joint so that movement can only occur there. Constant pressure is applied slowly and firmly to the segment distal to the joint. The tension should be maintained for at least 30 seconds, in which time the soft tissue tension will be felt to decrease. At this point the soft tissues may be stretched a little further. The procedure must be repeated regularly and full range of joint movement frequently takes several weeks to achieve in the case of congenital foot deformities.

Small children will invariably cry when this is performed and great sensitivity is needed on the part of the physiotherapist to what is a very distressing procedure for parents to watch and to undertake.

Active stretching

This may be used with older children who are able to participate in treatment. When soft tissue is actively stretched, the patient participates in the procedure assisting in elongation of the affected muscle by either its relaxation or inhibition of the muscle contraction. This method may only be used when a muscle is under the patient's conscious control; therefore it cannot be used for neurological conditions such as hypertonia.

An active stretch is usually applied using the

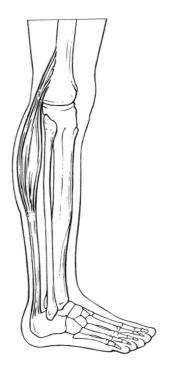

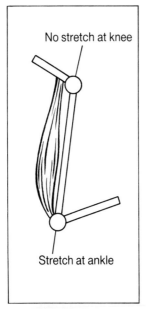

1. Over one joint

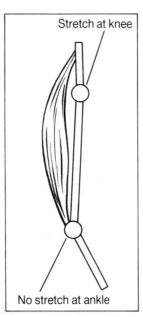

2. Over other joint

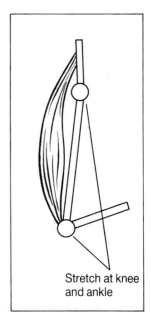

3. Over both joints

Figure 11.1   The gastrocnemius – sequence of muscle stretch.

hold–relax technique, which is one of a group known as proprioceptive neuromuscular facilitation (PNF) techniques. Hold–relax is designed to obtain a lengthening reaction in shortened muscle and thus produces an increased range of movement where muscle tightness is the limiting feature. The principle of the technique is that by producing a maximal contraction of agonist muscles at the limit of movement there will be reciprocal relaxation and thus lengthening of the tightened antagonists.

When there is muscle tightness in the plantarflexors, dorsiflexion will be limited. The ankle joint is taken to the limit of available dorsiflexion and maximal resistance is applied by the therapist to the plantarflexors, which are on a stretch. The patient is instructed to 'hold' the joint in that position, thereby achieving an isometric contraction of the plantarflexors. Once a maximal contraction has been achieved, the therapist then instructs the patient to 'let go' and waits 10–15 seconds to allow voluntary contraction of the muscles. When this has occurred the ankle joint is moved further into dorsiflexion brought about by the lengthened plantarflexors. The manoeuvre is then repeated to gain further range.

As the command given needs to be fairly specific, it may only be used with older children who enjoy the procedure, especially when the hold phase is viewed similarly to a show of strength as in arm wrestling, and the increased range is regularly measured to provide small achievable goals.

Mobilising exercises

Exercises to increase range of movement at one or more joints can only be used with older children and will only be successful when they have achievable goals and are entertaining. The patient must be positioned so that the limb can move through its full available range and is free from clothing. This ensures that the therapist can see how much range of movement is being achieved at the stiff joint and also which muscles are working.

The joint proximal to the joint to be mobilised must be fixed in order to prevent unwanted movement from occurring, e.g. when the aim is to increase range of movement

at the subtalar joint, the ankle joint must be fixed to prevent unwanted dorsiflexion and plantarflexion. Such fixation may be achieved by holding the relevant joint or a suitable position may be used to allow body weight or gravity to perform the task.

The joint should then be moved smoothly through the total available range of movement, taking care that the extremities of joint range are reached. This manoeuvre, the basis of mobilising exercises, should be repeated, the aim being to gain full range of movement at the joint. Mobilising exercises may be made more entertaining by the use of equipment such as balls, hoops and bean bags, and children thrive on achieving small goals set for them in the treatment programme. The following are a few examples of mobilising exercises for the lower limb that could be given to children, although the exercises given will depend upon which joints are limited in range. They are meant as an indication of the types of activities that may be performed, although the scope of mobilising exercises is endless.

Hip and knee. Position: lying on the floor on blanket with knee bent and soles of feet on floor.

1. Push body across the floor on the blanket by straightening hips and knees.
2. Pull body back across the floor by bending the hips and knees.
3. Rest one straightened leg on the blanket and roll the leg in and out, drawing a semicircle with the big toe.
4. Sitting on a high table, swing your legs as if you are dangling them in water; swing them forwards and backwards for the knees and side to side for the hips.
5. Lying on your stomach, bend your knees up so that you try to touch your bottom.

Foot and ankle. Position: sitting on a stool; feet in a sand pit or in warm water.

1. Curl and stretch toes (emphasising the stretch).
2. Open and close toes allowing sand to trickle through spaces.
3. Draw the biggest circle that you can in the sand/water.
4. Keeping knees together, try to get the soles of the feet to face each other.

5. Keeping knees together, try to get soles to face away from each other.
6. Standing up, try to jump as high as you can.

Mobilising techniques

Loss of joint mobility may be treated by the manual application of graded oscillatory force in order to mobilise the periarticular soft tissues and to increase the specific range of movement at that joint, usually termed as passive oscillatory movements. These techniques are not commonly used in paediatric foot conditions for several reasons: (i) with small children, any limitation of movement is often caused by soft tissue tightness and is most effectively treated with stretching and strapping; (ii) small children find it impossible to keep sufficiently still for oscillatory movements to be applied to a specific joint, nor are they able to report any alteration in the condition which this form of therapy has caused. However, it has been known for children of eight and over to be treated with passive oscillatory mobilisations when there is a musculoskeletal problem localised to an individual joint and when there are no other contraindications to the technique. These criteria are evaluated during initial assessment of the child's condition. Manual application of oscillatory movements at a joint are thought to:

1. Stimulate mechanoreceptors which in turn inhibit the passage of painful stimulus to the brain by blocking the 'pain gate'.[3]
2. Increase the movement of synovial fluid within the joint thus enhancing its nutrition.
3. Elongate shortened soft tissues.
4. Maintain or improve joint range of movement.

Passive oscillatory movements may be classified as either physiological or accessory. Physiological movements are those that normally occur at a joint and that can be performed by the patient, e.g. plantarflexion of the ankle. When limited, the therapist can achieve the same movements manually; e.g. in the case of plantarflexion by moving the talus on the tibia and fibula.

An accessory movement is one which must occur in order for normal joint movement to take place but which is not under the patient's control. A movement, such as dorsiflexion, may be limited by decreased gliding of the talus in the mortice. An anteroposterior movement of the talus which is performed manually by the therapist may resolve this problem.

There are very many different mobilising techniques for the joints of the foot and ankle and the success of their outcome is dependent upon the careful assessment of the patient and the skill of the physiotherapist performing the manoeuvre. It is impossible to cover this area in the necessary depth within this chapter, and it is suggested the reader refers to a specialised textbook.

Soft tissue massage

Massage in many forms has long been used for therapeutic purposes although the effects of such treatment have remained sketchy and open to interpretation. However, soft tissues may be mobilised and stretched by massage, the effects being considered as mechanical and physiological.

Mechanical effects. Massage to the body causes compression and distraction of the soft tissues as they are kneaded, squeezed and wrung. This leads to pressure on the thin walls of the veins and lymph vessels and increases venous and lymphatic return. The soft tissues are also manually lengthened by certain techniques and moved on underlying tissues or the skin. These actions tend to stretch any adhesions that may be present thus increasing soft tissue mobility.

Physiological effects. Most massage techniques produce a local hyperaemia which is brought about by the release of a histamine-like cell mediator from the tissues. This increase in circulation brings more oxygen and nutrients to the area thus aiding the healing process. Pain may also be relieved by massage as it is thought to have a sedative effect on the sensory nerve endings which consequently decreases protective muscle spasm. Massage techniques should not be used either over inflamed skin, in conditions such as eczema or unhealed wounds, or when there is malignancy or over deep vein thromboses, which most commonly occur in the calf.

The usual methods used in paediatric foot conditions are effleurage, kneading and deep transverse frictions.

Effleurage. The leg is elevated and firm strokes are applied to the leg from toes to knee or groin, each stroke ending with a small increase in pressure into the popliteal or femoral lymph nodes. This increases venous and lymphatic drainage and decreases oedema.

Kneading. Circular strokes are applied over the skin to mobilise the underlying tissues. Pressure is applied through a small part of the circle with the hands moving to cover the entire area. The whole hand may be used over larger areas such as the thigh or the posterior tibial muscles, whilst finger or thumb kneading may be more appropriate for localised areas such as the dorsum of the foot or around the malleoli.

Deep transverse frictions. A deep massage technique applied at 90 degrees to tendon or ligament fibres which have become fibrotic or shortened. This technique separates individual fibres from each other and from neighbouring structures. Although very effective in preventing and in treating contractures and adhesions, the process is usually uncomfortable and therefore is only recommended for use with older children.

Facilitation of normal movements

Normal functional ability of a child can only develop through normal movement. When a child walks on a plantarflexed foot without correction he or she will never acquire full functional gait including running, skipping and hopping. In addition, walking with a plantarflexed foot in effect lengthens the limb. Therefore there will be compensatory postures in the hip, knee and trunk, making gait more abnormal and thus decreasing function further.

Irrespective of the condition being treated, the physiotherapist aims to gain maximal function by encouraging as normal a movement pattern as possible. There will of course be situations when normality of movement must be forsaken in preference for function but this is a clinical decision made in individual cases.

Musculoskeletal disorders. Movements that are limited or muscles that are weak must be facilitated as early as possible by using recreational activities, movements and postures. From an early age, a child who is unable to dorsiflex fully, should be encouraged to kick, pull on the toes to try to reach the mouth with the foot, and to stand on the heels. In the case of rheumatological conditions, painful swollen joints must be protected by splints and appropriately treated whilst allowing the child to be as independent as possible.

Neurological disorders. Disorders of the nervous system may lead to abnormalities of muscle tone, sensation and coordination. These lead to other problems such as poor balance, posture, gait abnormalities and diminished function. When the nervous system is damaged, primitive reflexes may remain. Thus an older child may exhibit reflexes and movement patterns normally found in small infants and function will therefore be affected.

Muscle tone changes with an alteration of bony position and the therapist utilises this fact by positioning an affected child in such a way that either an increase or a decrease of tone is obtained. If the child is then ecouraged to move within the bounds of such a therapeutic position, tonal abnormalities and movement may be improved and thus function can be enhanced.

This concept will be discussed in greater detail when considering individual conditions.

Techniques to maintain or increase the strength of weakened muscle

The strength of a muscle or a muscle group may be defined as an increase in the amount of tension and thus in the resultant force that it can produce whether statically or dynamically. Under normal circumstances the child will develop muscle strength appropriate for normal activity. However, when there is a movement abnormality such as might occur with congenital foot deformities or juvenile chronic polyarthritis affecting the foot, certain muscle groups may produce inadequate muscular force or weakness. The following factors may lead to muscle weakness (Fig. 11.2).

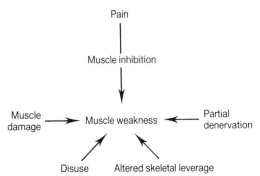

Figure 11.2   Factors leading to muscle weakness.

1. Pain. Pain on movement may lead to muscle inhibition; e.g. an acutely inflamed subtalar joint in a child with juvenile chronic polyarthritis will lead to inhibition of the invertors and evertors.

2. Denervation of the muscle. When motor impulses do not reach a muscle it will not contract. When only a few impulses reach the muscle, its contraction will be weakened.

3. Alteration in the muscles' normal skeletal leverage. For example, a soft tissue contracture of the plantarflexors will lead to weakness both of the plantar and of the dorsiflexors.

4. Disuse. A period of immobility may lead to atrophy. This may occur to the calf muscles when the lower leg has been immobilised in a below-knee plaster.

5. Muscle damage. Scar tissue formation within a muscle may prevent normal muscle contraction.

A muscle can work (i) isotonically where there is alteration in muscle length but not in muscle tone, or (ii) isometrically where there is an increase in tone but not in length. Both types of muscle work are employed when strengthening muscle.

Muscle strength may be measured in many ways. The following are often used:

Oxford scale

Grade 0 is no contraction.
Grade 1 is a flicker of a contraction.

Grade 2 is full range movement with gravity counterbalanced.
Grade 3 is full range movement against gravity.
Grade 4 is full range movement against gravity and with some resistance.
Grade 5 is normal strength.

Isometric strength tests

Resistance is applied to an isometric contraction by means of a weight or a spring. A poundage resistance is then noted when the muscle is working maximally. This may be measured at any part of the range of muscle contraction.

Dynamic strength tests

The affected muscle moves through its full range with a known weight resistance applied. The amount of weight that can be moved in this way smoothly 10 times is known as the 10 RM (repetition maximum) and is then used therapeutically.

Circumference measurements

These measurements are useful in smaller children and work on the premise that muscle strength is proportional to size; e.g. when a muscle is weak it will be atrophied and therefore will be smaller. This method may be useful for measuring calf or thigh bulk but it is rarely used in the lower leg and great care should be taken to ensure that oedema is not present since this may be confused with muscle hypertrophy.

Strength testing machines

Other methods of strength testing, e.g. myometers and isokinetic machines, are not commonly used with children.

The principle of muscle strengthening involves the application of specific resistance to a muscle contraction in order to either increase the size of muscle fibre or increase the number of motor units recruited. Thus the force of contraction (strength) is increased.

Care must be taken to ensure that strengthening techniques are not used when there is joint or muscle pain as these may be exacerbated and also that the muscle is allowed to relax completely between each contraction. The number of repetitions and speed of a strengthening technique will vary according to the individual needs of the patient. However, the technique is generally performed in a slow controlled manner until there is evidence that the muscle is tiring. After the muscle has rested the process will be repeated.

Muscle strengthening techniques

The following are the most commonly used methods of strengthening muscles in the lower limb.

Manual resistance

The therapist applies resistance manually to the distal part of the segment to be moved whilst fixing the area proximal to the joint over which the muscle works. The resistance may be lessened by resisting nearer the moving joint and made more difficult by moving the hands further away. The resistance is applied at 90 degrees to the moving bone throughout its arc of movement in order that the resistance alters throughout the range of movement. This resistance is applied to oppose the required movement, e.g. resistance is applied to the dorsum of the foot to resist dorsiflexion in order to strengthen the dorsiflexors of the ankle. The therapist determines how much resistance is required to strengthen a muscle but generally maximal resistance for that muscle is applied and the technique repeated until the muscle begins to fatigue.

This technique is valuable for use with fairly young children and with very weak muscles. When the child is instructed to 'push away' from the therapist the treatment may be used as an enjoyable game to play. It is useful that the child does not need to remain in a fixed position throughout the treatment, as the therapist can alter the application of the force as the child moves.

Mechanical resistance

The force used against the muscle contraction is produced by the application of weights, springs or pulleys. Although the resistance is measurable and easily progressed, the resistance is only maximal through part of the range of muscle contraction. Therefore it needs to be applied in such a way as to resist the weakest part of the range. This may need to be achieved by careful positioning of the child but this is often not possible with small children. This method is not suitable for either very weak muscles or for smaller muscles which may best be resisted manually.

As the amount of resistance is known, it is motivating for older children to note the increase in weight that they are lifting and thereby making the treatment into a personal competition.

Gravity resisted exercises

Muscles may be strengthened purely by contracting against the force that gravity may have on the body. An example of this might be a child standing on tip toes for a set number of times in order to strengthen the plantarflexors. Such an activity requires the muscle to move the weight of the body with gravity resisting such a movement.

PNF slow reversals

The technique of slow reversals is one of a group which are known as proprioceptive neuromuscular facilitation (PNF) techniques. The principle of slow reversals is that maximal manual resistance is applied to stronger muscle groups. This leads to facilitation of contraction of weaker groups of muscles. Therefore, there is a maximal contraction of muscles which produces a movement pattern and this is followed, without relaxation, by maximal manual resistance in the opposite weaker pattern. Mass motor patterns which are characteristic of normal movement are employed rather than individual movements. The patterns involve two angular movements and a rotatory component, e.g. one of the usual patterns of movement in the lower limb involves flexion, adduction and lateral rotation of the hip, with dorsiflexion, adduction and inversion of the foot and with the knee being either flexed or extended.

Re-education of balance and coordination

Maintenance of balance is an extremely complicated mechanism which is dependent upon integration between sensory input and a controlled motor response. This coordination is essential in the maintenance of balance.

When the body is displaced from its state of equilibrium there is stimulation of the sensory components such as the vestibular apparatus of the ear, the eyes, joint and muscle receptors. These impulses pass up to the central nervous system where various areas such as the cerebellum, basal ganglia and cerebral cortex are stimulated. The information thus obtained influences the adjustment of muscles and joints to produce a fine coordinated response in order to recover the original position.

In the adult, balance is almost entirely subconscious. However, the child learns to balance by repetition of an action, e.g. walking, until it is successful, coupled with progressive psychomotor maturation. Damage to one of these components leads to impaired balance and coordination and this may occur in neurological conditions, lower limb fractures, pain and specific muscle weakness.

Balance is essentially related to posture; e.g. the more unstable a posture is, the harder it is to maintain balance. The foot is an essential component of the balance mechanism as it not only adapts its shape to conform to the supporting surface, but it also alters the position of the line of gravity so that it is retained within the base of support. These actions are produced by the coordinated action of the foot and ankle musculature.

The physiotherapist must be aware of normal and abnormal balance reactions so that he may facilitate coordinated and efficient movements. Retraining balance is a continuous process and in principle it involves constant sensory reinforcement of movements which tend to unbalance the child and also those which lead to a regaining of a balanced posture. Initially the child starts to move from a relatively stable position such as half lying or sitting on a chair. The child must feel safe and well supported in the position or there will be an increase in muscular activity which will hinder fine balance correction. From this stable position the child may be moved slightly and may be guided to return to the balanced position again using normal balance reactions. Verbal, tactile and visual instructions are needed throughout the procedure and the use of a mirror gives greater sensory reinforcement as well as constant emphasis on the proprioceptive information that is being received from moving joints and muscles. When the child is able to maintain a balanced position despite small disturbances, trunk and limb movements are added so that the line of gravity moves further from the base. This may be achieved by the use of games, e.g. throwing objects such as bean bags into a bucket which is initially placed directly ahead of the child and which is then moved to one side or the other and finally behind the child so that trunk rotation is also incorporated into the activity. Throughout these movements there must be constant emphasis on the proprioceptive feedback that is produced by these movements. As balance is retrained, these stable positions may be exchanged for more unstable positions, e.g. standing, standing on a balance board, or even half standing, and all of these require a greater degree of neuromuscular coordination. Use of these positions will depend upon the child's specific problems and upon the stage of psychomotor development that he has reached. The role of the foot in these weightbearing positions is vital for the correction of balance.

Re-education of the proprioceptive mechanisms may be achieved by using the same methods as already discussed. Pushing the standing child backwards encourages the use of the dorsiflexors. Displacing the body weight further backwards will encourage the child to step backwards in order to recover his balance. Lateral weight transference encourages use of the invertors and the evertors in a similar way. The use of a balance board will facilitate reciprocal contraction of all muscles of the foot and ankle in order to maintain stability. Balance boards may move in one plane only to encourage either flexion and extension or inversion and eversion. Greater instability is achieved by the use of a balance board that moves in two planes at once. Such a balance board encourages co-contraction of all muscles around the ankle in order to maintain stability. In such unstable positions, most of the muscles of the feet will be contracting to some degree in order to maintain the foot in a plantigrade position.

In addition to the therapist manually displacing the child, activities may be used to achieve the same effect. Games could include throwing balls through high hoops in order to produce a backwards displacement, kicking balls whilst standing on one leg, and walking slowly across a line painted on the floor or on an upturned form. Final rehabilitation may include games such as dribbling balls through an obstacle course and running or hopping over uneven ground.

Re-education of gait and function

Before re-educating a normal gait pattern, careful assessment of the abnormal gait must be undertaken. When analysing the child's gait, the stage of psychomotor development should be borne in mind. When there is a degree of neurological disturbance which slows down the child's passage through the sequence, the therapist may concentrate on aiming to facilitate normal movement within the confines of the sequence before walking can be achieved.

The following factors will be investigated.

1. *Colour and temperature.* Acute inflammation is indicated by warmth and erythema.

2. *Areas of tenderness.* Are there any specific painful areas indicative of abnormal soft tissues, e.g. stretched ligaments, or acute joint involvement?

3. *Footwear.* Are the shoes worn uniformly or are there specific areas of wear?

4. *Foot posture.* Does the child stand with a neutral plantigrade foot? If not, is the malalignment caused by abnormal muscle tone, decreased range of movement or another factor?

5. *Muscle weakness.* Does there seem to be weakness of specific muscle groups or overactivity of others?

6. *Pain.* Is pain elicited by any activity; how long does it last and what relieves it?

7. *Limited movement.* Is there any limitation of specific physiological or of accessory joint range?

8. *Gait.* Is there an equal stride length, equal weightbearing and suitable size of the base of support? Individual aspects of the swing and stance phases should be analysed and reasons for any abnormality identified.

The overall objective of gait re-education is to provide the child with an efficient, economical and functional gait. When there is a specific problem which influences the walking pattern, e.g. an acutely painful knee, localised treatment such as ice, elevation and a walking aid must be combined with gait retraining in order that the most effective treatment possible is provided.

The principle of walking re-education is the use of therapeutic movement to diminish any movement abnormalities and to provide effective compensatory mechanisms where there is permanent disablement. All the exercise modalities so far discussed may be used to increase range of movement, muscle strength or balance and coordination.

Whilst a walking pattern is being re-educated, the child should either walk barefoot or wear sturdy shoes with non-slip soles. When there is any sensory impairment, barefoot training produces added sensory stimulus and this may be beneficial to the rehabilitation process. Gait progression must be carefully monitored and the therapist must be informed of any increase in pain such as may occur in children with juvenile chronic polyarthritis.

In the first instance gait re-education is performed within parallel bars which allow the child to bear a variable amount of weight through the arms thus ensuring the child's safety and confidence. Frequently a mirror is used to supply visual feedback of correct standing and walking posture. This helps to gain appreciation of any correction that has been made and to reinforce favourable patterns of movement. At this early stage the therapist may also need to support the child at the pelvis in order to maintain his stability.

As the child's balance and confidence progresses or as more weight can be taken through the lower limbs, walking re-education may be practised outside the parallel bars by the use of specific walking aids. There are a great many walking aids that may be supplied to a child and the type used will be dependent upon the age of the child, how much weight should be taken through the affected limb or limbs, and the nature of the condition. The type of aid given will also vary depending upon whether it is to be used permanently. Initially the child should only use the walking aid within the parallel bars until such time as the therapist is satisfied that the child is stable and then he should only use the aid with supervision.

Generally aids may be divided into the following categories.

1. Frames. These are stable provided the child leans forwards and bears weight through the frame. These may be used when a child is partial or non-weight bearing on one leg, or when he is able to bear weight through both legs. The frame may have wheels or ferrules, and may have gutter handles when the child has poor grip.

2. Crutches. Elbow crutches, which are less cumbersome, are most commonly used with children. These may be fitted with gutter handles and they are used in similar circumstances as frames, but when less stability is needed.

3. Quadropods or tripods. These aids are more stable than walking sticks but less so than crutches. They are awkward when stairs have to be climbed or in confined spaces. They should be used in pairs in order to prevent the development of a limp.

4. Walking sticks. The least stable walking aid, used when some relief of weight is required when the child is walking on both limbs. Such sticks should be used either in pairs in order to prevent the development of a limp or one only should be used on the non-affected side.

Other supports such as calipers may also be used in conjunction with walking aids and these are made to measure.

Hydrotherapy

Hydrotherapy is the therapeutic use of warm water to relieve weightbearing, to strengthen muscles, to increase range of movement and to aid relaxation, and it is especially useful in the treatment of children.

The pool is usually about 1.1 m deep although certain pools may have a sloped floor with a deep and a shallow end. The water temperature is usually maintained at between 35.5 °C and 36.6 °C. The therapeutic effects of immersion in warm water may be summarised as:

1. Relief of pain and of muscle spasm by the warmth of the water.
2. Inducement of relaxation.
3. Increased blood supply to muscles thus facilitating their contraction.
4. Support of the body by the water's buoyancy.
5. Ease of joint movement through the water due to this body support and to the relative weightlessness that it brings.
6. Gait re-education is easier due to the weight relief that is afforded by buoyancy.

The force of buoyancy acts in the opposite direction to that of gravity, i.e. upwards. Therefore it is easier to move a limb towards the surface of the water than away from it. Using this principle, joints may be mobilised when moving with buoyancy assisting them and muscles may be strengthened when such buoyancy is used as a resistance by moving in the opposite direction. When moving towards the surface of the water the addition of a float will make the activity easier. Thus weaker muscles may move a joint more easily through the water. When a float is added and the child is instructed to move the limb away from the surface of the water there will be added resistance and the activity will be more strengthening for the muscles involved.

Flippers may be added to the feet in order to make the limb less streamlined and thus to further increase muscle activity.

The principle of exercise in water is very similar to that on dry land. However, several factors must be borne in mind:

1. Due to decreased stability in water, greater fixation and support of the child generally, and specific joints in particular, will be necessary in order to gain maximal benefit from this form of therapy.
2. Care must be taken to prevent any falls or slips within the pool and the therapist should be aware of the depth of the water relative to the height of the child.

3. Exercise should always employ the force of buoyancy for maximal effectiveness and turbulence can be used when appropriate.

Initially a child may feel nervous at the prospect of treatment in the hydrotherapy pool and the use of pelvic, thoracic and neck floats to support the child and also a period of time adjusting to movement in the water will usually reassure and will provide him with confidence.

Hydrotherapy is a useful method of treatment in certain paediatric conditions. It is particularly valuable when treating children with juvenile chronic polyarthritis. Here the many joints involved will respond to the heat, whilst those that are being used will move with greater ease due to the therapeutic factors aforementioned. Therefore although the therapist's attention may be directed towards a few specific joints, there may be overall benefit. It is also a useful treatment for the child who has just had some form of fixation removed and when there may be considerable pain and muscle weakness. Specific methods may also be employed for the re-education of normal movement in children who have neurological impairment and who therefore may be able to move more freely in water than on dry land.

Gait re-education is especially effective in the hydrotherapy pool, as only the weight of the body above the water will pass through the lower limbs. Therefore the deeper the child is immersed, the less weight will be taken through the joints. This may be used as a method of gait progression with the child moving to shallower parts of the pool as he is more able to bear weight. Using this principle allows children who cannot weightbear on dry land, due most commonly to pain and muscle weakness, to begin to regain a normal gait pattern with the use of parallel bars and walking aids. These aids will assist in the strengthening of the appropriate musculature for the transition to gait rehabilitation on dry land.

Provision of Orthoses

An orthosis is an appliance which may be used to compensate for impaired tissue, e.g. structural malalignments in the foot which lead to pain or abnormal movement. Such orthoses aim to halt the progress of bony changes caused by faulty function and to reverse some of the soft tissue changes that occur. An orthosis achieves its function by virtue of the application of forces which are exerted upon the segments to which the orthosis is attached. The forces thus applied oppose the force of the abnormal movements and aim to gain a joint position from which maximal functional ability may be derived.

There is a very wide range of orthoses which may be employed in the correction of foot deformities. However, these are seldom used in the correction of paediatric foot conditions. Emphasis is usually placed on manual techniques in order to try to correct an abnormality and any orthosis required would need to be carefully modified and adjusted in order to produce a therapeutic effect on constantly growing and developing feet. However, when movement therapies alone are not effective, orthotic devices may be used under careful supervision.

Orthoses provide relief from pain in conditions such as juvenile chronic polyarthritis (JCP), where pads or supports relieve pressure from inflamed areas such as the metatarsal heads or from the heel. These supports are usually made of a padding or shock absorbing material.

Splints may also be used to correct a joint malalignment which has not been treated at birth, e.g. an older child diagnosed as having talipes equinovarus. Here greater control is required to correct the contracted soft tissues. When increased tone is present in the condition of cerebral palsy, an ankle–foot orthosis (AFO) may be used in order to encourage a plantigrade foot, thus significantly bringing about an improvement in gait. Orthoses are also used where a foot deformity is caused by abnormal muscle pull due to paralysis of individual muscle groups, e.g. in spina bifida.

The provision of special shoes may be necessary to provide comfort and support for a child. There are many different types of manufactured shoes for this purpose, e.g. shoes with extra wide fittings or with larger openings to accommodate the foot. In general, shoe modifications such as rocker bars and heel wedges are rarely used because much more emphasis is placed on treating the abnormality biomechanically, rather than by purely providing a compensatory mechanism for the foot. However, when this is not possible certain shoe modifications may be made.

Treatment of specific conditions

Talipes equinovarus (TEV)

Physiotherapy management should commence within the first few days of life and should continue until the child is walking. The bones and soft tissue will develop according to the stresses to which they are subjected. When treatment is delayed the abnormal stresses applied to the foot will increase the deformity and the longer treatment is delayed, the worse the outcome is likely to be.

Physiotherapeutic management consists of:

1. Manual correction of the deformity.
2. Active use of the affected muscles of the leg.

In severe cases where surgical intervention is necessary the therapist will be involved pre- and postoperatively.

Manual correction (Fig. 11.3)

There are many different manual correction techniques but all are based on the principle that the foot is overcorrected by passive stretching of the soft tissue. The therapist will teach the parents the technique that must be performed every time the child's foot is free from strapping or splintage. Initially the child's knee is flexed in order to prevent over-stretching of gastrocnemius and each component of the stretch is applied separately. It is suggested that each stretch lasts five minutes and that it is repeated at least three times a day.

1. To correct the heel: The heel and the gastrocnemius tendon is grasped between the thumb and forefinger and is then pulled down and laterally. This movement stretches the plantarflexors and the tissues on the medial side of the ankle.
2. To abduct the forefoot: The child's heel rests in the physiotherapist's hand whose thumb supports the lateral side of the lower

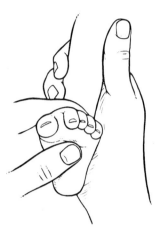

1 Position of operator's hands

Figure 11.3 Manual correction – position of operator's hands. Reproduced by permission of the Hospital for Sick Children, Great Ormond Street, London.

leg, with the index and middle fingers supporting the medial side. The foot is levered sideways using the carpometacarpal joint of the thumb as a fulcrum. The fingers of the therapist's other hand holds the toes.
3. To evert and dorsiflex: Once the foot is corrected it is pushed upwards and laterally so that the dorsum of the foot comes into contact with the lateral side of the lower leg. Care should be taken that this movement occurs at the ankle joint.

Maintenance of the corrected position. Certain methods of maintenance allow the foot to move into a favourable position which produces active correction while other methods hold the foot more rigidly. Certain splints are readily removable but others are semipermanent.

Strapping (Fig. 11.4). Initially the skin is prepared with compound tincture of benzoin in order to protect the infant's skin. Strips of zinc oxide tape are used and the lateral malleolus and the medial side of the great toe are protected by means of pieces of felt. Initially the strapping is reapplied or reinforced daily, but this timing progresses to every two or three days. Care must be taken to ensure that there is no circulatory disturbance and that the child is not allergic to the materials used. The

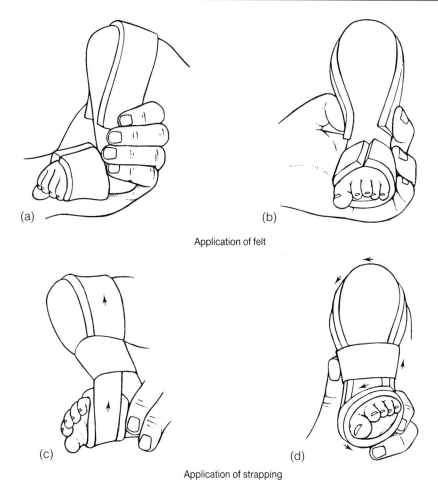

(a)

(b)

Application of felt

(c)

(d)

Application of strapping

Figure 11.4   a and b, Application of felt. c and d, Application of strapping. Reproduced by permission of the Hospital for Sick Children, Great Ormond Street, London.

parents are advised of these possibilities and are instructed to keep the strapping dry. Generally correction may be achieved in a few weeks when strapping is started early.

Splinting. This may be applied in the form of Denis Browne, plaster of Paris or plastic splints. Although the child will wear splints continuously and may possibly have a separate night splint, he should have part of each day to play and to kick without the splint. This time should also be used by the parents to maintain the mobility of the affected joints with the therapist's guidance.

Active correction

The child should be encouraged to dorsiflex

and to evert the foot. This may be facilitated by stroking the lateral aspect of the foot towards the heel. When it is possible for the foot to be in a plantigrade position the child may be 'stood' so that some weight is taken through the foot. Moving the child sideways, backwards and forwards from this position, without moving the feet, encourages contraction of specific muscle groups. As the child begins to play with the foot, parents should emphasise its lateral side, and should encourage play that directs movement towards dorsiflexion, eversion and abduction.

Talipes calcaneovalgus (TCV)

This deformity is characterised by dorsiflexion of the ankle, eversion of the hindfoot at the subtalar joint and abduction of the forefoot at the midtarsal joints. The prognosis is good when treatment is started early, but not so when there is a neurological cause.

The principles of treatment are the same as for talipes equinovarus.

Manual correction

Each component of the stretch is applied individually at first, with the full stretch applied as a progression. As the muscles involved do not pass over the knee, its position is not so important as in the TEV stretch.

The foot is gripped so that the calcaneus may be inverted as the foot is plantarflexed. The hand should be as near to the ankle joint as possible so that movement does not occur at the midtarsal joints. This position is maintained while the therapist's other hand everts the subtalar joint and adducts the forefoot.

Maintenance of the corrected position. A plaster of Paris splint may be made to fit the anterolateral aspect of the leg and also to include the calcaneus in order to correct the eversion element. The splint must be replaced every few days as correction is achieved, and it should be worn continuously until the condition improves.

Active correction

The child must be encouraged to point the toes. Stroking the sole of the foot and other such facilitatory techniques may be employed to emphasise plantarflexion, inversion and adduction. Play should be directed towards these movements as well.

Pes planus

A foot may be defined as flat when there is a decrease in the longitudinal arch. In young children this is always so until there is sufficient musculoskeletal development to maintain the arch. Occasionally such flatfeet persist and are frequently associated with cultural factors, and are usually asymptomatic and require no treatment since the joints are mobile and the muscles are sufficiently strong. An overpronated foot may also appear flattened and this is also common in children. The malalignment may be secondary to a more proximal problem such as knee malalignment or anteversion of the femoral neck, and ideally the more proximal problem should be treated first. Pes planus may be associated with specific muscle weakness or hypotonia in which case specific orthoses may need to be manufactured in order to prevent deterioration of the deformity. A flatfoot may also be brought about by increased tone in the plantarflexors and this leads to dorsiflexion of the forefoot and produces a plantigrade foot. Techniques to decrease the tone and to lengthen the tendocalcaneus may be used. These techniques include facilitation of normal movement patterns emphasising dorsiflexion, weightbearing through the foot when it is positioned in a favourable position, and even the application of a below-knee walking plaster.

The orthopaedic surgical patient

Surgery on the foot and on the lower leg may be undertaken for various conditions in the child: e.g.

- Correction of a persistent talipes equinovarus.
- Joint fusion.
- Metatarsal osteotomy.
- Tendon lengthening.
- Tendon transfer.

Irrespective of the surgical procedure undertaken generally the child will spend a period of time in fixation, e.g. plaster of Paris or some lighter material such as Baycast. This period of time will depend upon the surgical procedure undertaken and upon the wishes of the surgeon. Physiotherapy management may be divided into:

1. Preoperative management.
2. Postoperative management in fixation.
3. Postoperative management out of fixation.

1. Preoperative management. The therapist should make herself known to the child and to the parent and should explain her role in the postoperative management of the child. When the child is to be non-weightbearing after surgery, a frame or elbow crutches should be correctly measured in advance and also a wheelchair with leg support may be provided to assist the child to be mobile before he is able to walk with a suitable aid. All such aids should be explained to the family and the child should be given the opportunity to practise their use in advance.

2. Postoperative management in fixation. Following surgery it is likely that the surgical site will be immobilised in order to allow healing of cut bones and soft tissue. The duration of fixation will be variable as will its form.

It is not usually necessary to undertake exercises to maintain range of movement at unaffected joints as the child will soon be active and will be using all unaffected joints normally. However, when there is an underlying rheumatological condition, exercises to maintain range of movement may be necessary.

In order to maintain the strength of muscles which pass over immobilised joints, static muscle work will be employed. When the knee is immobilised, static quadriceps and hamstring contractions will be undertaken and similar activities for the muscle groups around the ankle joint will be performed when the ankle is temporarily fixed.

The parents should be advised as how to care for the method of fixation used and to encourage the child to be as functionally independent as possible. Small children will be given frames and those over the age of about six years will be able to use crutches. Trolleys may also be supplied so that the child may lie prone and may move around the floor. When a mobility aid is used the therapist must ensure that it is being used correctly and that the child is safe and stable before he is discharged. It is usually necessary to teach methods for climbing stairs using the mobility aid, although small children must obviously be carried.

3. Postoperative management out of fixation. Initially the child will require to use the walking aid in order to bear some body weight. However, as the joints become more mobile and the muscles become stronger, the support that the aid gives may be reduced and may finally be removed. The child will usually decide when it is right for him. Overall objectives of treatment will be to:

– Restore as much movement as is possible to the joints that have been immobile.
– Strengthen any muscles that are weakened, frequently those that pass over the site of surgery.
– Rehabilitate the child to as full functional ability as possible within the limits of ability and development.
– Educate the parents or guardians in maintenance of the child's condition and establish follow-up appointments as necessary.

Physical therapy for particular disorders

Juvenile chronic polyarthritis (JCP)

This term is used to describe a group of polyarthropathies that may occur before the age of 16, and which may frequently affect the foot. It is important that the therapist is involved from the earliest stage possible in the management of such a child. Physiotherapy plays a vital part in the management of these conditions coupled with drug therapy.

In the acute phase full bed rest should be avoided unless the child is febrile and systemically ill. Throughout this stage the therapist must aim to prevent contractures and to maintain soft tissue extensibility. These may be avoided by ensuring that each joint is moved through its full available range each day and pain relief may be afforded by the application of ice packs to inflamed joints. All joints of the feet may be affected in JCP but the most common deformities are flexion contractures of the long flexors of the toes, subluxation of the metatarsal heads, hallux abductovalgus and hindfoot varus or valgus deformity.[4] Therefore the physiotherapist must ensure that these joints are moved individually either actively or with assistance, daily. Great sensitivity and encouragement may be required to teach parents to perform these activities, which may cause some degree of pain to their child.

Resting splints may be applied to the feet and ankles in order to relieve pain and to prevent tightening of the tendo calcaneus. Such splints should aim to hold the foot in a neutral position and their use should be interspersed with movement.

In the acute stage, irrespective of whether the child is in hospital or at home, good posture should be emphasised. Parents should be advised that although putting a pillow under the child's knees may be more comfortable, this may lead to flexion contractures. Similarly a bed cradle should be used to avoid the weight of the covers pulling the foot into plantarflexion. Hydrotherapy may be used in the early stage in order to maintain joint range and to facilitate normal movement before this is possible on dry land. This is especially beneficial for re-education of gait because of the reduction in weightbearing that water provides.

When the child is ambulant, some form of walking aid with gutter handles to prevent extra strain on the hand joints should be provided.

As the joints become less acute more active movement may be undertaken and movement therapy should be progressed when appropriate. At this stage the child will be discharged home and the parents must be completely familiar with the movement regime that the therapist has initiated and they should be in regular contact with her in order to discuss any difficulties.

In the chronic phase when pain has subsided, the child may be left with stiffened joints, weakened muscles and some degree of deformity. Hydrotherapy is very valuable in improving range of movement with buoyancy assisted activities; such activities may be used to strengthen affected muscles. The child must perform a daily routine of exercises for all joints of the body and the parents should be trained to correct and to progress these exercises.

Serial splintage may be used to stretch contracted soft tissue; this form of splintage is more commonly required for the knee than for the foot and ankle. Orthoses or ultimately surgical intervention may be required to overcome deformity and to provide a functional foot position. The therapist should constantly liaise with the parents to ensure that no problems are arising and the child should attend for regular maintenance check-ups.

Spina bifida

Damage to the spinal cord may result when there is incomplete closure of the vertebral canal. In such an event there may be flaccid paraparesis of the muscles innervated by the affected nerve roots and spastic paraparesis of the muscles below the level of the lesion.

Flaccidity may be described as a decreased ability of contraction of a muscle due to damage of its peripheral nerve. This leads to paralysis of the muscle when there is no innervation, or severe weakness when there is partial innervation.

Spasticity or hypertonia is one form of increased muscle tone where there is increased sensitivity to stretch of a muscle due to a release of reflex activity from cortical inhibition. Such increased muscle tone tends to affect specific muscle groups rather than all muscles and a characteristic movement and limitation is then produced. This type of neurological lesion is often accompanied by spinal deformities which may lead to decreased respiratory function and to poor use of the upper limbs. Lower limb deformities may be caused by abnormal tone and muscle imbalance and should be treated as soon after birth as possible. As the child develops and maintains poor postures worsened by abnormal muscle tone, there is a danger that his deformities will worsen and that other bony changes may ensue. Such bony changes may include femoral antetorsion when there is prolonged increased tone in the hip flexors and adductors, or leg shortening when an asymmetrical posture is maintained. It is very important therefore that the therapist maintains soft tissue extensibility by the use of full range passive movements and techniques in order to normalise tone and educate posture. Parents should also be taught how these activities should be performed and they should also be advised of their importance.

The type of deformity that may occur in the lower limbs will depend upon which muscle actions are unopposed and upon any other external factors that may influence joint position. The following are examples of common deformities that may occur:[4]

1. Calcaneovalgus or varus deformity may be caused by weakness in the plantarflexors relative to the dorsiflexors.
2. Equinovarus deformity may be caused by weak evertors and dorsiflexors.

3. Flexion of the metatarsophalangeal joints may be caused by weak lumbricals.
4. A flexion deformity of the forefoot may be caused by an uncorrected calcaneal deformity with associated effects of gravity and pressure of bedclothes.
5. A flexion deformity of the knees may be caused by weakness of the knee extensors.
6. Hyperextension of the knee may occur by unopposed action of the quadriceps.

It may not be possible for physiotherapy to assist in the correction where deformities are brought about by abnormal muscle pull. In such cases orthotic management or orthopaedic surgery is indicated.

The physiotherapist will encourage the child to move through the development sequence beginning at a level appropriate for the child's abilities. Movement may be used to encourage head control at a very early age and this may lead on to assisted rolling or other activities. It must be remembered that there is likely to be altered tone below the level of the cord lesion and this makes the use of the lower limbs difficult and all body movements are therefore affected.

Some form of mobility aid will probably be required by the child with spina bifida. Such aids may be in the form of calipers (with or without pelvic and thoracic bands) and crutches, the level of support being dependent upon the level of the lesion. Most children should be ambulant with some form of aid. Irrespective of the walking aid used the child will require to develop the musculature in the upper limb, shoulder girdle and trunk in order to enable him to bear his body weight and to propel himself. The physiotherapist will therefore devise a suitable exercise regime to strengthen these affected muscles.

As with all paediatric conditions, it is very important that the parents are informed and are involved in the management of their child and that they are always aware that they can contact the physiotherapist for help and advice when problems arise. As there is likely to be some degree of sensory loss, parents must be made aware that the skin may be damaged and that pressure sores and ulcers may develop. The parents must be aware of the damage that may be caused by the pressure exerted by wrinkled socks or ill-fitting shoes, or by the use of excessively hot water when bathing.

Cerebral palsy (CP)

Cerebral palsy is thought to be due to damage or maldevelopment of the brain around the time of birth. This leads to abnormalities in muscle tone, sensation, balance and coordination and there may be associated speech, sight, and perceptual problems or epilepsy. As there are many manifestations of this condition, and as clinical features will depend upon the area of the brain involved and the severity of its damage, it is almost impossible to outline the role of the physiotherapist in its management. However, the condition may be broadly categorised as:

1. Prevention of deformities: these most commonly occur in the CP child with increased muscle tone since the muscles are rarely fully stretched. Treatment of deformities has already been discussed under spina bifida.
2. Facilitation of normal movement: normal movement may be only performed with normal tone and sensation. Therefore the therapist will aim to assist the child to move through the developmental sequence by trying to alter tone to a more normal level and techniques to improve sensory awareness will also be employed.
3. Re-education of gait: this may be undertaken only in conjunction with normal movement activities. Although there is always an emphasis on maximising function, walking on a hypertonic, inverted and plantarflexed foot will ultimately lead to an increase in tone and to greater deformity and to an even more abnormal gait pattern in an affected child.

References

1 Illingworth RS. *The Development of the Infant and Young Child*, 5th edn. Churchill Livingstone, 1972.
2 Kisner C, Colby LA. *Therapeutic Exercise. Foundations and Techniques*. Philadelphia, FA Davis Company, 1985.
3 Melzack R, Wall P. *The Challenge of Pain*. Penguin Education, 1982.
4 Shepherd R. *Physiotherapy in Paediatrics*. London, Heinemann, 1974.

Further reading

Downie PA. (ed) *Cash's Textbook of Neurology for Physiotherapists*, 4th edn. London, Faber and Faber, 1986.

Gassier J. *A Guide to the Psycho-Motor Development of the Child*. London, Churchill Livingstone, 1984.

Hall J, Bisson D, O'Hare P. *The Physiology of Immersion Physiotherapy*, 1990, Vol. 76. No. 9: 517–521.

Hunt G. (ed) *Physical Therapy of the Foot and Ankle*. Churchill Livingstone, 1988.

Maitland GD. *Peripheral Manipulation*. Butterworths, 1977.

McMennell J. *Foot Pain*. London, J and A Churchill, 1969.

Neale D, Adams I. (eds) *Common Foot Disorders*, 3rd edn. Churchill Livingstone, 1989.

Scrutton D, Gilbertson M. *Physiotherapy in Paediatric Practise*. Butterworths, 1975.

Skinner AT, Thomson AM. (eds) *Duffield's Exercise in Water*, 3rd edn. Baillière Tindall, 1983.

12 Orthotic Management

James Woodburn

In recent years many advances have been made in the field of paediatric biomechanics and gait analysis which have greatly improved our understanding of foot function. Coupled with this has been the introduction of new materials and techniques for orthosis production. The use of orthoses has made a significant contribution to the management of many congenital and early childhood lower limb and foot disorders. However, paediatric orthoses must be used selectively and with care. The podiatrist must take into consideration many factors when considering the use of orthoses in the treatment programme. These include:

1. The nature of the presenting condition.
2. The extent of the presenting condition.
3. The age of the patient.
4. The biomechanical function of lower limb and foot orthoses.
5. The characteristics of the orthoses available.
6. The manufacture of orthoses.

The nature of the presenting condition

The podiatrist must establish whether the disorder or deformity present is a localised condition or whether it is part of a more widespread generalised disorder, e.g. where joint instability presents as a feature of a neurological disorder. Will the instability improve or deteriorate? Will a regional orthosis stabilise the joint and improve function or will other measures be required?

The identification of the structures involved in the deformity is of major consideration. Differentiating between rigid and mobile deformity will influence the decision to use an orthosis and the choice of material for that orthosis.

The extent of the disorder present

The podiatrist must have a clear understanding of normal ontogenic development in the lower limb and foot.[1] The limits of normal variation seen during development must also be considered as apparent deformities, e.g. genu valgum, may be observed during phases of normal ontogenic development. Such deformities have no adverse long-term effects on foot function and intervention with orthoses is not indicated. Spontaneous correction is almost always seen.

Additional criteria which must be considered in the prescription of orthoses for children include, (i) the history of the presenting signs and symptoms; (ii) the progressive nature of the instability or deformity; (iii) the presence of pain in the leg or foot; and (iv) the presence of a family history. Disagreement exists between those who choose to intervene and prescribe orthoses and those who choose to monitor the condition looking for spontaneous correction. Obviously more research is required to address these issues. However, there are those who would suggest that monitoring alone is done at the expense of valuable weeks and months in which possible correction of a deformity may be obtained.

The age of the child

The podiatrist must be aware of ossification and epiphyseal plate closure times and of the possible harmful affects of orthoses on these processes. The mouldable soft tissue and ossifying structures of the foot may also be susceptible to damage from orthoses when they are prescribed at inappropriate times or when they are manufactured to incorrect specifications. Where corrective orthoses are prescribed developmental processes are of considerable importance. This is most apparent with deformities such as metatarsus adductovarus and calcaneovalgus which are only sensitive to manipulation at critical times.

Skeletal development and maturation in the

lower limb and foot are therefore critical factors when considering orthoses for children.

The biomechanical function of lower limb and foot orthoses

The podiatrist must have a clear understanding of the biomechanical function of the orthoses in current use. Lower limb and foot orthoses may be used for:

1. Stability: an orthosis which controls hypermobile joint states, e.g. heel cups, Shaffer plates and Whitman plates.
2. Correction: an orthosis which applies a force around a deformity with little or no involvement of normal structures to correct that deformity, e.g. silicone toe props, Hexelite night splints for metatarsus adductus and the Denis Browne splint.
3. Prevention: an orthosis which may be used for a temporary or prolonged period of time in order to prevent deformity, e.g. an anti-pronatory orthosis.

Directly or indirectly orthoses may also provide pain relief by reducing stresses on damaged or vulnerable tissues. In addition the range and direction of joint motion may be controlled by orthoses as in a foot with muscle imbalance due to neurological deficit, e.g. ankle–foot orthoses (AFO). Phasic muscle exercise may also be achieved with lower limb and foot orthoses. For the child this is important and may contribute to the improvement of stability in the foot.

The characteristics of the orthoses available[2]

Invariably the podiatrist is faced with a wide selection of orthoses which are suitable for use in a number of lower limb and foot problems. Any chosen orthosis should display the following ideal characteristics:

1. The orthosis must have a proven biomechanical effect.
2. The orthosis should be durable, lightweight, reliable in use and should be of high manufacturing standards.
3. The orthosis should be able to be easily and quickly repaired. Delay between supply times should be kept to a minimum.

4. The orthosis should be cosmetically pleasing, comfortable and hygienic.
5. The orthosis should be easy and safe to use. Instructions must be simple and easy to understand both for the child and for his parents.

The manufacture of orthoses

A significant number of podiatrists prescribe, manufacture and fit orthoses within their own department or practice. Certain paediatric orthotic techniques may be performed direct to the patient, e.g. direct splinting techniques in order to provide quick and effective orthoses. The choice and properties of materials used and the relative cost and availability of these materials will determine the type of orthoses that can be manufactured. The complexity of machining and finishing of devices must also be considered. The use of commercial orthotic laboratories and the employment of trained technicians within the health service has extended the range and quality of orthoses available to the podiatrist.

Materials

The range[3, 4] and quality of materials suitable for orthosis manufacture has improved significantly in recent years. Podiatrists can now manufacture orthoses to high finishing standards and as a consequence treatment outcomes have also improved both in terms of time and in the degree of stability or correction achieved.

Plastics form the largest category of materials used. The material is used for the manufacture of stabilising orthoses, corrective splints and for covering orthoses to reduce stresses at the foot/shoe interface. Plaster of Paris is extensively used as a splinting material for serial casting techniques and as an impression medium. Silicones are used for orthodigital splinting techniques. Traditional materials such as cork and felt still remain popular for insole manufacture, for wedges and for footwear padding and for splints.

Plastics

High temperature thermoplastics are almost exclusively used as rigid splint materials and as base or shell materials in the manufacture of plantar functional orthoses. Such materials soften when heated since this heating breaks the weak cross-linking bonds between the polymer molecules. These bonds reform as the material cools. The working temperature for these plastics ranges from 110 °C to 180 °C and therefore they are only suitable for moulding over impression models. The higher the working temperature the more cross-linking bonds there are and the greater the mechanical properties of the material. A hot air-circulating oven and a fully equipped laboratory facility are required when these materials are to be used. To produce a finished orthosis for a child may take some considerable time and several fitting appointments may be necessary. Optimum stability and correction are properties inherent to orthoses which are manufactured in high temperature thermoplastics.

High temperature thermoplastics are classified under several headings and trade names, as outlined below.

1. Polyvinyl chloride (PVC), e.g. Pacton

PVC has been successfully used for many types of functional and corrective orthoses for children. The material has high impact strength, rigidity and resistance to chemical damage. It is a safe material to use both for stabilising functional devices and for corrective night splints. The working temperature is between 110 °C and 130 °C. At 3–5 mm the material is rigid in use and it is a suitable alternative to acrylic glass such as Plexidur.

2. Polyethylene, e.g. Vitrathene, Northene, Ultranorthene

This material is available in sheet form and has been found to be entirely safe. Simple manufacturing techniques produce high quality orthoses. Pre-cut blanks are available which help to avoid many intermediary preparation procedures. Low density polythene based orthoses (Vitrathene) are semi-flexible and this property is often desirable for plantar functional orthoses for the young infant or where rigid control is not indicated. The working temperature for this material is 140 °C.

High molecular weight polythene (Northene) is a tougher, more rigid form of polythene. The use of this material is indicated for orthoses which offer rigid functional control or for those which are necessary to correct a deformity. Northene is also suitable for heavy children or for those who participate in sporting activities. The working temperature of this material is 165 °C. The material will lend itself to vacuum forming and has a working time of one minute in its malleable state.

Ultranorthene is a softer semi-rigid plastic sheet. The flexibility of the material makes it an ideal choice for ankle–foot orthoses (AFO).

3. Plastic foams, e.g. Plastazote, Evazote

Closed-cell, cross-linked polyethylene foam and ethyl vinyl acetate are available in various thicknesses and densities. For paediatric use high density versions of the materials may be employed in the manufacture of semi-flexible stabilising plantar orthoses. The material may also be used either as a base material for simple insole devices or as a lining material on orthoses.

4. Polymethylmethacrylate, e.g. Plexidur

This material belongs to the group of acrylic glasses. Plexidur has high strength, good toughness and a high rigidity factor. It is particularly suitable for rigid foot orthoses and splints.

For practical purposes low temperature thermoplastics are those which may be formed directly onto the patient. This is possible because of the low moulding temperatures of these plastics. Such materials are commonly used in the manufacture of paediatric splinting devices. Again this group of materials is available in different forms.

1. Plastic sheeting, e.g. San splint, San splint XR, Orthoplast, Aquaplast

These materials have activating temperatures of 60–80 °C which makes them suitable to heat in hot water when an oven is not available. The materials are in sheet form and may therefore be cut to the desired shape before application which may be direct to the skin over a thin protective cover such as stockingette. Setting times vary between 6 and 10 minutes. The materials are easy to mould and the finished devices may be adjusted as necessary with scissors. Semi-flexible and rigid splints may be readily manufactured from these materials.

2. Bandage materials, e.g. Hexelite

Hexelite is a low temperature, thermoplastic bandage material which may be used for direct forming. The material is readily cut to size and may be activated at a temperature of between 70 and 80 °C by using a hot water bath. The material is auto-adhesive and may be laminated to produce a rigid device with a hard porous mesh surface with a matt white finish. The material is useful in the manufacture of night splints and it may also be used as a splint in order to maintain correction after serial casting treatments or as a plaster of Paris cast protector.

Insoling materials and orthosis lining materials

Three types of insoling and lining materials are employed in paediatric care.

1. Closed cell cross-linked polythene foams

Plastazote is an effective insole base or lining material. Shock-absorption, insulation and dynamic friction reduction are some of the properties of this material which make it attractive to use.

2. Open cell polyurethane foams

Cleron, PPT and Poron 4000 may be used as simple arch supports incorporated onto an insole base. Additionally they may be used for heel pads, simple insoles or as a lining material. Such polyurethane foams exhibit good shock absorption properties and the foam has minimal compression set and good elastic memory. These materials also absorb moisture and this property may be important for the adolescent hyperhidrotic foot thus allowing the foot to remain dry, cool and comfortable.

3. Non-cellular polyurethane elastomers

Sorbothane and Viscolas demonstrate minimal compression set and excellent elastic memory. They offer cushioning by shock attenuation and are ideal for the sporting child or in heavier individuals.

Traditional materials

Cork heel wedges may be easily manufactured as temporary antipronatory devices. Birkocork is readily vacuum formed to impression casts for the manufacture of semi-flexible orthoses. Felt may be used for the manufacture of triplanar wedges and as padding material incorporated into a shoe in order to provide correction of metatarsus adductus.

Plaster of Paris

This is an extremely versatile material. In bandage form it is used in both serial and impression casting techniques. The material is easy to handle and to work. Finished casts are strong and will maintain a mobile deformity in a corrected position for moderate periods of time. The casts require regular replacement and also the use of soft cotton underwrap material to avoid soft tissue irritation. Although heavy the casts will seldom impair mobility in the active child. Attention must be given to the joints proximal and distal to the cast as the weight of the splint may adversely influence their position and development. This is a major concern around the knee when below-knee plaster serial casts are used to treat congenital and developmental foot deformities.

Plaster of Paris in powder form is used to obtain a positive model from a negative cast impression. This positive model is easy to adjust and to modify to individual specifications. A good surface finish may be achieved on the model to allow accurate forming of plastics during orthosis manufacture.

Silicones

Silicone rubber is a white viscid polymer which is converted to a stable resilient elastomer by the addition of a suitable catalyst. The addition of pigments can approximate the material near to skin colour. Plasticisers may be added in order to vary the softness of the finished product.

In paediatric care the use of silicone materials has been primarily for the correction of congenital and acquired toe deformities where they may be used alone or in conjunction with a stabilising foot orthosis. Other uses are protective devices, heel cups and prosthetics.

Many types of silicones are available although the dental elastomers such as Xantopren, Verone RS and Verone G, which were used extensively in the early years, have now been replaced by silicones such as Podiaform (KE 20) which have been manufactured specifically for podiatric use.

The properties of the silicones and their mixture with catalysts and plasticisers dictate the technique of application of the material. There are three basic silicone techniques.

1. Flow-on techniques. The silicone impression material, e.g. Podiaform (KE 20), is mixed with a catalyst according to the manufacturer's instructions. The mix is then quickly poured or spatulated onto the required area and allowed to set. The silicone may be manipulated in situ with the fingers whilst the foot is held in a functionally neutral position. This position should be maintained for about four minutes until the material sets. The flow-on technique is difficult to control, particularly when the area of interest is the toe region. Additionally, small skin ridges are cast on the surface of the device and these ridges may irritate the child's skin. Reactions to the catalyst may also occur. When flow-on techniques are used no plasticiser is incorporated into the mix. The finished device may be brittle and hard and subsequently young children may not tolerate them. The relative hardness required in a device to afford correction of a deformity may be lost at the expense of modifying the device for comfort. However, this technique is still useful where larger areas are to be covered, e.g. when making protective heel cups, and the device may be trimmed and adjusted as necessary.

2. Preforming techniques. In the preforming technique, the basic material is mixed with a plasticiser or emollient. The proportions are two parts silicone by volume to one part emollient/plasticiser by volume. When an emollient or plasticiser is used the volume of catalyst required is doubled in amount. The resulting mix may be transferred to the hands which should also be prepared with emollient or oil to prevent sticking. The mix may then be moulded to an approximate shape of the finished device and applied to the toe area.

The foot should also be prepared with emollient. The silicone may then be moulded to the desired shape and once again the foot should be appropriately referenced whilst the silicone sets. Setting will normally occur within 20–30 seconds depending upon the amount of silicone used. This technique produces well finished orthoses. The catalyst is absorbed before the material reaches the skin and therefore irritation is less likely to occur. The material performs well under shear and tensile stresses without distortion and any modification of finished devices may be carried out with ease. This technique is the one of choice especially where correction is required for children's toe deformities.

3. Silicone putty technique. Silicone putties, e.g. Otoform K and Podiaform 2, are by far the easiest of the silicone materials to use in clinical practice. The addition of fillers to the basic silicone produces a putty like substance which is easy to handle, mould and mix. However, such fillers reduce the amount of pure silicone in the mix and limit the amount of cross-linking available. A reduction in the amount of cross-linking reduces the ability of the material to resist deforming stresses. Silicone putty orthoses are quickly deformed under shear and tensile stress. Since orthoses frequently tear, their life span is invariably short.

When using silicone putties a mixing pad, dish or block is not required. The material is easily workable in the hands and a trial application may be attempted before the addition of the catalyst. The quality of the final orthosis will vary depending upon the amount of catalyst used. Soft, easily deformed devices occur when too little catalyst is used, whilst a silicone putty orthosis which is manufactured using too much catalyst, will fissure as maximal bonding will occur leaving free catalyst between bonding surfaces.

Silicone putties are easy, quick and cheap to manufacture. Without the addition of silicone elastomers to harden the structure, corrective orthoses for children's toe deformities cannot be made with silicone putties.

Paediatric impression casting techniques

Materials

1. Plaster of Paris bandage and powder.
2. Water and metal casting tray.
3. Emollient for child's skin.
4. Plaster separator for negative:positive cast interface.
5. Abrasive pads/paper.

Impression casting techniques serve to capture the foot in the most functionally stable position. From a positive impression cast a suitable orthosis is then designed.

In children below the age of three impression casting for the manufacture of orthoses is not always necessary. The cartilaginous nature of the foot at this age and the absence of ossification at the navicular means that generalised rather than custom-made orthoses can be supplied. The child above the age of three will require custom designed orthoses manufactured on accurate representative impression models. In addition to providing optimal support and control, orthoses designed to individual impression casts must not damage immature osseous structures in the foot. Ontogenic development within individual bones and the alignment between the bones are sensitive to the external forces applied around these structures (Wolff's law and the Heuter–Volkmann principle). Therefore when an inaccurate, malaligned cast is taken the subsequent orthosis designed to that cast may damage the young foot. Stability and correction must not be obtained at the expense of normal osseous development of the foot.

The criteria for impression casting in children at all ages are:

1. The calcaneus is captured in a neutral or vertical position.
2. The metatarsals are captured on the same plane perpendicular to or in slight valgus to the vertical bisection of the calcaneus.
3. The medial longitudinal arch profile is obtained.

Any impression casting technique adapted for children should be quick to perform with little or no discomfort to the child.

Three techniques for impression casting are available and the choice of technique is based upon the age of the child and upon the associated skeletal development. The criteria aforementioned should where possible be realised.

The Root neutral position casting technique[5]

For this technique plaster of Paris bandage is applied to the child's foot which is then held in an anatomically referenced position until the plaster sets. This is a non-weightbearing technique where the child may lie prone or supine. The anatomical referencing for this technique is:

– The knee joint fully extended.
– The ankle joint dorsiflexed to resistance.
– The subtalar joint in neutral position.
– The forefoot locked against the hindfoot about the midtarsal joint (either by pushing up on the fourth and fifth metatarsal heads or by using the toe suspension technique).

When the cast has set it is removed from the foot and is allowed to dry. The cast is then assessed for errors particularly when a false pronated or supinated position is captured. An orthosis manufactured from such a cast would be extremely detrimental to foot function in the child. A positive model is prepared from the negative cast in the usual manner. Surface flaws on the plaster model may then be removed with abrasive paper or pads in order to leave a smooth surface. The model is then ready for the reception of a mouldable plastic material for the manufacture of an appropriate orthosis.

Advantages of this technique

1. The plantar soft tissue contours can be captured in a non-weightbearing position (where the toe suspension technique is used).
2. A single individual can manipulate the foot and can maintain it in the neutral position whilst the plaster sets.
3. A valid forefoot/hindfoot relationship is captured.

4. Minimum alteration of the positive cast is required.

Disadvantages of this technique

1. This technique is only suitable for children above the age of 10. In children under this age calcaneal varus and forefoot varus are present. The extent of the varus alignment of the foot is age dependent. Natural ontogenic development should realise a parallel forefoot/hindfoot and a perpendicular calcaneus by the age of 8. However, development in certain individuals may continue up to the age of 10–12. When an orthosis is manufactured to a positive cast of a child's foot captured in the neutral position, forefoot posting has to be incorporated into the design of the orthosis in order to maintain the foot in a functionally stable position. The possible consequences of the use of this orthosis would be the prevention of a proportion of compensatory motion, i.e. pronation at the expense of encouraging the retention of up to five degrees or more of forefoot varus. Although a hindfoot post of two degrees may be allowed, forefoot posting should be avoided.[6] Therefore this technique may only be suitable for adults and older children.[1]
2. The accurate alignment of bone segments during this five minute procedure in the child who is easily distracted or distressed cannot always be maintained. In certain instances the child's attention may be held by means of a suitable toy or doll.

Non-weightbearing semi-referenced casting technique

This technique incorporates certain of the features of the Root neutral casting technique. The child may adopt a supine, prone or sitting position with the legs dangling over an examination couch. Plaster of Paris bandage is applied in the usual way. The principal aim of this technique is to manipulate the position of the forefoot in such a way that all the metatarsals lie on the same plane whilst the calcaneus is placed in the vertical or neutral position. Correction of the forefoot position may be achieved by grasping the forefoot with the thumb placed on the dorsum and the forefinger on the plantar surface spanning all five metatarsals. A valgus rotation of the forefoot on the hindfoot may then be applied. It is important to maintain the vertical or neutral position of the calcaneus whilst the forefoot is corrected. An excessive forefoot valgus position should be avoided. Less emphasis is placed on the ankle and knee position although the ankle should not be in equinus.

Advantages of this technique

1. The plantar arch contours are captured in the cast.
2. Correction of the forefoot position may be achieved. An orthosis designed to the cast would not adversely affect normal ontogenic development. The orthosis would provide heel, medial and plantar support and would therefore be suitable for the child above the age of three who had developed a propulsive gait.

Disadvantages of this technique

1. In the irritable or restless child active correction may be difficult to maintain whilst waiting for the plaster to set. Again the child may require to be distracted by means of a suitable toy or doll. Where the corrected forefoot/hindfoot position is not guaranteed the foot once more may be subjected to undesirable forces from a functionally unsuitable orthosis.
2. The positive cast requires adjusting and finishing due to the thumb and forefinger print which remains from the forefoot manipulation.
3. As with the Root neutral technique a heel expansion may be required to accommodate the soft tissues of this region.

The semi-weightbearing casting technique[1,7]

This technique may be the most appropriate for the child under the age of 10. With this technique the child adopts a sitting position, the height of which is altered so that the knee and ankle joints are at 90 degrees and the foot rests on the floor. The plaster bandage is applied and the foot is manipulated as follows. Internal or external rotation is applied around the leg in order to bring the calcaneus to the vertical. The child can help with this. While the leg and hindfoot position is maintained the opposite hand of the clinician is placed over the dorsum of the foot spanning all five metatarsals. Downward pressure is applied in order to bring all the metatarsals into ground contact in the same plane. With the calcaneus held in a vertical position the plane of the forefoot will be perpendicular to the calcaneal bisection. The foot is maintained in this position until the plaster sets. Particular attention should be placed on moulding the plaster to the arch region. This is achieved much more easily by moulding the plaster to the foot before the foot is placed in ground contact. A polished plastic board should be used between the foot and the weightbearing surface. This board may be easily cleaned and it prevents the cast from sticking to the floor. Additionally the use of a raised plinth for the child to sit on allows the clinician easy access to the leg and foot.

Advantages of this technique

1. The corrected position of the forefoot is easy to achieve with this technique. The opposing force from the ground is uniform and therefore 'bunching' of the metatarsals is avoided. The metatarsals may be maintained in the same plane parallel to that of the hindfoot and perpendicular to the calcaneal bisection. An orthosis designed to such a cast will offer individualised midtarsal support whilst maintaining vertical heel position. It will not adversely affect foot function or ontogenic development.
2. This technique is suitable for children of all ages and it is also a suitable alternative to the use of the Root technique for the older child or adolescent.
3. The semi-weightbearing technique allows natural soft-tissue expansion to be captured in the cast. This negates the need for positive cast alteration such as expansions.
4. This technique is more suited for the uncooperative child. The sitting position 'locks' the foot to the ground whilst the leg and forefoot is held. The child is not frightened by lying down and the parents can hold the child's attention or distract him more easily.

Disadvantages of this technique

1. There may be difficulty in maintaining the leg and foot in the corrected position during casting. This can be improved by having two clinicians involved and by practising the technique with the child before the plaster is applied. Additionally the plaster can be allowed to achieve a considerable amount of setting before the foot is placed to the ground.
2. An arch profile may be difficult to obtain. A ridge in the plaster material frequently occurs where the lowest aspect of the arch in the midfoot region meets the ground. This ridge will subsequently appear on the positive cast and therefore some alteration to the cast will be required in order to ensure that the orthosis is comfortable.

The choice of casting technique is often a matter of individual preference. The criteria for impression casting must be met when a technique is adopted or is modified for children. An accurate impression cast is the basis for safe effective orthosis manufacture. When considering the possible damage that orthoses may do on immature structures, attention to technique is critical for impression casting.

Paediatric lower limb and foot orthoses

Devices for the hypermobile/ hyperpronated flatfoot

Heel stabilisers (Fig. 12.1)

A corrective heel seat device for the treatment of the valgus heel was described by Helfet in 1956.[8] The heel cup holds the heel vertical or slightly inverted and allows the metatarsals to fall to the supporting surface. Helfet believed that the device had an advantage over more distal arch supports in that the heel seat created a valgus relationship in the forefoot which in turn created the arch.

There are many types of commercial prefabricated heel cups available to control prona-

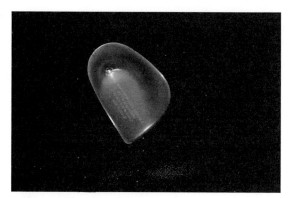

Figure 12.1   Heel stabiliser.

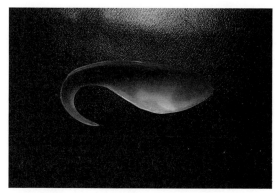

Figure 12.2   Rose–Schwartz heel meniscus.

tion in the child's foot. Additionally a device may be easily constructed by moulding a suitable high temperature thermoplastic over a positive model of the heel region. It is essential for the manufacture of heel cups that the cast is taken in a weightbearing position. A square sectional appearance to the orthosis is important in order to allow the turning of vertical forces through a right angle. This will allow effective transformation of the body weight into a horizontal corrective force.

Heel stabilisers may be indicated in cases of excessive pronation where hypermobility is coexistent and where the child will tend to pronate off a standard plantar device. In the child below the age of three who has yet to develop a propulsive gait the heel stabiliser may also be used. Here the excessive motion is eliminated rather than redirected.

The disadvantage of the heel seat is that the device tends to significantly reduce or even fully limit most of the subtalar joint motion. In use the heel seat also tends to rotate horizontally thus allowing the lateral border of the device to press uncomfortably against the lateral side of the foot.

Heel menisci (Fig. 12.2)

The Rose–Schwartz meniscus[2] was designed to prevent the inward rolling of the calcaneus. This meniscus consists of a medial flange which conforms to the arch profile and acts as a medial wedge. A shorter lateral flange extends from the heel cup and prevents the heel from slipping laterally. The device was originally constructed from fibreglass. Modifications for additional control include filling the

gap between the two flanges with a thin membrane.

A Rose–Schwartz meniscus may be constructed over a positive cast of the foot using rigid thermoplastic. Its use is indicated in children of all ages who exhibit moderate degrees of excessive calcaneal pronation and a valgus heel. The device should be monitored every three months and should be replaced as the child's foot grows. The meniscus may be prone, like heel stabilisers, to rotate medially under horizontal torsional forces. The use of the device should be withdrawn where this occurs and where stability is not achieved.

Shaffer plate (Fig. 12.3)

The Shaffer plate is a plantar shoe inlay and is used to provide plantar support and to control excessive pronation. Commonly constructed in metal the device comprises a small posterior

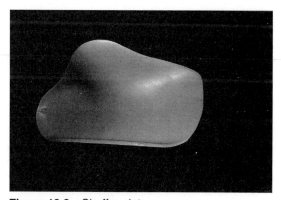

Figure 12.3   Shaffer plate.

heel cup which extends forward to just behind the metatarsophalangeal joints. The device has a medial longitudinal arch flange which extends up to the navicular.

A Shaffer shaped semi-soft orthosis manufactured in a flexible thermoplastic material may be used to control pronation in the 18 month to 3 year old child.[7] When used in a rigid shank stiff-countered shoe the device is provided with adequate rigidity in the arch contours. Above the age of three the Shaffer plate may be used in combination with a rigid shoe where mild excessive pronation is present.

Whitman plate

This rigid device was designed by Royal S. Whitman in 1907 and is intended to be used with the flexible but severely pronated foot. The device consists of a medial longitudinal arch support without a posterior heel cup. A small rectangular flange on the lateral border of the device extends upwards to just below the lateral malleolus. During gait, eversion of the heel causes pressure against the lateral rectangular flange. As the foot rolls, the medial flange is raised and this creates pressure on the soft tissues of the medial longitudinal arch. It was assumed that the pressure and pain caused would result in a reactionary and voluntary inversion of the foot away from the medial flange. When adequate muscle tone was achieved the orthoses would be discarded.

The device was originally constructed in metal but this is seldom used nowadays because of the pain produced. The device has been modified with the addition of a heel cup and with the extension and modification of the lateral flange. The modifications give the device the appearance of a Shaffer plate. The device may be manufactured in thermoplastic materials.

Roberts plate

Percy Willard Roberts originally designed this rigid orthosis to be attached to a leg brace in order to control a corrected clubfoot. The device has been extensively modified over the years but the original design consisted of a lateral and a medial flange and a longitudinal arch support. The flanges forced and held the calcaneus in an inverted position and the forefoot in an everted position. Again the orthosis was designed to be discontinued once the primary muscle weakness had corrected.

Modified Roberts–Whitman orthosis

The typical orthosis used to control pronation in both children and adults resembles a modified Roberts–Whitman device[6] and is often referred to as the Root functional foot orthosis. The orthosis consists of a high medial and lateral flange and a posterior heel cup. The rounded plantar heel section is stabilised using a level heel seat. With this device the subtalar and midtarsal joints are stabilised. The peroneus longus muscle is allowed to function about a stable cuboid in order to allow normal plantar flexion of the first ray. Tax[1] recommends a modification to this device whereby the area under the first metatarsal of the orthosis is cut out in order to allow normal articulation of the first ray around the metatarsal/cuneiform complex. The heel seat and forefoot may be posted when necessary in order to enhance the effectiveness of the device. The problems associated with using posting techniques where children are concerned and the need for a flattened posterior plantar heel region to aid in transmitting the body weight into a corrective force can be avoided when the device is constructed to a semi-weightbearing model of the foot.

UCBL shoe insert (Fig. 12.4)

This is a semi-rigid plastic laminate foot support designed by the University of California Biomechanics Laboratory. The orthosis is designed to a plaster model of the foot which is captured in a semi-weightbearing corrected position. The device consists of medial and lateral flanges which join at the heel in order to provide a deep heel cup. The flanges are high and extend to a position just proximal to the metatarsal heads. The device holds the calcaneus in a neutral position and the forefoot everted about the tarsometatarsal joints thereby elevating the medial longitudinal arch.

Semi-flexible prefabricated orthoses

In the child below the age of three, custom

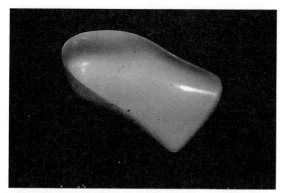

Figure 12.4   Shoe insert (University of California Biomechanics Laboratory – UCBL).

casted orthoses are unnecessary. Generalised foot support may be achieved by using pre-fabricated orthosis manufactured from average foot proportions. The orthoses should not have forefoot posting and where used the talo-navicular complex should be raised whilst the metatarsals lie on the same weightbearing plane. This plane should be perpendicular to the vertical bisection of the calcaneus. Such orthoses are available from commercial orthotic laboratories.

Valgus pads (navicular pads, arch cookies) (Fig. 12.5)

These may be quickly and easily constructed from felt or from modern insoling materials such as PPT or Cleron. The support may either

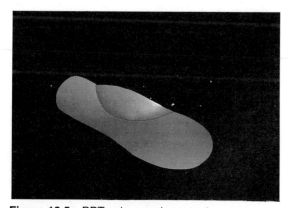

Figure 12.5   PPT valgus arch support.

be added to a template to fit the shoe or be cemented into the shoe. These may be used for children of any age and may be supplemented with a triplanar or medial heel wedge. In children who have developed a heel–toe propul-sive gait the use of a functional orthosis is indicated rather than the use of a simple arch support.

Triplanar wedges

The triplanar wedge[9] may be used to control excessive pronation in the child at an early age (24–36 months). The wedge is a supinatory pad which is fitted to the medial heel region of the shoe and it may be constructed from cork or dense felt. The felt is tapered in order to leave a high point to support the distal–medial aspect of the calcaneus.

The effectiveness of these orthoses is deter-mined not only by the design of the orthosis but by the footwear in which it will be used. For the child, such orthoses should be used in shoes which have a rigid shank, a stiff counter and a flexible forefoot in order to encourage propulsion. In cases of mild excessive prona-tion, shoes exhibiting these features may alone control the problems. In the severe pronating foot additional features such as a Thomas heel or medial heel wedge should be considered as necessary modifications in order to assist the action of the orthosis.

Regular review is necessary when utilising functional orthoses to manage excessive pro-nation in the child. The effectiveness of the orthosis should also be reviewed. Modifi-cations of the treatment plan may then be implemented at the earliest opportunity when necessary.

Other indications for the use of plantar functional orthoses

Pes cavus

Neurological pes cavus may be controlled functionally by using a plantar foot orthosis which controls the heel in its neutral position of varus. Additionally the orthosis should sup-port the longitudinal arch and evert the fore-foot. The Roberts plate was originally designed for use in the pes cavus foot. A modified Roberts–Whitman device which supports the foot is suitable in the management of this foot type. Stability of the foot is essential in order to slow the progression of the deformity and most importantly to reduce the risk of secondary soft tissue and osseous complications.

Osteochondritis

Calcaneal apophysitis, Frieberg's infarction and Kohler's disease of the navicular may manifest as pain in the foot. Although orthoses cannot alter the pathological processes involved, their use is important in stabilising the foot in order to reduce the stresses around these painful areas. In calcaneal apophysitis, for example, the use of orthoses is aimed at the removal or the reduction of traction forces on the apophysis. A semi-flexible orthosis with medial arch support and a heel lift will reduce the traction forces from the tendo Achillis by reducing subtalar or midtarsal pronation and by maintaining foot function around the neutral position.

Peroneal spastic flatfoot

The painful peroneal flatfoot may be aided by the use of a semi-flexible soft orthosis manufactured on a cast of the pronated foot position. Symptomatic relief is said to be more readily achieved by the use of orthoses when a calcaneonavicular bar is present.[7] The use of conservative orthosis management alone will be ineffective when a posterior or medial facet talocalcaneal bar is present.

The use of orthoses in the management of metatarsus adductovarus

The conservative management of metatarsus adductovarus is determined by the age of the child and by the extent of the deformity. Serial casting, although not strictly an orthosis, is the most effective method of treatment available for the moderate and severe flexible and functional forms of the deformity. The use of serial casting is supplemented by passive stretching, footwear therapy and by appropriate night-

splints. Serial casting is most effective in the pre-walking child but may be used selectively up to the age of two to three. Where there is present a mild form of metatarsus adductus, passive stretching and footwear therapy alone is usually effective.

Passive stretching

The parents are taught the following procedure:[10]

1. The subtalar joint is held in neutral or slight inversion (demonstrate a pronated position and warn about avoiding this position). The ankle joint should be held at 90 degrees or slightly plantarflexed.
2. The forefoot is grasped behind the metatarsal heads with the thumb and forefinger anchoring the metatarsals on a straight plane.
3. The forefoot is maximally abducted whilst the subtalar joint position is maintained. This position is held for 10 seconds and is repeated 10 times per session. Ten stretching sessions are advised each day. Nappy changes and after feeding are the most appropriate times for performing these stretches.

Footwear therapy[1]

A straight last shoe, with simple modifications, forms an effective splinting technique for mild, flexible metatarsus adductovarus. Optimum results are obtained in children below the age of 10 months.

The shoe is worn continually night and day for one week. Padding is then added in the following fashion:

1. A dense felt strip is applied from the distal medial tip of the front of the shoe to the base of the first metatarsal. This strip exerts an abductory force around the forefoot.
2. In order to counter this force, further padding is added over the lateral mid-aspect of the shoe corresponding to the cuboid region.
3. The abductory forces exerted around the forefoot from the shoe and the padding can unlock and sublux the midtarsal joint and pronate the hindfoot. This may not be a problem in infants who are not yet bearing

weight but the further measures required to counteract this problem are so simple that they should be included in the procedure. A felt medial varus wedge may be added to the shoe. Additionally the heel counter of the shoe when a close fit, should further prevent subtalar joint pronation.

The padded footwear therapy is used in conjunction with passive stretching exercises. The child should be reviewed regularly in order to replace compressed padding or to add extra padding to further influence correction. When correction is achieved, the padded shoes should be continued for a period twice as long as the time taken to correct the deformity. Shoes are renewed when the child outgrows them. The straight last shoes should be continued unpadded for a further two years. Night splints when required may also be used.

Serial casting

Serial casting is reserved for children who have moderate to severe deformity. Such casting is most useful in the pre-walker but where a degree of flexibility exists around a deformity the technique may be used selectively up to the age of two to three.

Procedure

1. Passive stretching exercises as previously described are implemented for 1–2 weeks prior to casting.
2. Before a cast is applied, 10 minutes is taken to manipulate the foot into a corrected position. In order to achieve this position an abductory force is applied around the forefoot whilst maintaining the subtalar joint in a neutral or slightly inverted position (the technique for passive stretching).
3. An underwrap is added in order to protect the leg and foot from the plaster bandage. Stockingette and Tubigrip are used between the skin and the underwrap material before the plaster bandage is applied. These materials are easy to use but they may allow excessive movement of the cast and this will either irritate the skin or will slip off. An alternative method is to paint compound tincture of benzoin onto the skin to which the underwrap material is applied directly

before the plaster bandage is used. The benzoin protects the skin and its tacky nature holds the underwrap material closely to the skin. When the plaster cast is applied it will not slip off nor will it move sufficiently to irritate the skin. The underwrap material is applied over the area to be casted. The material should extend beyond the proximal and distal ends of the cast in order to protect the skin from abrasions. One layer of underwrap is sufficient but further protective layers should be added over the first metatarsal head, the cuboid region, the head of the fibula and the posterior and plantar heel region.

4. A plaster cast is then applied to the leg and foot. A below knee cast may be applied but the weight of the cast may be sufficient to create excessive motion around the knee joint. This is more likely to occur when the child bears weight or when he walks with the cast but it may also occur in the pre-walker. A medial genicular position may be avoided when an above-knee cast is used. The cast may either be applied in sections positioning or correcting each region as the plaster is added or the cast may be applied as one unit and the deformity then corrected.
5. As the plaster dries the following manipulations should be performed:

   (a) When an above-knee cast is used the knee joint should be captured in 60 degrees of flexion.
   (b) The ankle joint should be held in neutral or in slight plantarflexion.
   (c) The calcaneus should be held in neutral or in slight inversion.
   (d) The metatarsals are held and manipulated into maximum abduction.

The corrected position is held until the plaster sets. Further layers of plaster bandage may be added in order to strengthen the cast. Walking heels and moulded Hexelite may also be used to protect the cast.

A return period of one week should be given to infants below the age of one year. Above this age 10–14 days is usually sufficient. The casts are replaced until correction is achieved (usually four casts at an average time of 4–6 weeks). When correction is achieved two further casts are applied to maintain the correction. After serial casting, night splints are used for 10–12 weeks. During the day the child should wear straight last shoes. The use of such shoes should be continued for up to two years after the serial casting.

Complications

1. Pressure sores from casts which have been applied too tightly. Such sores are more commonly seen around the heel, the cuboid region and the head of the first and fifth metatarsals.
2. A valgus hindfoot when the calcaneus is not held in neutral.
3. Internal positional changes around the knee from a heavy below knee cast.
4. Restriction of movement for the child; difficulties for the parents when bathing and dressing their children; sleeplessness and restlessness in the infant.
5. Common peroneal nerve irritation from the proximal end of a below knee cast. This problem is exceptionally rare and may be avoided by the use of appropriate protective padding to the area.

In the rigid or more severe forms of metatarsus adductus referral for an orthopaedic opinion should be sought or when no correction has been achieved after four or five casts.

Night splints

Mild and moderate flexible metatarsus adductus may be treated using night splints and passive muscle stretching exercises. Prefabricated commercially produced splints such as the Langer counter rotational device[11] and the Ganley splint[12, 13] are excellent devices to use. The split forefoot to hindfoot plates on these devices allow safe effective control of the foot whilst correction is maintained.

The podiatrist can manufacture corrective night splints after taking an impression cast of the foot in a corrected position. A rigid high temperature thermoplastic material may then be vacuum formed over the cast. The splint must extend around and above the heel. Adequate material must extend high and around onto the dorsomedial aspect of the foot and also distally to beyond the first metatarsophalangeal joint in order to hold the foot in the corrected position. The material must extend beyond the first metatarsophalangeal joint in order to avoid subluxing this joint. The abductory correcting force from the medial flange of the splint must be counteracted by a similar high lateral flange. The splint may be lined for comfort and Velcro straps attached in order to retain the splint on the foot. The device should be used at night and during naps. Combined with stretching exercises such an orthosis may be a primary form of treatment or it may be used following serial casting management.

Orthoses for torsional or rotational problems

Positional and rotational disorders of the lower limb and foot may be corrected by the use of bars and splints. Several of these devices are also effective for maintaining the corrected position of a deformity after serial casting. As a rule positional problems respond better than torsional problems. The conditions which respond best to the use of bar and splint devices are medial genicular rotation, internal femoral position, internal tibial torsion, talipes calcaneovalgus and metatarsus adductus.[13]

Care must be taken to apply the correcting force in a controlled manner when using bars and splints, e.g. transverse plane deformities should be corrected by no more than five degrees over a period of one month. Additional care should be given to the joints proximal and distal to the deformity. Where possible the correcting force must be transmitted as close to the deformity as possible without other joints being affected. A device used on the feet to correct a deformity around the hip transmits forces through the midtarsal joint, the subtalar joint, the ankle joint and the knee joint before affecting the hip. These joints must remain stable under such forces.

Bars and splints are used on children between the ages of three months and five years. They may be used at night or during the day whilst the child sleeps. Recent developments such as the Langer counter rotational system (CRS) allow active and uncomplicated movement for the child when the device is in place. Patient and parent compliance must be considered when these devices are used.

The link between the splint and bar is frequently a shoe and these are orthopaedic in type. When the child's own shoes are to be used high top shoes are advisable in order to prevent the child pulling his feet out of the shoes. In both instances the foot must be controlled within the shoe. Varus wedges are frequently added to prevent subtalar and midtarsal subluxation.

The Denis Browne orthosis, the Fillauer bar, the Uni-Bar, the Ganley splint, the Langer counter rotational system, the Friedman counter splint, the Stevens abduction splint and the Brachmann talipes splint are all well documented but the podiatrist need not have all of these devices at his disposal. Several devices should be available which may be used on the majority of lower limb or foot positional or torsional problems.

The Denis Browne splint (Fig. 12.6)

The Denis Browne splint was originally designed for the treatment of talipes calcaneovalgus. The device consists of a spreader bar and two metal plates or brackets to which the shoes are attached. Rotational adjustments

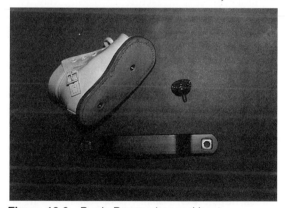

Figure 12.6   Denis Browne bar and boot.

may be made to the attachment plate as correction is obtained. The width of the bar should not exceed that of the pelvis otherwise a genu valgum deformity may arise. An inverted 'V' bend may be made in the centre of the bar in order to prevent pronatory foot problems.

The Denis Browne splint is not recommended for torsional hip problems but peri-articular soft tissue tightness will usually respond to treatment with this splint. The

Denis Browne bar is effective in cases of rotational disorders below the knee, e.g. internal tibiofibular rotation. The splint is still effectively used as originally intended for maintaining correction achieved after clubfoot surgery.

Lack of patient and parent compliance presents a major treatment problem with this splint. The device may be difficult to place on the child and the restricted movement that it creates is sometimes distressing to the child.

The splint is tolerated best in children below the age of four and is used as a night splint and also when the child sleeps during the day. Its use is continued until the deformity is corrected.

The Fillauer bar and the Uni-Bar are proprietary names for the Denis Browne splint. Such devices have been modified by employing clamps rather than screws on the footplate in order to allow easier fitting of the shoes and also the bar section can be fitted and adjusted with ease.

The Ganley splint[12, 14]

The Ganley splint consists of two forefoot and hindfoot plates which are connected by a central bar. The device is extremely versatile as the forefoot and hindfoot plates on the bar may be rotated on the frontal plane. Transverse rotations may also be achieved and the connecting bar can be altered to size. A varus bend in the bar may be set to avoid subluxations. Shoes which are split across the sole at the level of the tarsometatarsal joint are attached to the plates and are used where correction of a metatarsus adductus or calcaneovalgus deformity is required. The splint may also be used for the treatment of internal or external femoral position, internal tibial torsion or medial genicular rotation.

The paediatric counter rotation system (CRS)[10] (see Fig. 3.9)

This system has recently been developed by the Langer Biomechanics Group. Initial reports confirm the effectiveness and versatility of this device. When a single splinting device is required in a clinic then the CRS may fulfil all splinting requirements. The CRS is a modular device manufactured in high strength plastic.

It consists of a series of hinged and rotational joints which allow normal independent leg movement when the system is in place. The CRS allows the child to remain mobile whilst correction is achieved. An obliquely cut split forefoot again provides forefoot to hindfoot control.

The CRS modular unit is applied in three steps:

1. The patient's shoes are glued to the foot-plates.
2. The intoe or out-toe angle is set by means of an adjustable screw on each footplate.
3. The shoes are put on the child and the CRS unit is snapped onto place on the footplates which are attached to the foot.

This system is recommended for a variety of intoe and out-toe disorders and it may be used for post serial casting or as a primary form of therapy, e.g. for metatarsus adductus. The infant is able to crawl without difficulty and greater comfort is reported when the child is sleeping. The device has been designed in order to avoid secondary complications such as hip dislocation, lateral tibial torsion, genu valgum and pronated feet which very oc-casionally are reported with other splinting devices.

Gait plates[15]

Gait plates may be used on children above the age of two years who present with intoeing or out-toeing gaits. The gait plate is essentially a modified Shaffer type plate with an added dis-tal extension. Rigid high temperature thermo-plastic or acrylic materials are best employed. For intoeing gaits, the plate is extended later-ally over the fourth and fifth metatarsal heads to the toe cleft area. The medial portion remains behind the first metatarsal head. For out-toeing gaits the device is extended medially to under the first metatarsal head with the lateral portion proximal to the fourth and fifth metatarsal heads. This is often termed a reverse gait plate.

Gait plates are designed to function at the propulsive stage of the stance phase of gait. Therefore the gait of the child must be closely analysed in order to ensure that a propulsive heel–toe gait has developed. For maximum effect the plates function best in shoes which are flexible around the metatarsophalangeal joint area. Sports shoes are an ideal choice for children. When the gait plate is worn the shoe is unable to break at a right angle to the line of forward progression, unless the foot out-toes. Additionally part of the influence of the gait plate is lost during the swing phase. During stance phase improvements of 5–20 degrees of transverse rotation may be achieved. Gait plates may be used successfully in internal or external femoral positions and where internal and external tibiofibular segment rotation is present. When excessive pronation exists alongside the transverse rotational problem then this too should be addressed simul-taneously. The gait plates tend to be ineffective when the child intoes greater than 40 degrees.

References

1 Tax HR. *Podopediatrics*, 2nd edn. Williams and Wilkins, 1985.
2 Rose GK. *Orthotics, Principles and Practice.* London, Heinemann Medical, 1986.
3 Kippen CK. Insoling materials in foot orthosis manufacture – a review. *Chiropodist* May, 1989; 83–88.
4 Kippen CK. A review of plastic materials used in foot orthotic manufacture. *Chiropodist* May, 1989; 90–95.
5 Root ML, Orien WP, Weed JH. *Neutral Position Casting Techniques*, Vol. III. Los Angeles, Clinical Biomechanics Corp, 1978.
6 D'Amico JC. Developmental flatfoot. *Clin Podiatry* 1984; 1(3): 535–46.
7 Spencer AM, Person VA. Casting and orthotics for children. *Clin Podiatry* 1984; 1(3): 621–9.
8 Helfet AJ. A new way of treating flat feet in children. *Lancet* 1956; i: 262–4.
9 Valmassy RL, Terrafranca N. The triplane wedge: An adjunctive treatment modality in pediatric biomechanics. *J Am Podiatry Assoc* 1986; 76(12): 672–5.
10 Tachdjian MO. *Pediatric Orthopedics*, Vol. II. WB Saunders Company, 1972.
11 CRS. *Counter Rotation System.* Clinical Prospec-tus. Langer Biomechanics Group (UK) Ltd.
12 Lynch FR. The Ganley Splint. *Clin Podiatry* 1984; 1(3): 517–34.
13 Valmassy RL, Lipe L, Falconer R. Pediatric treat-ment modalities of the lower extremity. *J Am Podiatry Assoc* 1988; 78(2): 69–80.
14 Shoenhaus HD, Poss KD. The clinical and practi-cal aspects in treating torsional problems in chil-dren. *J Am Podiatry Assoc* 1977; 67(9): 620–7.
15 Schuster RO. A device to influence the angle of gait. *J Am Podiatry Assoc* 1967; 57(6): 269–70.

13 The Child in Dance and Sport

Thomas M. Novella, Kit Woods and
Ian Stother

Children of all ages should participate in sport or dance especially when they, as individuals, want to. It is important that outside pressure, e.g. from parents, from other children or from athletic coaches, does not force any child to pursue athletic activity to excess – either in quantity or in quality.

The individual child may obtain personal satisfaction from prowess in an athletic pastime, and have a natural aptitude for an individual sport, such as tennis, much as another child may excel at an academic subject. Such prowess is often rewarded by prizes gained in competition in schools and clubs and this recognition may also be a source of satisfaction to the child.

Team sports are an important means of developing interpersonal relationships. Such sports are one of the ways in which the developing individual learns how his rights also involve him in obligations, both to peers and to the society group in which he or she participates.

Many team sports involve physical contact with opponents, e.g. in rugby and association football. Those who are concerned with the organisation of such sports need to be aware of the risks to the participants. It is important also that parents of the players fully realise the potential dangers of sports. In contact sports it is important that teams compete only with other teams of similar age and weight. In schoolboy rugby, for example, serious neck injuries are much commoner when teams are not matched for age and weight. Therefore games against 'Old Boys' are potentially more dangerous.

Most children undergo an adolescent 'growth spurt'. This may occur from the age of about 10 years up to the age of about 16 years. This spurt tends to be earlier in girls than in boys and any child who has grown considerably recently is at a greater risk than usual of suffering from minor sprains of the joints and muscles. Recurrent injuries in an adolescent who has grown rapidly may really only be treated by rest. In certain instances the sufferer may need to abandon competitive athletics for up to a year.

As a child grows his or her physique alters and at a very variable point an individual changes from a child into a young adult. Most obvious are the changes in secondary sexual characteristics. Changes also occur in muscle bulk and power. Generally as the individual matures and puts on weight his or her power-to-weight ratio tends to fall so that peak performance may do likewise, although endurance may be improved, e.g. for long distance running.

At the same time as these physical changes occur, the mental attitude of the individual also alters. Young people often rebel at this stage of their development and they may lose their dedication towards activities which they previously enjoyed.

For some professional sports and for dancing as a career, it is important to try to predict the youngster's eventual height and weight but this is very difficult to do. Older brothers and sisters may serve as a useful guide, as may parents, but both genetic and environmental factors play a part in accurate estimations of an individual's eventual height and weight.

Childhood illnesses must be recognised and treated appropriately and it is important for trainers and coaches to be aware of chronic conditions, such as asthma, diabetes and epilepsy. For each of these conditions, exertion may precipitate symptoms which were previously well controlled. Obviously some conditions such as brittle bone disease and haemophilia effectively exclude the sufferers from many contact sports.

Any child wishing to consider dancing as a career will eventually undergo an audition at one of the dance schools. The precise details of the audition will vary from school to school and also with the type of dance in which the student wishes to major.

Physical examination of dance students

The physical examination of dance students assesses the whole child.

The precise details of the 'ideal' dancer are a matter of opinion. For most types of dancing boys need more power than joint mobility whilst girls need more mobility than power (because in many forms of dance the males support the females).

The following remarks apply especially to ballet dancers but many of the points apply to other forms of dance as well.

When the dancer stands he should be symmetrical. The head should be held straight and not tilted and the shoulders and the hips should be level.

Neck

The neck should be neither very long nor very short and should be flexible with a full range of flexion, extension, tilting and rotation; i.e. the dancer should be able to look downwards to approximate his chin onto his chest, to look upwards to the ceiling, to tilt each ear to the shoulder and to look 90 degrees to the left and to the right. Good neck movement is important in order to compensate for the rotation of the trunk which occurs in most dancing.

Shoulders

The shoulders should be level and the shoulder blades should be symmetrical and at the same height. Shoulder movement should be full with a normal anatomical range which allows:

1. The backs of the hands to be touched above the head with the elbows straight.
2. Both hands to be placed behind the back between the shoulder blades.
3. Both hands to be held with palms facing forwards with the elbows bent.

Upper limbs

Girls' hands require to be elegant but boys' hands must be strong. At the elbow too much recurvatum must be avoided. At the wrist it is important that there is a good range of dorsiflexion: it should be possible to bend the hand back to about 90 degrees. This is important when the hands are used to support other dancers overhead or when handstands, cartwheels or other more gymnastic movements are being performed.

Spine

A strong spine with normal posture is essential. There should be no scoliosis. Scoliosis in the upper spine may be detected as a rib hump. With the knees straight the child is asked to touch his toes. When the spine is curved the ribs will be more prominent on one side than on the other.

Scoliosis in the lower spine presents as a fullness of the muscles on one side of the spine itself.

Any child with either of these abnormalities should be referred to an orthopaedic surgeon.

Certain children possess an exaggerated normal anteroposterior curve of the spine. Their shoulders are rounded and the hollow in the lumbar spine is increased. Frequently such children have poor spinal muscles and they may require close supervision and spinal muscle exercises if they are to avoid spinal injuries when lifting and bending.

All dancers should possess a full range of spinal movement and they should be able to touch their toes and to lean backwards by a slightly smaller amount.

Hip joint

Hip movement is very important in ballet dancers. Any potential dancer must have good 'turnout' at the hips. In anatomical terms, turnout is external rotation of the hip joint in the extended position. This feature is important because in the five basic foot ballet positions, the feet are turned out to 90 degrees. For a dancer to avoid foot and knee problems it is important that the whole lower limb is turned out from the hip downwards.

The 'ideal dancer' has 90 degrees of turnout at each hip joint but this is very rare and girls show more turnout than boys. Rotation of the hip joint may be measured in a number of ways. Perhaps the easiest way is to have the patient on a firm couch with the knees bent over the end. The external rotation of the hips may then be measured as shown in Fig. 13.1. In this method of measurement turnout over

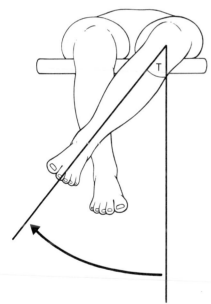

Figure 13.1 Measurement of hip turnout over the end of the bench. The angle 'T' measures the angle of external rotation at the extended hip joint ('turnout').

45 degrees is satisfactory. It is useful to measure the range of internal rotation as well and usually this is much less than the range of external rotation in a dancer with good physique.

There should be no fixed deformities in either hip joint and the hips should be symmetrical.

Knees

There should be no severe knock knee or bow leg deformity since bow leg deformity may be difficult to conceal during dancing. However, a small degree of knock knee deformity is common in girls.

The alignment of the hips, knees and feet should be good. With the feet facing forwards, the knee caps should also face forwards. The knees should not hyperextend to any significant degree (i.e. they should go straight but not far beyond straight). Students with knock knee deformity, hyperextension and knee caps which face laterally are at risk of developing dislocation of the patellae.

While testing the knees, the quadriceps muscles should be inspected. The thigh muscles should be well developed. At the same time a check should be made for hamstring tightness, i.e. with the student lying on his back and with the knees straight it should be possible to elevate the leg to the vertical position.

Feet and ankles

The ideal dancer's foot is one with a large range of movement in all of the many joints and also with good muscle power to control this range. The general foot posture should be normal with a straight heel, moderate longitudinal arch and no evidence of callosities on the sole of the foot.

The hallux should be straight. A second toe as long as the hallux gives extra support for girls 'en pointe'. Hallux abductovalgus should be regarded with suspicion since it is likely to worsen, especially in ballet dancers. Extension of the hallux should also be good because any stiffness here will produce problems on 'demi-pointe' (Fig. 13.2).

The small toes should not be too curly nor have any fixed deformities. The intrinsic muscles controlling separation of the toes should be well developed (but these rarely are).

The student who is pursuing a career in ballet should be able to point the foot in such a

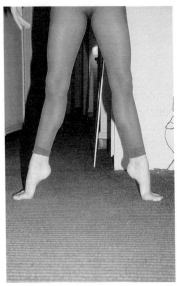

Figure 13.2   Demi-pointe.

way that its upper surface is straight and parallel with the shin. Similarly a good range of ankle dorsiflexion without any hamstring or Achilles tightness is important for the 'plie' (Fig. 13.3).

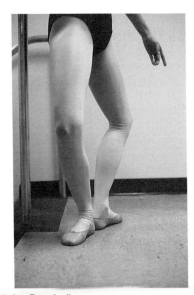

Figure 13.3   Demi-plie.

In assessing the physique of a potential dancer it is important to consider the whole body. Unless localised physical abnormalities are very gross they are unlikely to prevent the

enthusiastic student from pursuing a successful dancing career. However, where physical problems are noticed it is important that dance teachers and physiotherapists recognise these problems and subsequently teach the student how to cope with them and thus avoid potential chronic problems.

Role of the physiotherapist in preventing injury

The young athlete or dancer requires advice not only when he starts his career, but frequently thereafter as to ways in which injury may be avoided. The physiotherapist should work in close consultation at all times with all those involved in the coaching or training programme.

Warm-up

It is important that coaches and athletes alike understand the necessity for sufficient time to be devoted to a warm-up period which is then followed by appropriate stretching techniques specific to their own particular sport. During stretching it is advisable to demonstrate how to progressively stretch a muscle. Consideration should be given as to how the muscles work stressing, for example, their function as a group rather than on an individual basis.

Muscle strength

This is important when precision and coordination are required. Frequently there may be a complaint of tightness in a particular joint and it will be evident after examination that the restriction in range of movement is due merely to weakness of muscle groups controlling that area. Therefore it is important to demonstrate a progressive programme of active exercises for the affected area. Usually this will lead on to the use of weights which will normally be approximately two to five kilograms. Two methods are usually employed. The first is a high weight with a low repetition; the second is a low weight with a high repetition. The latter is normally considered more advantageous. It must be remembered that in order to obtain an increase in muscle strength, the muscles must be exercised to the point of fatigue.

Development of coordination

It is vital to encourage the motion of the body as a whole. When there is difficulty, e.g. in maintaining the hip in turnout, inrolling of the foot will arise and pain in the longitudinal arch will ensue. It is wise to consider not only how to strengthen the intrinsic muscles of the foot, but also how to control effectively the turnout at the hip joint.

The preservation of cardiac fitness

Frequently the athlete or dancer exercises to such an extent that he soon possesses the required level of physiological fitness for his heart, i.e. his body will be ready to respond effectively when necessary with regard to cardiac output. It is important that this fitness should be maintained even whilst on vacation, or perhaps even when he is recuperating from an injury. Emphasis should be put on activities which will not affect the injured area, but which will still preserve cardiac fitness, e.g. stomach and back exercises and also the use of weights for the trunk.

Healthy diet

A healthy balanced diet is of great value, especially for girls since at the age of puberty they are sometimes over concerned about possible weight increase. Such girls are already aware of the need for carbohydrates and minerals to be included in a balanced way in their dietary intake because of their nutritional importance with regard to performance in sport. These young people must also learn which foods are appropriate for them after exercise in order that their glycogen stores may be replaced to their original level. It is vital that this instruction is given at an early age so that when they proceed into the professional side of their sport they will already have formed healthy eating habits. Advice should also be given as to the type of food which may be eaten prior to a performance and immediately afterwards.

Advice on footwear

It is imperative that footwear fits correctly as incorrect fitting may damage the future growth pattern of the young athlete. The dancer should be advised as to where correct fitting of their dance shoes will be carried out and they should continue to patronise the same supplier throughout the growth period since the particulars of the first examination should still be available to facilitate further fittings.

Other equipment

Supports are of value in areas where overuse of a tendon might occur. Their main value is in their ability to take over the function of the muscle which may be under strain. However, the use of supports should be limited since they might lead to weakness if over reliance were to be placed upon them.

Common causes of dance injuries

Prior to treatment the cause of injury must be determined. If this were not done symptoms alone would be treated and would simply re-manifest themselves at a later stage.

1. *Anatomical (i.e. not possessing a perfect physique).* It is important here to enable the student to understand his physical limitations and how best to deal with them. Graduated exercises on a regular basis would normally be recommended.

2. *Poor understanding of dance technique.* Educating the student is principally done by the dance teacher but when it is suspected that the difficulty is arising from a technical problem, then it would be wise to alert the teacher in order that the instruction may be modified.

3. *Failure to apply correct technique.* This may be due to either tiredness and lack of concentration or perhaps even to an over enthusiastic choreographer/trainer. Poor technique may result in awkward movements or perhaps the

participant may be required to use muscle groups which are unaccustomed to this type of movement.

4. Environmental. (a) Temperature: problems may arise when the participant is not adequately warmed up. Similarly, when the room temperature is too high, problems of dehydration may occur and the participant has to be encouraged to maintain the normal level of body fluids in order to avoid muscle cramps and spasms. (b) Floor: the best situation is a well-sprung wooden floor. Frequently the floor is concrete and this may give rise to foot injuries, shin splints and lumbar spine problems. For sporting activities shock absorbing insoles should be worn within training shoes in an effort to minimise the problem. The dancer may also face the problem of a raked stage. Whilst excellent from the audience's point of view, this type of stage may cause difficulties for the dancer. It presents a weight back situation and may often lead to an injury becoming chronic.

Types of dance injury

Dance injuries may be classified as follows:

1. Acute major injuries, e.g. a ruptured anterior cruciate ligament in the knee following a severe fall on landing.
2. Chronic overuse injuries, e.g. a stress fracture.

Spinal injuries

These should be rare. However, dance does involve bending and on occasion lifting and thus much strain is placed on the lumbar spine. Prevention of spinal problems is by insistence on good posture, proper warm-up and ensuring that dancing partners are of a similar weight and physique.

Prolapsed intervertebral disc and sciatica

The intervertebral discs act as shock absorbers between the bodies of the spinal vertebrae.

When the tough outer layer of the disc tears then the soft centre bulges outwards. This may cause local back pain and muscle spasm. The normal lumbar lordosis is lost and the young patient will not flex the spine forwards. However, they may be able to touch their toes by flexing their hips.

When the disc presses on one of the spinal nerve roots then sciatica results, i.e. pain which radiates down the leg. Young patients often have no loss of ankle reflex but they hold their spine very rigidly in a sideways tilted position (sciatic scoliosis) in order to try to minimise pressure on the affected nerve root. There may be numbness and paraesthesia either on the outer aspect of the leg down to the big toe from pressure on the fifth lumbar nerve root, or down the back of the calf to the little toe from pressure on the first sacral nerve root. When severe, there may be loss of muscle bulk in the calf, together with either weakness of plantar flexion of the ankle or weakness of the hallux extensor.

Any patient suspected of having a disc problem should have radiographs of the lumbar spine taken. These radiographs may show the spinal tilt but in acute disc prolapses they are otherwise normal. It is important to remember that the discs themselves cannot be seen on a normal radiograph.

Any disc problem is potentially serious and initial treatment should be bed rest in order to unload the disc and also to avoid spinal flexion. As the repair heals the spine will straighten and the paraesthesia in the leg will settle. Muscle strengthening exercises for the spine may then be started and the patient may gradually mobilise by starting to get up for short periods of time, e.g. only standing and sitting initially.

Swimming and hydrotherapy are useful at this stage. When pain in the leg recurs, the exercise level must be reduced temporarily. When the symptoms persist further investigation, usually in the form of a computed tomography (CT) scan or nuclear magnetic resonance (NMR) scan to define the disc bulge, is necessary following referral to an orthopaedic surgeon.

When pain is severe surgery may be indicated to decompress the nerve root. It is important to realise three points regarding surgery:

1. Most patients do not require surgery.
2. Surgery does not necessarily speed up the recovery.
3. Surgery is indicated for problems in the legs and *not* for back pain.

After any lumbar disc problem the student is unlikely to return to full activity for at least six months.

Spondylolisthesis

This is a defect of the spine and it may be congenital or it may be due to a stress fracture. The patient usually complains of low back pain radiating down one or both thighs. Spinal mobility is frequently full and lower limb neurology normal.

Clinical examination reveals only local tenderness over the lower lumbar spine.

Diagnosis is by X-ray and the defect is seen on oblique views of the spine.

Treatment is by rest, followed by gradual mobilisation with emphasis on good spinal posture and abdominal exercises. When symptoms recur or do not settle, surgery to stabilise the spine is the only alternative.

Hips

It is rare for the hips to be injured during dancing. However, the common childhood disorders of the hip may present in dancers and may cause a limp which is often accompanied by thigh and knee pain. The two conditions that must be considered are:

1. Perthes' disease in children aged 4–12 years.
2. Slipping of the upper femoral epiphysis in children aged 8–16 years.

In both conditions hip movement is reduced and the final diagnosis is by X-ray.

Stress fractures of the femoral neck have been reported in break dancers. The risk of such a fracture is increased in people with abnormal diets, e.g. certain vegetarians. A stress fracture of the femoral neck presents with hip and knee pain and a limp, and again diagnosis is by X-ray.

Pelvic injuries

Groin injuries are common in adults. In young dancers these groin strains are replaced by avulsion fractures of the equivalent muscles from the pelvic bone. They may be minimised by good warm-up and by avoiding dancing when fatigued.

When the large muscles which attach to the pelvis are overloaded, the young dancer develops pain typically in the groin for an adductor avulsion, over the ischium for a proximal hamstring avulsion, or over the front of the pelvis for a rectus femoris avulsion.

These avulsion fractures may be confirmed with appropriate X-ray. Initial treatment is by rest. Local ultrasound is contraindicated as this may cause severe pain at the fracture site. The majority of avulsion fractures heal with conservative measures but may take six to eight weeks to do so.

Recurrence is a risk and training and dancing regimes may need to be modified to minimise this risk.

Thigh and knee injuries

Thigh injuries are rare in young dancers. Hamstring tears occur which produce pain on the back of the thigh, just above the knee joint. These injuries should be treated as for a muscle strain.

Injuries to the quadriceps apparatus (Fig. 13.4) are more common. The muscles themselves are rarely damaged. The two common problems are partial avulsions of the patellar tendon, either proximally (jumper's knee) or distally (Osgood–Schlatter disease).

There is pain and stiffness with exercise, and examination reveals very localised tenderness.

Radiographs usually confirm the bony lesion.

Treatment is difficult and recurrence is common. These are essentially overuse injuries and any attempt to return rapidly to previous activity levels will fail. In older patients surgical exploration is occasionally useful.

Patellar dislocation/subluxation

This is primarily a problem in girls – especially when they are 'double jointed', knock kneed and have recurvatum at the knee joint. They complain that the knee gives way on landing

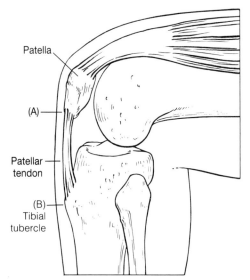

Figure 13.4 The quadriceps mechanism (viewed from the side). (A) Site of damage of patellar tendon in 'jumper's knee'. (B) Site of patellar tendon in Osgood–Schlatter disease.

and turning. When the patella has actually dislocated the dancer usually describes this as 'the knee dislocating'. The patella almost always spontaneously reduces to its normal position.

Initially treatment is to build up the quadriceps muscles. When this fails, surgery to release or to realign the muscles may be necessary.

Ligament injuries of the knee

Ligament injuries of the knee occur as a result of major incidents rather than overuse problems. All knee ligaments are very strong and require major violence to damage them. Therefore there is always a history of a fall, a bad landing or some sort of collision. After any such incident the dancer should seek orthopaedic advice at an early stage.

Chronic (missed) ligament injuries may cause giving way of the knee. The most common injury is to the anterior cruciate ligament. Dancers with suspected ligamentous instability require examination under anaesthetic and arthroscopy, and an orthopaedic surgeon must assess and treat the damage.

The initial treatment of long-standing anterior cruciate ligament injuries is conservative with emphasis on hamstring exercises in order to allow the hamstring muscles to take over the ligament function. Surgical reconstruction of the ligament may be helpful but any young athlete with an anterior cruciate ligament rupture should probably be advised against pursuing a professional athletic career.

Meniscus (cartilage) injuries

In young people these injuries usually occur as a result of a major twist or fall and may occur at the same time as a rupture of the anterior cruciate ligament. The dancer is usually unable to continue after the injury.

A torn meniscus may 'jam' the knee so that it will not extend fully. The knee usually swells over several hours. There is tenderness over the joint line over the torn meniscus and this tenderness is usually to be found on the inside of the joint. When the initial symptoms settle the torn meniscus subsequently jams the joint thus making it give way under load in an unpredictable fashion and causing pain on exercise.

The initial treatment consists of the use of ice and quadriceps exercises. Definitive treatment follows referral to an orthopaedic surgeon when the damaged part of the meniscus may be excised (meniscectomy) or repaired (meniscus suture). After arthroscopic meniscectomy recovery is usually rapid with return to activity over two to three weeks. After meniscus suture, recovery takes about three months. The advantage of meniscus suture is that it restores the knee more nearly to its pre-injury state.

The Role of the Podiatrist

Patellofemoral malalignment syndromes

These are most frequently observed in adolescent, competitive female runners and less frequently seen in males.[1] The condition may also be found in female dancers, especially those who begin rigorous training after the onset of the menses, when a gynaecoid (wider) rather than an android pelvis may well be present. A wider pelvis brings about an increased lateral pull on the patella during leg extension. Basketball players or other jumpers or cyclists may also be affected.

Early on in the injury, pain or discomfort is present only during the most taxing part of the sports activity, e.g. at the end of a particularly long run, during sprints or during the part of the ballet class when the dancer is called upon to leap (allegro). The injury may proceed to involve all aspects of sports activity, however gentle, and may be followed by discomfort when climbing stairs, hills or even with ordinary walking. Supporting shoes appear to help, but flimsy or higher-heeled shoes are not well tolerated. Certain patients describe a lateral giving way (subluxation) of their kneecap, particularly when climbing or jumping or otherwise ballistically stressing the quadriceps mechanism.

Tenderness is frequently palpable at the superolateral or inferomedial patellar pole and the infrapetellar tendon may be tender. There may be an apprehension sign in patients whose kneecaps readily sublux. Crepitation may also be present.

Several factors may produce problems with the patellofemoral mechanism, e.g. weakness in the quadriceps, particularly vastus medialis; tightness in the retinaculum; inflexibility in the hamstrings or psoas; dysfunction in the sacro-iliac joint which will produce a high riding patella; tibial varum; genu valgum; previous meniscal or collateral ligament injury; direct blow or stress fracture of the patella; synovial plicae; retinacular laxity; shallow condylar grooves; or tight fitting patellae in the condylar groove. Such factors are treated by the physiotherapist and the orthopaedic surgeon. The chief factor to be considered by the podiatrist is the relationship between changes in foot alignment and changes in knee alignment.

Chondromalacia patellae

This is a condition in which the joint surface on the back of the patella becomes softened. In severe cases the surface may break up completely. It is usually the result of overload and often there is a serious injury to start the problem.

The dancer complains of anterior knee pain, especially after exercise and on ascend-

ing and descending stairs. Arising from the squatting position is also very difficult. The knee may also grate and grind during full flexion.

The condition needs to be distinguished from other causes of anterior knee pain, e.g. Osgood–Schlatter disease, jumper's knee and certain meniscus tears. Referral to an orthopaedic surgeon is appropriate when anterior knee pain persists after initial conservative treatment.

Treatment of chondromalacia patellae consists of modifying exercises to avoid load with the knee bent. Non-steroidal anti-inflammatory drugs may be helpful in the short term coupled with anti-inflammatory treatment from a physiotherapist and also with static quadriceps exercises. It is important to realise that there is no long-term cure. Severe chondromalacia patellae precludes a career as a dancer.

Shin splints

This term is used to describe a variety of conditions which cause pain in the region of the shin. The two common causes are:

1. Stress fracture.
2. Tibialis posterior syndrome. (See below.)

Achilles tendinitis

Presentations include the adolescent male, particularly those who are engaged in jumping sports and who are in the throes of a growth spurt. Achilles tendinitis often accompanies heel pain syndromes,[2] e.g. Sever's disease,[3] a condition (Fig. 13.5) most frequently affecting young males. This may result from a compensatory overuse of the Achilles tendon in order to soften painful heel contact. The condition may also be observed in the mid-adolescent ballerina whose obligations to execute more pointe work are increasing. Achilles tendinitis is not unusual in dancers who return to pointe too soon after a long vacation or after an injury layoff and they should take two weeks of non-pointe class before resuming pointe in order to build up strength and to improve technique.

Pain in the Achilles region most commonly

occurs while jumping or running but it may also occur during casual walking. Pain is often present when descending stairs, when the momentum of the body's weight ballistically recruits the Achilles tendon. This fact helps to differentiate Achilles pain from pure posterior impingement pain (discussed later), although these may coexist.

The major muscles of the calf use the tendo Achillis to lift the body's weight onto the toe, and to ease the weight back down to the ground. Thus the calf muscles act both as an accelerator at take-off as well as a shock absorber while landing.

Certain jumpers, particularly dancers or basketball players, during rapid, repetitive leaps do not possess the stamina, proprioception or simply the time to allow heel-to-floor contact after each leap. Therefore instead of the calf muscles absorbing shock by eccentrically contracting, the Achilles tendon is subjected to increased ballistic tension and thus it begins to fray, at first microscopically and later more significantly.

Load on the tendon increases when it is used to lift and land overweight individuals, or when it is asked to do too much too soon. The Achilles tendon must also absorb more shock on hard surfaces such as concrete.

When a patient is on a growth spurt his long bones may be growing at a rate faster than his calf flexibility can accommodate. The tension on his Achilles tendon thus increases via a first-class lever action at plantigrade stance.

Finally, in heel pain syndromes the Achilles tendon is often involved, e.g. Sever's disease,[3] which is an avascular necrosis of the calcaneal apophysis.

With the patient kneeling or preferably lying prone the examiner locates the upper margin of the os calcis at the Achilles juncture and begins meticulously to palpate the tendinous or 'watershed' region of the Achilles which extends for 4 to 6 cm proximal to the heel. The tendon is then palpated for tenderness, swelling and interstitial or superficial defects and the location and estimated size of the pathology is noted. Judging the portion of the palpable cross-section involved helps to estimate the tensile strength of the remaining tendon. This helps in deciding when and to how much activity the patient may return. However, the

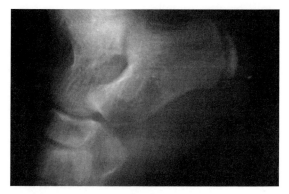

Figure 13.5   Sever's disease.

degree of tenderness of the Achilles to palpation is not an accurate gauge of its tensile strength. Squeezing of an Achilles tendon may well be painful for a year or more even after the patient has resumed full, robust, pain-free function. Once everyday activities are asymptomatic, the best way to determine the load the tendon may bear is to gradually add more strenuous activity to the schedule and to monitor carefully for either subjective or objective signs.

Infrequently the Achilles paratenon becomes involved, but when it is involved symptoms very similar to Achilles tendinitis are present. However, the main difference is that the examiner does not palpate either any frank thickening or any defect along the tendon. The symptoms are most evident when the patient actively dorsiflexes the foot while the knee is extended. Meticulous palpation of the tendo Achillis reveals the typical crepitance and pain of a paratenosynovitis. Overuse, especially in combination with direct pressure as in a ballerina with a too tight shoe, may produce these symptoms. When this happens the feet must be measured to ascertain whether they differ in length.

The effectiveness of the treatment for any microtrauma is directly proportional to the degree to which the underlying cause is eliminated. When an injury is treated early and when tissue damage is not significant, little hands-on physiotherapy is needed and after a brief rest the patient may return to sport within gradual, judicious guidelines. When a growth spurt is coincident, a mitigated activity level should be prescribed until calf flexibility improves. When this course is not followed the tendon could partially tear and activity thereafter could be restricted.

When a calcaneal apophysitis is present, soft heel pads coupled with moderate activity until the disorder self-remits (usually 6 to 18 months) is often helpful. Calf stretching exercises may not be tolerable until the lesion settles. A reduction rather than an increase in walking pain should be the guide to prescribing calf stretches in this instance.

Technique, i.e. having a dancer work closely with her instructor and with her practising bringing her heel all the way down in landing, is very important. This is easier for the dancer to perform when she has an adequately strong calf for the rigours of dance. Strengthening may also have to wait until the inflammation subsides.

Local care for Achilles tendinitis includes 15–20 minutes of ice massage (wrap the ice cube in a plastic ziploc bag and then in a wet washcloth) every 2–6 hours in the acute stage, as indicated. Transverse friction massage is very helpful when carried out by a competent physiotherapist but such friction may exacerbate paratenosynovitis. In more severe cases ultrasound treatments may be helpful but radiographs should be taken to rule out open growth plates in the vicinity as the presence of these would be a contraindication for such treatment.

The prognosis is dependent upon the estimated tissue damage. It is unwise to allow a youngster to continue sport when he is suffering from a pain-producing injury, e.g. a tendinitis, since lifelong sequelae could result. However, children usually heal more quickly than adults.

Sprained ankles

Sprained ankles may be observed almost exclusively in mid to late adolescence, as the malleolar growth plates close. Twisting violence imparted to younger ankles will most frequently produce avulsion at the growth plate rather than a sprained ligament, although Vahvanen et al.[4] have reported sprains in the 5 to 15 year age group. All paediatric ankle sprains require radiographs to confirm diagnosis.

Sprained ankles occur more frequently in females,[5] e.g. in ballet, especially in pointe class; in boys in advanced ballet when they are involved in intricate combinations and heroic leaps; in basketball; in gymnastics; in soccer; and less frequently in cross country or track running.

The primary complaint is pain in the anterolateral aspect of the ankle and this pain is usually accompanied by stiffness. Occasionally the patient may express a feeling of instability in the injured ankle. The patient may or may not present with limping but he will invariably recall a specific incident where the foot twisted under. However, one should not instantly arrive at a diagnosis of sprained ankle as the problem may be impingement syndrome, a stress fracture, or capsular sprain. The patient may report one or even frequent previous inversion sprains and this information should be sought when the joint is rather lax or when there is the possibility that the injury has been inadequately or incorrectly cared for. Ankle sprains are common in tired individuals, e.g. dancers who have been overworking.

The anterior talofibular ligament provides anterior and lateral stability to the ankle while the foot is plantarflexed,[6] e.g. in pointe, demi-pointe, or in the initial stage of foot contact when landing from a leap. The calcaneofibular ligament provides lateral stability to the ankle when it is in the plantigrade position.[5] The peroneus longus and peroneus brevis muscles provide lateral stability to the ankle when the feet are in the plantigrade or plantarflexed positions.

The variety of reasons that may produce an ankle sprain indicates why this is such a common injury. Peroneal weakness, either primary or induced, is a very common cause. Induced peroneal weakness is frequently due to a previous ankle sprain which may then lead to an increased likelihood of another tear in the ligament.[7–9] Sprained ankles may also result from a diminished purchase of the peroneal tendons in their fibular groove and this occurs when the ballerina's foot points too much. This has been called the 'too good foot' by Hamilton.[10] It is obvious that ligamentous instability is a cause of recurrent sprained ankles. Proprioceptive deficit, although it may be primary, may also be induced in much the same way as peroneal weakness. People with proprioceptive deficits frequently trip or lose balance or are called 'clumsy'.

A forefoot valgus or plantarflexed first metatarsal or hyperadduction available to the oblique axis of the midtarsal joint, findings which are frequently observed in pes cavus, can be the cause of a sprained ankle. Short lateral metatarsals, a first metatarsophalangeal joint which has inadequate dorsiflexion, or compensation for a sesamoiditis bringing about a lateral weight-shift to clear heel-off, often accompany ankle sprains. Distal tibial or ankle mortise varum may be other possible structural causes of this injury, as well as athletic shoes which are worn out from the lateral heel right through to the midsole. Sticky dance floors or irregular turf are obvious possible predisposing causes. Supinative in-shoe orthoses which are supplied to a patient for, e.g. patellofemoral subluxation, and which do not take these factors into consideration may increase the risk of a sprained ankle.

Most injuries involve simple inversion or inversion/plantarflexion of the ankle. Occasionally the lateral malleolus strikes the ground thus effecting an impact-induced periostitis which must be differentiated from an avulsion or fracture.

When the patient demonstrates any other mechanism of injury, e.g. eversion, adduction or dorsiflexion, the condition may be more severe.

Typically there is swelling in the anterolateral ankle in the acute stage. If the injury is not recent there may still be a little swelling, but it is important to ask where and how extensive the initial swelling was, so that the location and extent of ligamentous damage may be determined. A change of colour should slightly increase the suggestion that a fracture is present. Unusual anatomical angles or 'extra bumps' point to fracture, avulsion or dislocation.

The colour of the distal aspect of the foot including the nail beds should be normal except perhaps for some lateral ecchymosis which may drain toward the metatarsophalangeal joints. The dorsalis pedis pulse should be palpated. It is not uncommon for one foot to be cooler compared to the other following an ankle sprain, but the remainder of the aforementioned vascular signs should

be nominal. The joint line should be gently palpated for tenderness, swelling, defects, or other irregularities anteriorly, posteriorly, medially and laterally. The malleoli should be meticulously palpated as is tolerable and also the length of the fibula in order to look for a more proximal fracture. The appearance of the fifth metatarsal should be checked (swelling, redness, ecchymosis, angulation) and any undue tenderness to palpation or gentle motion should be noted. The fifth metatarsal is a common fracture site after an inversion injury. Such fractures vary from minimal avulsion injuries to displacements which will require open reduction. Unless the practitioner is familiar with their management an orthopaedic surgeon should be consulted.

The area of the instep just distal to the anterior talofibular ligament region is important because when it is swollen, bruised, or tender to motion stress a sprain of the bifurcated ligament or avulsion fracture of the anterior calcaneal process may be indicated. Such an injury is frequently completely overlooked.[11, 12]

The range of motion at the midfoot should be assessed and this is achieved by stabilising the calcaneus and by attempting to carefully invert/plantarflex and evert/dorsiflex the forefoot. It is important to resist dorsiflexion of the lesser digits. When either of these tests produces pain in the region beneath the extensor digitorum brevis muscle belly, or when the area is tender to palpation, there exists either a sprain of the bifurcate ligament or an avulsion fracture of the anterior calcaneal process. This evaluation should be halted at the slightest sign of apprehension or pain, and radiographs (AP, lateral, and 45 degree medial oblique) of the anterior calcaneal process (Fig. 13.6) should be evaluated. The treatment of an avulsion fracture of the anterior calcaneal process is below-knee immobilisation. The treatment of the mild to moderate ankle sprain is rarely if ever complete immobilisation.

Tests for joint instability include the following:

1. The 'drawer test', in which the os calcis is drawn forward by cupping behind the heel and by pulling the mildly plantar flexed foot forward in the direction of the toes, while

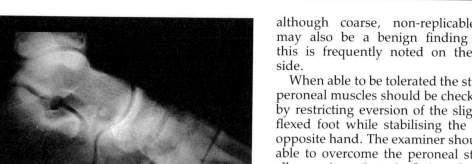

Figure 13.6   Avulsion fracture of the anterior calcaneal process.

the other hand stabilises the tibia at its distal anterior aspect. The test is carried out on the uninvolved ankle for comparisons. The extent to which the heel can be drawn forward indicates the degree of anterior ligamentous damage. This is corroborated and quantified via the lateral view stress radiographs.

2. The shift test, in which an attempt is made to displace the talus medially and laterally in its mortise. Here too a comparison is made with the uninvolved side. This may be corroborated via AP stress radiographs and will indicate damage to the ligaments which bind together the distal tibiofibular mortise. When excessive inversion is available to the os calcis, significant damage has been done to the calcaneofibular ligament. Stress views are not routinely obtained by all practitioners unless there is reasonable suspicion of a significant rupture. The plates usually taken for a sprained ankle include the AP, lateral and oblique views. Any previous sprains to either the ankle in question or the comparator ankle must be taken into account in any assessment of laxity caused by the current injury.

When passively plantarflexing/inverting the ankle causes anterior–lateral pain, damage to these ligaments is indicated. When posterior ankle pain is produced an os trigonum may have been fractured.

Crepitance may be an ominous sign of an intra-articular or transchondral fracture, although coarse, non-replicable crepitance may also be a benign finding and in fact this is frequently noted on the uninvolved side.

When able to be tolerated the strength of the peroneal muscles should be checked manually by restricting eversion of the slightly plantar-flexed foot while stabilising the leg with the opposite hand. The examiner should hardly be able to overcome the peroneal strength, if at all, even in patients in their early teens. Often it is all too easy to overpower the patient's strength which is a sign of weakness in the muscles which stabilise the ankle against inversion.

When it is suspected that a complete tear of an ankle ligament or epiphyseal damage has occurred it is best to refer the patient to an orthopaedist who is experienced in children's foot trauma. Early surgical repair of a 'ruptured' ankle ligament may provide the best long-term stability and also the shortest recovery time. In other cases, inversion ankle sprains should be managed bearing two factors in mind. First, the ankle should be stabilised sufficiently in order to prevent further tearing, but not so strictly that muscle atrophy and joint stiffness result. Taping, air splints and the initial use of weight-bearing devices such as canes and crutches should be provided in order to allow ambulation with minimal if any pain. Canes and crutches are not necessary when there is no weightbearing pain. In some cases an elastic bandage and a high top sneaker suffice.

Ballet and gymnastics patients present a special problem when it comes to using ankle tapings. The performer's ankle must be supple through a tremendous range of plantarflexion and dorsiflexion. Most appliques which are robust enough to secure an ankle at the apex of pointe will not allow the dancer to achieve adequate demi-plie. This situation is frustrating not only choreographically, but it could also lead to another injury, such as Achilles tendinitis.

The next consideration must be when the youngster can resume everyday and then sports activities. A return to activities is again based upon the ankle-intensity of the target sport, and the degree of tear, as well as the patient's response to physiotherapy and in particular strengthening. For example, a ballerina aged 16, who sustains a grade I sprain of the anterior talofibular ligament, and who upon examination displays minimal signs of laxity or tissue damage or muscular weakness, may expect to return to most of her rigorous work within 14 days, once she begins concerted remedial strengthening of the peroneals and does not do anything in the interim to worsen the tear. On the other hand, a basketball player aged 16 who presents having sustained only the last of several grade I tears, although the acute tissue damage may not be severe, may have accumulated significant grade II or even grade III laxity. (Soft tissue tears may be divided into three broad categories of severity which are based on the cross-sectional area of the lesion. A grade I tear is one from a microscopic to a tiny nick; a grade II tear is a significant but not a complete rend; and a grade III sprain is a complete tear.) Unfortunately, significant laxity tends to prolong the time required to strengthen the ankle muscles and to gain proprioception. In such cases the return to activity is difficult to predict. Therefore muscular strength should be evaluated every two weeks or so as when this strength returns a gradual resumption of activities is indicated. Rijke *et al.*[13] present a strong argument for surgical repair in such cases.

Rehabilitation is the second broad category in the conservative approach to management of the sprained ankle. Included here is physiotherapy when necessary in order to reduce swelling and subsequent stiffness via massage and galvanic stimulation. Other objectives are to reduce accumulation of fibrous tissue via massage and (when the growth plates are closed) ultrasound, to restore proprioception and the range of motion via balance exercises or balance boards, and most importantly, to supervise and later to instruct the patient in a home exercise programme in order to spot-train the peroneals and other leg muscles in an attempt to restore the muscular strength which has been lost as a result of the trauma. Indeed 'normal' strength is frequently not sufficient for a lax ankle. Such ankles usually require supernormal strength by means of regular ankle exercises thereafter in the athletic career.

Posterior tibial tendinitis

Posterior tibial tendinitis frequently occurs in males in mid-adolescence. Here the posterior tibial tendon undergoes both a considerable intensification of organised overuse activities and also a long bone growth spurt. However, it may also be observed in any child who overpronates at the foot/ankle or who engages in over accelerated activity.

Consistently the older child will describe pain on weightbearing in the arch of one or of both feet. The discomfort is often greatest when activity commences, only to slightly ease and then worsen again as the activity continues. Pain may be worse when standing rather than when walking. Certain children may not complain but may simply lag behind the others in sports or may be reluctant to engage in play which requires weightbearing.

The posterior tibial tendon is an anti-pronator which in concert with the peroneus longus imparts stability to the midfoot.[14]

As the posterior tibial muscle is firing to counteract pronation of the foot and ankle, the foot and ankle must be able to accept supination or the tendon may suffer. In certain adolescent males whose legs are growing at a rate of several centimetres per year, the gastrocnemius muscle finds its origin–insertion distance rapidly increasing. The distance may increase so rapidly that the gastrocnemius is unable to keep up, and thus a shortage (equinus) is brought about. The lever arm for the Achilles tendon is overwhelmingly skewed in its favour to overpower any other foot/ankle supinator.[15] In the presence of a gastrocnemius equinus, a foot has absolutely no other choice but to pronate in order to achieve a plantigrade position and any pronation caused by an unaddressed equinus cannot be overcome by an extrinsic device, e.g. an arch support which children may well find uncomfortable and in consequence will not wear.

An uncommon mechanical cause of posterior tibial tendinitis in children is hypermobility without the equinus which may be seen in a child who presents with excessive eversion of the calcaneus and hypermobility of the midtarsal joints.

The most striking finding in most children

who have posterior tibial tendinitis is a marked flatfoot. However, flatfoot is not always symptomatic and it does not have to be pronounced to contribute to this condition. There may be acute tenderness to palpation of the tendon and this is usually inferior to the tuberosity of the navicular in the long arch of the foot. Sometimes no palpable tenderness is present, but pain in the region of the posterior tibial tendon may be elicited by resisting inversion of the somewhat plantarflexed foot. Pain at this site may just arise from a simple shoe bruise, particularly in those children who demonstrate radiographic evidence of a pronounced navicular tuberosity, or an accessory ossicle at this site (os tibial externum). Such patients frequently have tendon pain which is due not only to pronation but also to instability of this important fulcrum.[16] A stress fracture, though rare, will show up on X-ray after a period of some weeks and will appear as a sagittally oriented lucency which is more in the body of the navicular. Such fractures are usually accompanied by much pain, swelling and distress.

Where pure hypermobility without equinus is present orthoses in the shoe are extremely helpful. Such cases usually do not require long-term supervised physical therapy. Children with mild equinus benefit from daily calf stretching exercises with or without orthoses. Where a moderate equinus presents, calf stretches and orthoses with a relatively high arch will be helpful, but the orthoses must incorporate heel lifts in order to obviate the need for full plantigrade stance. When marked equinus presents, particularly in those who are experiencing an accelerated growth spurt, calf stretches may not achieve results until the growing slows down. Most youngsters in this group would benefit from a temporary halt to athletic activity to allow their symptoms to subside.

Individuals with mild symptoms early in life may sometimes reap benefits as adults since they had been guided into flexibility routines or footwear selection criteria. The congenital problems which may benefit the most from a carefully selected plan of management in childhood are those which combine ligamentous laxity with gastrocnemius equinus.

Flexor hallucis longus tendinopathy

This condition occurs primarily in female dancers who are undertaking a considerably increased amount of pointe work (on the tips of the toes). This shift from mainly taking class in soft or ballet slippers (in which the dancer does not releve (lift the heels) to the very tips of the toes) to mainly pointe work usually begins around the age of 15 or 16. This injury is not seen in any other paediatric group except occasionally gymnasts.

The child complains of unilateral or perhaps posteromedial ankle pain, deep in the soft tissues. This pain is frequently worse at the commencement of class. As the class proceeds the pain will ease and towards the end of the class it will reintensify. Sometimes, even in the under 18 year old, the patient may demonstrate palpable or audible retromalleolar crepitance during active toe motion. Unless the injury is more extensive, pain is present only during dancing, but this pain may also be experienced immediately following class. This lack of walking pain helps to differentiate it from posterior tibial and Achilles tendinitis.

Flexor hallucis longus is the primary medial stabiliser of the ankle in the fully pointed position.[17] It is also an accessory plantarflexor of the ankle and an accessory supinator of the subtalar joint.[18]

A rapid increase in the amount of pointe work may cause microtrauma to the flexor hallucis longus (FHL) tendon. In addition the interface between this motor unit and its retinaculum in the posterior ankle may cause it to fibrose, fray and spindle.[17] This is particularly the case when the muscular fibres of the FHL extend sufficiently close down the course of the tendon towards its insertion to produce the common phenomenon called 'functional hallux limitus'. This is a painful limitation of dorsiflexion at the first metatarsophalangeal joint (MPJ) not due to pathology at the joint itself, but to entrapment of the widened FHL musculotendinous structures in the retinaculum behind the ankle. This injury particularly manifests itself in grande-plie when both the ankle and the great toe are maximally dorsiflexed and thus pull the muscle fibres of the FHL forcefully into its retinaculum.

Dancers who require to overpronate while dancing, e.g. in the presence of a short or 'Morton's' first metatarsal, or where lateral ankle weakness causes compensatory medial overshift, may strain their FHL muscle. Relative weakness in the soleus or gastrocnemius may also cause the FHL to be over-recruited in jumping.

The patient experiences tenderness to palpation along the medial and posterior malleolar course of the FHL tendon. This pain is accentuated with resisted plantarflexion of the hallux and is also accompanied by palpable crepitance in this region while the first MPJ is being actively/passively taken through its full range of motion. In particular, local palpable tenderness as the dancer releves and descends from releve is pathognomonic, but this must be differentiated from pain in full locked pointe and full tendu (posterior impingement syndrome) and at the bottom of demi-plie (pseudo posterior impingement syndrome). (A tendu is a gesturing of the foot into a downward pointing position in which the toes lightly touch the floor without bearing the full body weight.) Although any or all of these conditions may occur in conjunction, each must be differentiated as precisely as possible since their treatments differ markedly.

The first criterion here is rest. Physical therapy should be directed to the local pathology as well as the underlying cause. Thus modalities such as friction massage, ice and ultrasound are indicated. Again, pre-emptive radiographs should be taken if ultrasound will be used to rule out any open growth plates. Any lateral ankle weakness, instability, and proprioceptive deficit which would cause medial weight shift as a 'safe' compensation should be assessed. Here the dancer may have developed poor technical habits which require the assistance of a specialised dance teacher.

The sooner a strained tendon is rested, the sooner a remedial strengthening programme is begun, and the more gradual the dancer resumes her pointe work, the quicker the injury will heal. When such children have adequate supervision they become significantly stronger in a matter of two to three weeks. Subsequently they may be reintroduced to their pointe work. When the tissue pathology has proceeded to a weakening of the tendon and an amassing of scar tissue, the injury will resurrect and worsen throughout the dancer's career.

Impingement syndromes about the ankle

1. Anterior impingement syndrome[19]

This is most often observed in dancers, although anterior ankle pain in the absence of an acute incident should arouse suspicion of impingement in all patients. In ballet the incidence is slightly higher in females. Ballet dancers usually present with this and most other injuries in their mid teens, when organised dance suddenly becomes more rigorous.

The patient complains of pain in the anterior or particularly anterolateral aspect of the ankle joint. The dancer is frequently of the opinion that she 'must have sprained' her ankle, although she has no recollection of such an incident. However, further investigation may reveal that the ankle is not particularly unstable or weak. Anterior impingement is most noticeable at the very end of a leap, when the dancer decelerates to the bottom of a demi-plie. When descending stairs pain may also be reported, since this activity produces weight-bearing on the dorsiflexed anterior ankle joint line.

When a dancer jumps she firstly initiates demi-plie then leaps, then lands and proceeds into a shock-absorbing (via eccentric calf muscle contraction) demi-plie. Thus the foot dorsiflexes. The plantar surface of the foot should be able to attain a 30 to 35 degree angle with the anterior aspect of the tibia in order to provide the triceps surae with sufficient decelerative range to absorb shock when landing from a leap.

When more than 30 to 35 degrees is available, the centre of mass of the body falls so far forward of the ankle that the triceps surae and other posterior muscular and ankle capsular structures are inadequately strong in order to decelerate forward momentum. This first brings about complaints at the front of the ankle due to impingement. In more advanced cases, the force generated at the anterior impingement fulcrum due to an unimpeded demi-plie causes a strain of the posterior capsular structures. This may be visualised by taking a weightbearing lateral radiograph of the ankle in full demi-plie. Even here it will be noted that there is an appreciable widening of the posterior joint space which indicates a posterior sprain. This spraining of the posterior capsular structures of the ankle produces pain there, both in plie and in releve, presumably as inflamed tissue is pinched at the posterior ankle joint line.

When much less than 30 to 35 degrees of ankle dorsiflexion is available, the dancer cannot plie sufficiently deeply in order to fully decelerate the momentum of the leap. In adults this problem is often caused by the proliferation of osteophytes at the talar neck or at the anterior lip of the tibia. In children the impingement is most frequently noted in cases of pes cavus. Intrinsically this cavoid type of foot has less available dorsiflexion in the ankle.

Occasionally a child will have sustained much previous trauma to the ankle and this will have brought about fibrosis. This fibrosis may impede distal tibiofibular diastasis, which is necessary to allow adequate dorsiflexion of the talus.

A disconcerting factor during the examination of the patient is the lack of physical signs compared to the degree of disability that this injury produces. This results because the range of motion that is required of the ankle with normal walking does not usually challenge this injury. Meticulous palpation along the anterolateral ankle joint may elicit tenderness. Visible signs such as erythema, ecchymosis or swelling are rarely present in non-fractures (stress or otherwise).

The patient should lie supine upon a flat examination table in order to determine the available dorsiflexion of the foot upon the tibia. Using one hand, the foot should be dorsiflexed upon the tibia whilst the examiner's other hand supports the patient's flexed knee. A perpendicular angle should be maintained between the sole of the foot and the examining surface. This represents the floor as if she were standing and executing a demi-plie. When, as the knee continues to flex, the angle between the sole and tibia becomes significantly more than 35 degrees, too much demi-plie exists. When, as the knee flexes, it pushes the sole of the foot out of a perpendicular before the tibia reaches a 30 to 35 degree angle with the examining surface, an excessively shallow demi-plie is present. Either of these findings represents a potentially pathological range of motion.

Radiographs usually do not demonstrate tissue pathology in the child who has anterior impingement syndrome. A bone scan will show a stress fracture in the most acute cases.

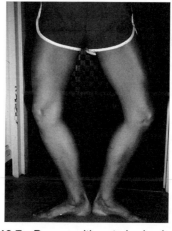

Figure 13.7   Dancer with anterior impingement of the ankle in first position demi-plie. The figure illustrates, on the affected side: limited dorsiflexion in the ankle; less tone in the soleus muscle; flattened arch in foot and valgus rotation of the hallux.

Regardless of whether an anterior impingement is due to too much or too little demi-plie, the primary long-term therapy involves eccentric strengthening of the soleus (Fig. 13.7). The amount of rest depends upon the tissue impinged. When anterior talar neck or tibial margin stress fracture has occurred, the patient is facing a protracted rest period of usually 10 to 12 weeks. When soft tissue only is involved, the rest period depends upon the extent of the synovitis. It is unusual for this to be at all massive in children, but when it is, the rest period may be even longer than that for a stress fracture even in spite of systemic and/or local anti-inflammatory treatment.

When a more mild inflammation exists, the rest period is very brief, and activity may resume gradually when strength has improved. Ice and where necessary systemic anti-inflammatory drugs will help soft tissue involvement. Heel lifts may be helpful, particularly in the non-dancer. With an impingement due to inadequate demi-plie the practitioner will observe that the longitudinal arch flattens when the dancer demonstrates this movement and he should not hurriedly provide in-shoe arch supports because the forces that are crushing the arch of the foot are far stronger than any orthosis which could be sufficiently flexible to allow dance. Thus the orthosis would only result in pain due to the relentless counterpressure from the advancing tibia. Indeed supinating the foot via any means inhibits the retreat of the talus from the tibia and exacerbates this type of impingement.

The prognosis is far better for those with too much rather than too little dorsiflexion at the ankle. In the latter case, the hindrance may eventually be compensated for by a progressive loosening of the midfoot and posterior ankle to a degree which allows sufficient demi-plie but which does not produce other symptoms. When a nominal amount of compensation does not occur it is doubtful that the child will wish to pursue a dance career.

2. Posterior impingement syndrome[17, 19–21]

Posterior impingement syndrome is a microtraumatic injury which is fairly unique to the dance population.

The young dancer complains of pain in the back of the ankle but only when pointing the foot. It is unusual for the injury to cause much walking discomfort even in the event of a posterior ossicle fracture. Although palpable tenderness may be present in the Achilles (from trying to force pointe through a blockage) a thorough examination must still be carried out when a dancer or gymnast complains of posterior ankle pain, until impingement is ruled out.

Dancers who have been born with an accessory bone on the posteromedial aspect of the talus (os trigonum; Stieda's process) (Figs. 13.8 and 13.9) have an object the size of a pea which impedes talar plantarflexion and which is impinged when the dancer tries to force pointe (this may cause an Achilles tendinitis). Such dancers will be able to plantarflex to less than 180 degrees.

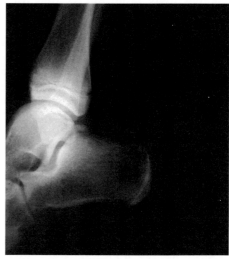

Figure 13.8   Os trigonum – in posterior joint space causing posterior impingement on pointe.

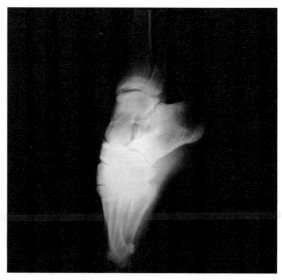

Figure 13.9   Stieda's process (posterior talar tubercle), causing posterior impingement on pointe.

Dancers with rather marked pes planus frequently simply lack plantar-flexory range of motion in the ankle joint. Similarly individuals with pes cavus may lack the ability to dorsiflex.

Posterior ankle pain which may be elicited on maximum passive plantarflexion of the foot by the examiner is pathognomonic.[22] There may be deep tenderness upon palpation. A singular pronounced crepitation during passive plantarflexion may indicate the fractured ossicle. Crepitation may be an ominous sign of a transchondral fracture of the talar dome or it may be a benign finding also present on the uninvolved side. Radiographs should be taken, particularly lateral views of the posterior ankle while the dancer is weightbearing in full pointe or high demi-pointe. The radiographs may confirm that impingement is taking place and also which type of impingement is occurring. A bone scan may show a stress fracture.

In cases of stress fracture a no-jump, no-releve period of three months allows a gradual return to dance. In cases of accessory bones, a stress fracture may also be present and this would require such rest. However, the dancer may experience a recurrence of symptoms once sustained vigorous dancing is resumed. Such instances require a very important decision: should aspirations be directed towards another career or should the offending ossicles be removed surgically? Posterior impingement syndrome probably causes more young dancers to abandon a serious career than any other dance related injury.

Stress fractures

In the paediatric group stress fractures of the lower extremities occur in the lesser metatarsals, particularly the second metatarsal of ballerinas or of runners who are in their mid to late teens. Mid shaft stress fractures are more common than basal stress fractures. Tibial stress fractures are frequently observed in teenagers who engage in long distance running and there is a greater frequency of these fractures in females. Fibular stress fractures are most often seen in teenage ballerinas while stress fractures of the hallux sesamoids are seen in dancers

and runners in their late teens. Navicular stress fractures are less common, as are stress fractures of the cuboid cuneiforms. First metatarsal stress fractures are extremely uncommon but they do occur. Talar dome stress fractures are less common than talar neck fractures. Os trigonum stress fractures are not uncommon in ballerinas who are in their mid to late teens. Calcaneal tuberosity stress fractures are rarely seen in the paediatric group, although the common Sever's calcaneal apophysitis, which is usually observed in adolescent males, closely mimics the symptoms of adult type calcaneal stress fractures.

Metatarsal stress fractures

Metatarsal stress fractures may only cause discomfort during jumping or other heavy impact activities in their early stages. As the injury advances, descending stairs begins to produce pain and eventually everyday walking becomes painful. Pain is usually not present during non-weightbearing. When pain or throbbing is reported consistently during non-weightbearing, a simple fracture or Freiburg's infarction should be discounted.

Each of the lesser metatarsals bears a certain percentage of the torsional stress which is applied after forefoot contact when landing from a leap or from jumping. As the incidence of stress increases, the metatarsal cortices thicken in order to sustain the loading forces imparted by more and more sport or dance.[23]

Unlike a simple fracture, where a complete partition occurs and can be demonstrated on X-ray, stress fracture is a more microscopic or interstitial lesion which does not shear through completely (thus plaster immobilisation is not usually necessary). There are three main causes of stress fracture:

1. Before a bone has completed its adaptation to the increased microstresses of sports, it follows a remodelling pattern which includes continuous mineralisation and demineralisation to fortify and to somewhat repattern cortical and trabecular calcium deposition.[24] It is postulated that a stress fracture occurs at the interval be-

tween the demineralisation which results from a microfracture and its potential re-mineralisation, since the bone is not yet able to sustain the loading forces when it has had insufficient time to supermineral-ise.[25]

2. Structural considerations. A dancer or runner who has a very mobile foot, a flat-foot or a hallux abductovalgus imparts greater stress upon the lesser metatarsals. Since the medial segment of the foot may readily fail here when subjected to impact, the lesser metatarsals bear increased load-ing.[26] Another injury or a weakness pro-ducing a technique change may develop into a stress fracture due to compensation, e.g. a weakened calf may not have the sta-mina to totally lower the heel to ground contact following several successive leaps. Thus the dancer may hop along on a more rigid foot making contact with the ball of the foot only and this will overstress the metatarsals.

3. Metabolic considerations. It is well docu-mented that intense athletics may delay the onset of menses. It is also known that oes-trogen, which is suppressed in the absence of the menses,[27] is the hormone respon-sible for retaining ossific calcium. Thus the very group which most requires strong bones, is disadvantaged by a hormonal twist of fate.

Metatarsal stress fractures are nearly always accompanied by tenderness to palpation in the dorsal and occasionally plantar aspect of the shaft. Palpation should be meticulous and sys-tematic and the opposite foot should be simul-taneously and similarly examined until the small but exquisitely tender site is located. In early cases little or no swelling may be noted. Ecchymosis almost always indicates a simple and not a stress fracture. As the injury matures the swelling becomes rather more generalised and also slightly erythematous over the metatarsus. Later the swelling begins to resolve into a more palpable mass at the fracture site. This mass is in effect bony callus. Occasionally no frank palpable tenderness is present and pain may only occur when the dancer releves or jumps in class. However, the examiner may elicit the typical tenderness of the injury by asking the patient to actively plantarflex the ankle while plantarflexion is resisted by the examiner placing his crossed thumbs beneath the involved metatarsal's MPJ only. Radiographs taken prior to two and in some cases up to four weeks after the onset of the injury may be absolutely negative for path-ology. This is due to the fact that stress frac-tures themselves do not show up on X-ray but only the evidence of their healing. This evi-dence of healing is the bony callus proliferat-ing, and it shows up eventually as a focus of periosteal elevation which is sometimes ac-companied by increased endosteal organis-ation, to a wispy, cotton-like appearance around the trauma site.

The primary goal of stress fracture treatment is to reduce sufficiently the impact and the weightbearing forces in order that limited weightbearing (i.e. easy walking) rapidly drops to being pain free or near pain free. Sim-ultaneously the cause of the injury must be addressed. Is the muscle weak? Is there a tech-nique fault on the part of the dancer/gymnast? Is there a hormonal imbalance? Is the dancer/gymnast over training?

When treated early lesser metatarsal stress fractures may become pain free to allow walk-ing in three weeks and may be completely healed in six weeks. Most tibial stress fractures become pain free in four weeks and should be healed in eight weeks. Fibular stress fractures may well be pain free in six weeks and healed in twelve weeks.

Frequently youngsters are pressured from outside influences to return as quickly as possible to their activities. Those who return immediately after the walking pain abates will experience a quick recurrence of their stress fracture. Therefore it must be emphasised that even although everyday walking pain has been relieved, it is vitally important to exer-cise caution in the resumption of athletic activities.

Less common stress fractures

The principles covered under metatarsal stress fractures apply to all lower extremity stress fractures. However, there are certain stress fractures which deserve special con-sideration.

1. Stress fractures of the hallux sesamoids[28]

present acutely with a limping distressed patient. Pain may be elicited on passive or resisted range of motion of the first MPJ coupled with exquisite tenderness to palpation of the involved sesamoid. Radiographs are usually of little help.

Treatment is two weeks off weightbearing via crutches, followed where tolerable by a gradual resumption of assisted weightbearing by means of a cane and wooden-soled shoe. Special in-shoe orthoses may provide symptomatic relief by distributing pressure away from the involved area.[29] Where treatment is delayed the injury may last 6 to 18 months or longer.

2. Tibial stress fractures present with pain which is usually in the distal medial third of the tibia. This pain is differentiated from the pain of shin splints as it occurs not only with activity but also simply with standing. The condition occurs most frequently in runners and in basketball players. The point of tenderness (usually about 2 cm in breadth) on palpation is generally between 7 and 14 cm proximal to the medial malleolus on the bony medial tibial margin. Viscoelastic heel pads inserted into soft shoes help in mild cases. Initially air splints or crutches are occasionally necessary.

3. Fibular stress fractures occur in the lower lateral leg at the fibular isthmus. Such fractures are distressing and the patient often presents on crutches. The condition is frequently accompanied by erythema and swelling. Tenderness on palpation is more exquisite and is not as focal as in the case of tibial stress fractures. The treatment of fibular stress fractures is similar to that of tibial stress fractures. Fibular stress fractures often develop while exercising through another painful injury which requires a compensatory weight-shift.

4. Talar neck stress fractures occur in dancers who have weak soleus muscles or who demonstrate extremely deep demi-plie, or in youngsters who exhibit pes cavus coupled with little available ankle dorsiflexion. Such fractures represent the more advanced stage of anterior ankle impingement syndrome previously discussed.

Talar neck stress fractures require about three months' cessation of perpetuating activities in order to heal, plus concurrent soleus strengthening.

Treatment of soft tissue injuries

Rest

Rest is necessary in the acute stage so that excessive pain and swelling may be avoided. Advice is also given on 'active rest', i.e. the patient is encouraged to exercise other areas of the body which will not produce a direct effect on the injury. This is carried out to maintain the rest of the body in the peak of condition and thus cardiovascular fitness and a general increase in circulation are promoted.

Encouragement of increase in blood flow

This will bring nutrients to the area and so assist in the healing process. This is effected by appropriate exercises and by the use of, for example, ultrasound and interferential equipment.

Rehabilitation exercises

A graduated programme of rehabilitation exercises is introduced as healing occurs and this should achieve the restoration of full range of movement. This is then followed by strengthening techniques. Advice must also be given to the dancer or athlete as to how and when their training programme should be advanced. Careful consideration should be given to the duration of absence from activity.

Management in the acute stage

Swelling is one of the first signs of injury and in order to minimise the problem the following methods are employed:

1. Ice. This is always used in the first 36 hours following injury in order to arrest bleeding into the tissues. If heat were to be used at this stage there would be a resulting increase in circulation which would encourage further bleeding into the injured area. However, the ice has a direct effect on the blood vessels and causes a vasoconstriction which in turn reduces bleeding and swelling. A piece of wet material is usually applied with the ice pack superimposed. By doing this the skin is protected from any possibility of an ice burn.

2. Compression. This technique may prevent bleeding which occurs at the site of injury. The time span is usually in the region of 10 to 15 minutes.

3. Elevation. In conjunction with these techniques elevation may be advantageous since the effect of gravity will assist in the drainage of fluid and thus will serve to reduce swelling.

In the acute stage the main symptoms are pain, swelling and muscle spasm. These symptoms are indications of the need for rest from the activity. Since the body's protective mechanism is coming into operation at this stage, the use of cold sprays, analgesic drugs and strapping has to be viewed with caution initially until the area has been fully examined and any suspicion of serious underlying injury has been eliminated.

References

1 Dehaven KE, Lintner DM. Athletic injuries: Comparison by age, sport and gender. *Am J Sports Med* 1986; 14: 218–24.
2 Jorgensen U. Achillodynia and loss of heel pad shock absorbency. *Am J Sports Med* 1985; 13: 2 March/April.
3 Sever JG. Apophysitis of the os calcis. *NY J Med* 1912; 95: 1025
4 Vahvanen V, Westerlund M, Kajanti M. Sprained ankle in children – a clinical follow-up study of 90 children treated conservatively and by surgery. *Ann Chir Gynaecol* 1983; 72: 71–5.
5 Watson MD, Dimartino PP. Incidence of injuries in high school track and field athletes and its relation to performance ability. *Am J Sports Med* 1987; 15: 252.
6 Inman VT. *Joints of the Ankle.* Baltimore 1976.
7 Allman FL. Rehabilitations following athletic injuries. In *Treatment of Injuries to Athletes*, 3rd edn. (Ed O'Donaghue), Philadelphia, WB Saunders, 1976.
8 Gleim GW, Nicholas JA, Webb JN. Isokinetic evaluation following leg injuries. *Phys Sports Med* 1978; 6: 8.
9 Hamilton WG. Post traumatic peroneal tendon weakness in classical ballet dancers. AOSSM Meeting, Lake Placid NY, July, 1978.
10 Hamilton WG. Sprained ankles in ballet dancers. *Foot Ankle* 1982; 3(22): 99–102.
11 Degan TJ, Morrey BF, Braun DP. Surgical excision for anterior process fractures of the calcaneus. *J Bone Joint Surg* 1982; 64A: 519–24.
12 Harburn TE, Ross HE. Avulsion fracture of the anterior calcaneal process. *Phys Sports Med* 1987; 15(4): 73–80.
13 Rijke AM, Jones B, Vierhout P. Injuries to the lateral ankle ligaments of athletes. *Am J Sports Med* 1988; 16: 3 May/June.
14 Root JL, Orien WP, Weed JH. *Clinical Biomechanics, Volume II: Normal and Abnormal Mechanics of the Foot.* Los Angeles, Clinical Biomechanics Corporation, 1977, pp 203–5.
15 Kapandji IA. *The Physiology of the Joints, Vol II: Lower Limb.* Edinburgh, Churchill Livingstone, 1970, pp 216–17.
16 Bromberg M. The role of the os tibiale externum in pathomechanical disorders of the foot. *J Am Podiatry Assoc* 1960; 50: 378–81.
17 Hamilton WG. Stenosing tenosynovitis of the flexor hallucis longus tendon and posterior impingement upon the os trigonum in ballet dancers. *Foot Ankle* 1982; 3(2): 74–80.
18 Root ML, Orien WP, Weed JH. *Clinical Biomechanics, Volume II. Normal and Abnormal Function of the Foot.* Los Angeles, Clinical Biomechanics Corporation, 1977, pp 207–8.
19 Thomasen E. *Diseases and Injuries of Ballet Dancers.* Universitets-forlaget, I. Arhus, 1982.
20 Fond D. Flexor hallucis longus tendinitis – a case of mistaken identity and posterior impingement syndrome in dancers: evaluation and management. *J Orth Sports Physical Ther* 1983; 5: 204–6.
21 Brodsky AE, Momtaz AK. Talar compression syndrome. *Foot Ankle* 1987; 7: 338–44.
22 Cyriax JH, Cyriax PJ. *Illustrated Handbook of Orthopaedic Medicine.* London, Butterworths, 1983, p 121.
23 Wolff J. *Gesetz der Transformation der Knochen.* Berlin, Aug. Hirschwald, 1892.
24 Clancy WG Jr. Lower extremity injuries in the

jogger and distance runner. *Phys Sports Med* 1974; 2: 47.

25 Devas M. *Stress Fractures*. Edinburgh, Churchill Livingstone, 1975.

26 Kelikian H. *Hallux Valgus, Allied Deformities of the Forefoot and Metatarsals*. Philadelphia, Saunders, 1965.

27 Millar AL, Hunter D. Osteopenia: Its relation to menstrual disorders in female athletes. *J Orth Sports Physical Ther* 1990; 11(8), February.

28 Van Hal ME, Keene JS, Lange TA, Clancy WG. Stress fractures of the great toe sesamoids. *Foot Ankle* 1982; 10: 122–8.

29 Novella TM. Dancers' shoes and footcare. *Dance Medicine*. Pluribus Press, Chicago, 1987.

14 Health Education

Caroline Pollacchi and Fay Crawford

Of the work undertaken by the paediatric podiatrist not all will be in the area of diagnosing and treating pathologies. Podiatrists also spend their time attempting to prevent foot deformities by encouraging individuals to adopt positive foot health.

In this chapter certain of the basic issues and methods behind young people's foot health education will be considered. Such education aims to inform individuals about health, thus enabling them to make informed decisions about their own health, and it encompasses issues such as self-empowerment, decision-making skills and assertiveness.

The relationship between footwear and foot health has been recognised for many years by podiatrists. Maintaining and improving healthy feet against their strong opponents, e.g. fashion and inappropriate footwear, is and will continue to be a major battle for those who seek to promote positive foot health.

Young people are surrounded by role models, e.g. parents, siblings and teachers, who may have developed unhealthy habits during the course of their lives and who will have tremendous influence upon the impressionable young. The advertising industry together with television programmes and the images portrayed in comics and magazines provide influential information about life-styles, values and beliefs.

These 'media messages' may contradict the message from the health educator and provide obstacles which must be overcome as part of an effective health education programme. When attempting to change behaviour the school podiatrist needs to identify measures which will gain support from those individuals and groups who are influential with the target group and whose support will contribute to the positive foot health of young people. Such groups will include teachers, pupils, parents, footwear manufacturers, shoe distributors and the fashion industry.

There are a number of models which the health educator will find useful, e.g. medical, educational, informational and radical models,[1] but these have individual advantages and disadvantages. The podiatrist should aim to provide young people with the knowledge and skills to make decisions about their own feet, and positive foot health messages are more likely to be accepted by the target group than negative ones. It would be naive and unrealistic for the health educator to believe that knowledge and skills acquisition in themselves are sufficient to ensure an increase in positive foot health behaviour. Foot health educators must market the concept of positive foot health and promote these ideas with the target audience.

This means that the health educator must have effective communication skills. Such skills may be enhanced by a formal training in health education or by teacher training. The effective communication of the health education messages may be approached in a number of ways, e.g. the lecture, group work, one-to-one and written or visual material. A combination of these types of communication may be employed to convey the health message.

Each method does have its own limitations. *Lectures/talks* may be used to convey knowledge and facts to a large audience. However, these methods are mainly a one-way form of communication with limited feedback provided in the form of question and answer sessions.

While the lecture is useful in conveying much information to the target audience in a limited period of time it is unlikely to affect the attitudes and the foot health behaviour of the audience. This stems largely from the lecture's failure to foster skills development. For example, it would be impossible to train an individual to practise podiatry simply from several years of lectures on the principles and practice of such a profession. By contrast *group work* is very definitely a two-way process where the health educator's role is that of facilitator. Here the group members use their own knowledge and skills as well as those provided by the health educator in order to explore the issues concerning foot health. Group work may use role play, brain storming and group exercises which are designed to allow the group members to consider the issues and decisions that may arise in a real-life situation. Group members may role play by, for example, going to purchase a pair of shoes. The group will require knowledge about styles, foot shape, materials and life-skills such as assertiveness, negotiation and assessment of footwear in terms of fit, in order to be able to purchase footwear that is compatible with the healthy foot. The limitations of group work are the availability of time, the provision of space and the skills of the health educator in facilitating group work successfully. One disadvantage with group work is that mistakes or misconceptions may not be corrected at the time. It is therefore important that the health educator has clear aims for this type of session.

In contrast to either of these types of communication is the *one-to-one* session. Most podiatrists are already familiar with the one-to-one type of communication[2] as they will already use a part of their consultation providing information to patients. In this situation the health educator is able to deal specifically with the issues that are relevant to that patient. This may be particularly useful when the patient has problems which are not commonly experienced by the majority of people; e.g. a young insulin-dependent diabetic will require particular health advice that would not be appropriate to the non-diabetic pupils in the class. In fact it may be confusing to attempt to include information about diabetic neuropathy when giving general health education as it may lead to individuals believing that the advice given was to be followed by everyone.

The health educator needs to be able to listen to the patient and to adapt the health message appropriately to the circumstances of the individual patient, while remembering that it is not helpful to present people with a list of 'don'ts'. The disadvantage of one-to-one communication is that it is costly in terms of time and effort on the part of the health educator.

Other methods of health education are often necessary as time does not permit large numbers of one-to-one consultations. Personality clashes are likely to be more significant in one-to-one communication; when the podiatrist is unable to establish a relationship with the patient the patient may choose to ignore appropriate health advice.

Health education messages may be reinforced by using written materials. These may be in the form of leaflets, posters, hand-outs and notes. When written resources are given to young people such resources may influence parents, guardians, siblings and other family members.

All written material should be clear, concise, relevant and have a reading age of no more than seven years of age. There are several indices of readability available.[3,4] When producing material it is important not only to test the readability level but also to organise a pre-test of the literature. The pre-test should involve a cross-section of the target audience in order to review the materials. This should include individuals from a range of social backgrounds and should cover a range of educational levels and reading ages.

Beware of including medical terminology[5] that is not understood by the target audience. Phrases such as 'loss of feeling in your feet' should be used in preference to terms such as peripheral neuropathy.

Resource lists are available from local health promotion units and from the Foot Health Council. Resources are also available from certain drug companies. Written resources are particularly useful when much new information is being conveyed. Individuals have a limited memory for new information and may find written information helpful to read over at their convenience.

Presentation skills

Presentation skills are a vital asset to health educators. Advertising companies spend a great deal of money producing first class presentation materials in order to sell their products. The general public now expect to see well presented materials and are unlikely to be impressed by badly written leaflets or by acetates that have been written before the session.

Presentation skills include the planning, timing and content of a presentation thus creating a favourable learning environment; the use of audio-visual aids, verbal and non-verbal communication and marketing. Health educators may undertake 'presentation skills' as part of a more general health education course but there are also a number of specific short courses available which will enhance or improve this technique.

Negotiation

Negotiation is also an integral part of the planning process. It serves to ensure the smooth running of the campaign and greatly influences its effectiveness. It is necessary to use negotiation as a means of achieving a budget, resources and a venue. In order to obtain the cooperation of teachers, parents and pupils it will be necessary to negotiate the final programme. The foot health programme must be sufficiently flexible in order to fit in with the differing needs and demands of individual schools whilst still ensuring that the main elements of the programme are retained.

Planning

In the planning stage it is important to identify the aims, the target population and the key individuals who will influence the foot health behaviour of young people. At this stage negotiation should take place with individuals such as the District Health Education Officer, teachers, parents and youth workers.

It is important to establish details such as budgetary requirements, availability of resources and the acceptability of the materials and programme content to the recipients. The relevance of the materials should be carefully considered.

Once the programme has been planned and the support of the individuals involved with the programme has been achieved then the planned programme can be implemented and the designed activities undertaken. The type of activities will of course have been designed specifically for the target group and should have taken account of certain group characteristics, e.g. age, race and existing knowledge.

Examples of such activities might include surveys of staff footwear styles compared to pupil footwear styles or of the type of footwear provided by local shoe shops.

Content

A foot health education programme for young people should include functions of the foot and footwear, the influence of fashion on foot health, criteria for sensible footwear (from both the health educator and the wearer's point of view), footwear materials, style and costs, assertiveness, negotiation and self-identity as well as hygiene, nail cutting and general care of the feet.

In secondary schools these may be tackled opportunistically within the curriculum, e.g.:

Science: investigations into (i) the properties of materials used in footwear manufacture; (ii) functions of footwear; (iii) micro-organisms affecting the foot.
History: history of footwear through the ages.
Geography: footwear in different countries.
Art: advertising – how to market sensible footwear.
Physical education: footcare and hygiene; first aid for the sporting foot.

In primary schools it may be possible to be more flexible about the subject headings although the same types of activities are applicable taking into account the age of the pupils and the greater possibility of experiential learning.

Publicity

Usually it is helpful to obtain local press coverage when planning foot health education events. This publicity is popular with the school and the pupils themselves and will encourage them to participate in the foot health events such as essay or poster competitions especially when it can be arranged for the winning essay to be published in the local newspaper. Press coverage should also help the local shoe shops to become interested in the project, e.g. a survey which shows their stock favourably will be good for business and may influence shops with a poor supply of suitable footwear to increase their stock.

A particularly effective method of publicity is a press release which may be produced by the podiatrist in conjunction with the press officer of the local health authority. A press release should be no more than two sides of A4 paper; it should be double-spaced type and should contain the main points of interest as well as a contact name and address.

The use of media personalities to reinforce health messages in other health education campaigns, e.g. National No Smoking Day and Say No To Drugs campaign, has increased the profile of such campaigns.

There are many role models, e.g. pop stars, parents, siblings, peers, teachers and sports personalities, whose health behaviour may have a positive or negative influence on the young person. The foot health educator should act as a positive role model and should encourage other role models to display positive foot health behaviour.

Venue

The school is one of a number of settings that allows the foot health educator to target young people. Other settings include youth clubs, play groups, nurseries and in the home. However, the school is the more common setting for health education as it allows the health educator to contact large numbers of young people on site and to ensure the attendance of young people at foot health education sessions. The school setting is also a suitable environment within which to screen for foot disorders and therefore initiate early intervention in both structural and acquired foot deformities.

Evaluation

The evaluation of any foot health education is desirable as it provides the health educator with an indication of the effectiveness of the foot health programme. Evaluation should be based on the measurable objectives identified in the planning process. Reasons should be sought for any variances between expected and actual results.

Measurable objectives may be evaluated either qualitatively or quantitatively. Quantitative measures include the use of questionnaires and surveys in order to measure levels of knowledge and/or changes in behaviour whereas qualitative measures may be more subjective and usually involve interviewing a few people and asking them more open questions about how they feel about the programme.

Many organisations and funding bodies favour quantitative measures and may demand quantitative measures of effectiveness.

The role of the school podiatrist is to act both as an initiator and as a coordinator of foot health education within the school environment. It is the role of the podiatrist to ensure that foot health education is on the agenda of the school and to provide support and advice as well as resources to those involved in foot health education. This coordinating role will allow the podiatrist to utilise the skills of other professionals, e.g. school nurses and teachers, thereby increasing the total amount of health education being undertaken within the district or region. In order to fulfil this coordinating role the podiatrist may require to reduce his total classroom contact with young people in order to support other professionals who are undertaking foot health education. This may result in the podiatist developing new skills in the area of facilitation and training.

References

1 Ewles L, Simmnet I. *Promoting Health*. Chichester, Wiley, 1985; pp 30.
2 Kippen C. Foot health education – an observational analysis. *Chiropodist* April, 1988; 57–60.
3 Flesch R. A new readability yardstick. *J Appl Psychol* 1948; 32: 211–13.
4 Lanese R, Thrush R. Measuring the readability of health education literature. *J Am Dietet Assoc* 1963; 42: 214–17.
5 Cole R. The understanding of medical terminology used in printed health education materials. *Health Ed J* 1979; 38(4): 111–121.

Further reading

Gatherer A *et al. Is Health Education Effective?* Health Education Council Monograph No. 2, 1979.

Seedhouse D. *Health – The Foundations for Achievement.* Wiley, 1986.

Tucket D. Work, life chances and life-styles. In *An Introduction to Medical Sociology.* (Ed. D. Tucket). London, Tavistock, 1976.

Appendix I
Special Investigations

Laboratory investigations may be required to make or to confirm a clinical diagnosis. Most haematological, bacteriological or radiological procedures are not unique to dermatology and will not be discussed. However, there are some which require an extra knowledge in order to obtain valid results.

1. Mycology specimens

An active area of the lesion, usually the outer border, should be selected. When it shows signs of being contaminated with ointments it should first be cleaned using surgical spirit. Scrapings should be taken using a clean scalpel blade held at right angles to the surface. Care should be taken not to draw the blade longitudinally or a cut will ensue. A blade with a round end, e.g. a no. 15, helps to avoid the point causing damage. The scrapings should be collected in folded paper and should not be put in universal containers as the static makes it very difficult for the laboratory to remove them adequately. Black paper makes it easier to find the small scrapings. Commercial packs are available, although expensive, e.g. Dermapack.

Adhesive tape, e.g. Sellotape, may be used and it is particularly useful in awkward sites or when the patient will not stay sufficiently still to allow a blade to be used safely. The specimen may be posted to the laboratory taped to a slide or doubled back on itself, although the latter is more difficult to handle.

Swabs have little place in the diagnosis of dermatophytes although they can be used for moist areas where *Candida* is suspected. More rapid transport is required for these.

Nail samples may be obtained by scalpel blade scrapings from under the nail or from the dorsum, depending upon the type. A chiropody drill with vacuum extraction may be used. Nail clippings may also be sent. As proximal a specimen as possible should be obtained.

All specimens may be sent to the laboratory by ordinary post. Apart from the swab, they will not deteriorate within this time scale. The laboratory will normally carry out a direct examination and will try to culture a specimen within three to four weeks.

The practitioner can examine scrapings under a microscope on site. The specimen is placed upon an ordinary microscope slide and a drop or two of potassium hydroxide 10–30% added. A cover slip is added. Ideally the preparation should be left for approximately 20 minutes (much longer for nails) but warming the slide, although not boiling the potash, may speed it up. Slight pressure on the cover slip helps to squash out the preparation. In the optimum the keratin cells are single thickness and any hyphae may be seen traversing their boundaries. Spores may also be seen. The same technique may be used for other diseases, e.g. scabies, molluscum contagiosum.

Certain forms of fungi can be diagnosed using a Wood's light, which is an ultraviolet light from which most of the visible rays are removed by filters. Cheap hand-held battery types are available and have largely replaced the cumbersome machines of the past. The Wood's light's main use is in scalp ringworm which fluoresces when the light is shone upon it in a dark room. Care must be taken not to confuse the non-specific fluorescence of ointments.

2. Biopsy

A skin biopsy is a common procedure and is not usually technically difficult. However, unless one or two points are remembered, the specimen may well be useless for diagnosis. There are two main types: (i) an elliptical biopsy and (ii) a punch biopsy. The elliptical biopsy traverses the margin of the skin lesion, thus allowing the pathologist to look at some normal skin and then progress to the abnormal skin. This zone may be vitally important in diagnosis and is, therefore, usually the preferred option. It must be remembered that a skin biopsy is an elective procedure and the aim is to obtain a specimen without causing any disfigurement. Therefore, it should be carried out in an aseptic manner in an appropriate area. The operator should scrub up, mask and gown, and wear sterile gloves. A suitable lesion should be chosen and a suitable line of excision should be planned, weighing up the importance of the specimen with the ultimate cosmetic result. Where possible, the long axis of the excision should be parallel to the line of one of the skin markings. Langer's lines were used in the past but it is perhaps better simply to try pinching the skin between the forefinger and thumb and see in which direction there is most 'material'. The area should be cleansed and the local anaesthetic instilled; usually 1% lignocaine is satisfactory. In very vascular areas lignocaine with adrenaline may be used but this should be avoided around the digits. In order to obtain satisfactory analgesia in thickened areas, e.g. the palm or the sole, the addition of some hyaluronidase may help spreading and thus speed up the anaesthetic effect.

Once the area is anaesthetised the ellipse should be cut out. It is best to use a D-shaped blade such as a no. 15. This allows the instrument to be held in a more pencil-like position and a more vertical cut through the skin will be obtained. It is best to try to make the cut in one firm movement in order to avoid ragged ends. The incision should then be extended to an adequate depth. The specimen of skin should not be removed with forceps as this procedure will traumatise cells and make them look abnormal and the pathologist may therefore be unable to determine whether there are malignant cells or not. A skin hook should be used to gently tease the ellipse out which is then freed from its base. The next vitally important point is for the specimen to be placed on a small square of blotting paper. This will stop it from twisting in the formalin and will allow the pathologist to view the correct orientation of all the layers of the epidermis and also their relation to the dermis. Once again, this is of the utmost importance in making the diagnosis.

Thereafter, the wound should be sutured depending upon the size of the area; deep vessels may require to be tied off and subcutaneous stitches may be required. The skin is then stitched in the conventional manner.

A quicker method of skin biopsy is to use a punch. Disposable skin biopsy punches are available in sizes varying from 2 to 6 mm. The punch is really a circular blade, rather like an apple corer. It is more difficult to get an adequate biopsy of a transitional zone and the orientation of the subsequent specimen can be much more difficult. However, they are very useful in biopsying a solid tumour or a large plaque. Once again care should be taken with asepsis. Analgesia is obtained as before and the punch is rotated with some firm pressure until it has reached full depth. The small core specimen should again be treated gently and should be removed by means of a skin hook. When this is not available, gently teasing it out with a needle may be successful and then cutting the base. Under no circumstances should forceps be used or crush artefacts may be caused. Again, the specimen should be placed upon blotting paper and, after a few minutes, should be transferred to the formalin fixative. It is important that the specimen is on the blotting paper when it enters the formalin. If it subsequently floats off this does not matter. With the 2 mm punch, a stitch may not be necessary, although with the larger punches one or two stitches are usually required.

3. Immunofluorescence

Immunofluorescence is used for detecting the location and the extent of substances in the skin, e.g. antibodies and antigens. It is of great use in the diagnosis of many skin conditions of which the most important would be the blistering skin conditions. The specimens are obtained by the same means as, and often in conjunction with, a conventional skin biopsy. It may therefore be possible to dissect the specimen either before removal from the patient or immediately thereafter. The specimen for immunofluorescence should be snap-frozen, which is usually achieved using dry ice or carbon dioxide snow, and then transported to the laboratory.

4. Immunoperoxidase methods (immuno-enzymes)

This technique depends upon the antigen on site in the skin being made to react with a reagent antibody to which has been attached an enzyme with peroxidase. The ensuing reaction may be demonstrated as dark brown deposits. Its great advantage is that it can be used on many fixed specimens and that a non-facing preparation can be obtained.

Appendix II
Examples of Recognised Human Teratogens

Aminopterin/ Methotrexate	Facial anomalies Microcephaly Mesomelia (short forearms) Talipes equinovarus Hypodactyly
Phenytoin	Cardiac defects Limb defects Growth retardation Nail hypoplasia
Sodium valproate	Facial anomalies Spina bifida Developmental delay Long, thin fingers and toes Hyperconvex finger nails
Thalidomide	Phocomelia Anomalies of teeth, gut and eyes
Warfarin	Short digits Stippled epiphyses Hypoplasia of nails Nasal hypoplasia Mental deficiency
Alcohol	Intrauterine growth retardation Microcephaly Mental deficiency Cardiac defects Flexion contractures Characteristic facies
Lead	Cognitive impairment
Smoking	Intrauterine growth retardation ? Abnormal facies at birth
Methyl mercury	Mental deficiency Microcephaly Spasticity
Iodides	Goitre Neonatal hypothyroidism

Maternal disorders

Maternal cytomegalovirus infection	Microcephaly Mental deficiency Chorioretinitis Neonatal hepatitis
Maternal diabetes mellitus	Cardiac defects Sacral agenesis Spina bifida
Maternal HIV infection	Microcephaly ? Characteristic facies Growth failure
Maternal phenylketonuria	Anencephaly Mental deficiency Microcephaly Cardiac defects
Maternal rubella	Cardiac defects Microcephaly Cataracts Deafness Mental deficiency Neonatal hepatitis Chorioretinitis
Maternal systemic lupus erythematosus	Congenital heart block
Congenital toxoplasmosis	Microcephaly Megalencephaly Microphthalmia Mental deficiency Neonatal hepatitis Chorioretinitis
Varicella	Skin scars Limb hypoplasia Microphthalmia Cataracts Mental deficiency

Appendix III
Autosomal Dominant Disorders

Achondroplasia	Short limb dwarfism Microcephaly Frontal bossing Short stubby trident hand	Epidermolysis bullosa simplex	Non-scarring intra-epidermal blisters; prognosis good
Adams–Oliver syndrome	Aplasia cutis of posterior parietal region Terminal transverse limb defects	Fibrodysplasia ossificans progressiv syndrome	Short hallux Fibrous dysplasia with ossification of muscles and subcutaneous tissues
Apert's syndrome	Acrocephaly Syndactyly Hypertelorism Midfacial hypoplasia Mental retardation	Freeman–Sheldon ('whistling face') syndrome	Microstomia/puckered mouth; grooved chin; flat mid face Talipes equinovarus/ulnar deviation of fingers
Beal's syndrome	Contractural arachnodactyly 'Crumpled ears'	Greig cephalopolysyndactyly syndrome	Frontal bossing Polydactyly Syndactyly
Brachydactyly syndrome	Short metacarpals Brachydactyly Short stature	Hereditary spherocytosis	Recurrent haemolytic anaemia Splenomegaly Acholuric jaundice
Clouston syndrome	Nail dystrophy Dyskeratotic palms and soles Hair hypoplasia	Hypohidrotic ectodermal dysplasia (Rapp–Hodgkin type)	Hypohidrosis Oral clefts Dysplastic nails
Distichiasis–Lymphoedema syndrome	Double row of eyelashes Below knee lymphoedema	Hypochondroplasia	Short limb dwarfism Near normal craniofacial appearance Caudal narrowing of spine
Dystrophia myotonica (Steinert's syndrome)	Myotonia Severe neonatal hypotonia with talipes Frontal alopecia Cataracts Variable mental retardation	Huntington's chorea	Progressive involuntary movements (choreoathetosis) Dementia
Ectrodactyly–ectodermal dysplasia–clefting syndrome (EEC)	Cleft lip/palate Ectodermal dysplasia Ectrodactyly (total or partial absence of fingers or toes)	Langer mesomelic dysplasia	Mesomelic (mid portion) Dwarfism Rudimentary fibula Micrognathia
Ehlers–Danlos syndrome	Neonatal hypotonia Blue sclera Hyperextensible skin Hypermobile joints Poor wound healing	Leri–Weill dyschondrosteosis	Short forearms Madelung's deformity Short lower legs

Marfan's syndrome	Arachnodactyly Pes planus Hyperextensible joints Lens dislocation Aortic aneurysm	Robinow (fetal face) syndrome	Flat facial profile Short forearms Hypoplastic genitalia Broad thumbs and toes Hypoplastic middle and terminal phalanges of fingers and toes
Nail patella syndrome	Absent/hypoplastic nails and patellae Limited elbow mobility	Spondylo-epiphyseal dysplasia	Short trunk Lag in epiphyseal mineralisation Myopia
Neurofibromatosis (Von Recklinghausen's disease)	Multiple café au lait spots Axillary intertriginous freckles Multiple neurofibromas Hemihypertrophy Many neurological complications	Stickler syndrome	Flat facies Myopia Lag in mineralisation of epiphyses
Oculodentodigital syndrome	Microphthalmos Enamel hypoplasia Camptodactyly of fifth finger Syndactyly of third/ fourth toes	Treacher Collins syndrome	Malar hypoplasia Antimongolian slant of palpable fissures Defect of lower limb Malformation of external ear
Osteogenesis imperfecta type one	Fragile bones Blue sclera Hyperextensibility and/ or odontogenesis imperfecta	Trichodento-osseous syndrome	Kinky hair Enamel hypoplasia Sclerotic bone Brittle nails with superficial peeling
Pachyonychia congenita syndrome	Thick nails Hyperkeratosis Foot blisters	Tuberous sclerosis	Facial angiofibromas Depigmented macules of skin Subungual fibromas Seizures Variable mental handicap
Pfeiffer syndrome	Turricephaly/ brachycephaly Broad thumbs and toes Syndactyly Proptosis Strabismus Midfacial hypoplasia	Von Willebrand's disease	Decreased factor 8 (clotting factor) Decrease platelet adhesiveness

Appendix IV
Autosomal Recessive Disorders

Acromesomelic dysplasia
Short distal limbs
Frontal prominence
Low thoracic kyphosis
Short hands and feet
Progressive multiple joint contractures

Ataxia telangiectasia (Louis-Bar syndrome)
Conjunctival and cutaneous telangiectasiae
Café au lait spots
Sclerodermatous changes
Progressive neurological deterioration with involuntary movements
Immune incompetence

Autosomal recessive muscular dystrophy
Pseudohypertrophic type of muscular dystrophy
Progressive weakness affecting both sexes

Chondroectodermal dysplasia (Ellis–van Creveld syndrome)
Short distal extremities
Polydactyly
Nail hypoplasia

Cotten syndrome
Hypotonia
Obesity
Prominent incisors
Narrow hands and feet
Short metacarpals and metatarsals

Epidermolysis bullosa letalis
Blistering skin lesions from birth
Secondary infection common
Defective dentition
Secondary nail dystrophy
Prognosis poor

Escobar syndrome
Multiple pterygia
Camptodactyly (flexion deformities of fingers)
Syndactyly
Talipes equinovarus
Rockerbottom feet

Geleophysic dysplasia
Short stature
Round face
'Pleasant, happy natured' appearance

Haemoglobinopathies (sickle cell anaemia and thalassaemia)
Recurrent haemolytic anaemia secondary to abnormal haemoglobin

Homocystinuria
Mental deficiency
Arachnodactyly
Pes planus
Subluxation of lens
Malar flush

Mohr syndrome
Cleft tongue
Conductive deafness
Partial reduplication of hallux

Mucopolysaccharidosis Types 1, 3, 4, 5, 6, 7
Variable effects of mucopolysaccharide storage in bone, viscera, skin and CNS

Phenylketonuria
Blond hair, blue eyes
Mental retardation
Eczema
Mousey odour in untreated individuals

Radial aplasia/thrombocytopenia syndrome
Absent/hypoplastic radius
Associated ulnar hypoplasia and defects of hands and feet
Severe thrombocytopenia

Rothmund–Thomson syndrome
Poikiloderma (marbling and hypoplasia of skin)
Cataract
Ectodermal dysplasia
Small dystrophic nails and hyperkeratosis of palms and soles

Sjögren–Larsson syndrome
Ichthyosis
Spasticity
Mental retardation

Weill–Marchesani syndrome
Brachydactyly
Small spherical lens
Short stature

| Werdnig–Hoffmann syndrome | Early onset spinal muscular atrophy
Progressive weakness | and lower motor neuron paresis
Death in early infancy |

Appendix V
X-linked Disorders

Albright hereditary osteodystrophy (pseudohypopara-thyroidism)	Short metacarpals and metatarsals Rounded facies Hypocalcaemia and osteoporosis		Deficiency of steroid sulphatase enzymes (less severe dominant type and more severe recessive type also described)
Child syndrome	Unilateral hypomelia Skin hypoplasia Cardiac defect	Oral-facial-digital syndrome	Oral frenula and clefts Hypoplastic alae nasi Asymmetrical shortening of digits and polydactyly of feet Fatal in utero in male
Duchenne muscular dystrophy	Pseudohypertrophic type of progressive muscular dystrophy		
Dyskeratosis congenita syndrome	Hyperpigmentation of skin Leukoplakia and nail dystrophy Pancytopenia	Oto-palatal-digital syndrome	Deafness Cleft palate Broad distal digits with short nails Hallucal nail dystrophy Syndactyly of toes
Glucose-6-phosphate dehydrogenase deficiency	Recurrent haemolytic anaemia	Vitamin D resistant rickets	Genetic rickets resistant to large dose of Vitamin D
Haemophilia A and B	Recurrent bleeding due to factor 8 or 9 deficiency		Bow legs and waddling gait
Hypohidrotic ectodermal dysplasia	Defective sweating Alopecia Hypodontia Eczema Nail dystrophy	X-linked agammaglobulinaemia (Bruton type)	Recurrent pyogenic infection Bronchiectasis Eczema Increased incidence of malignancy
Ichthyosis	Scaling skin of scalp, neck, face, anterior trunk and limbs		

Appendix VI
Developmental Milestones

Birth. When the child lies prone the head is turned to one side and there is flexion of the hips and knees so that the infant's legs are tucked under his chest. Head control is absent and there is general flexion of the upper and lower limbs. The walking reflex is apparent but is lost by the end of the first month. This reflex may be demonstrated by holding the child so that its feet are placed on a hard surface such as a table. This leads to a reciprocal flexion and extension of the lower limbs and simulates gait. This movement does not continue for very long as the activity of the hip adductors leads to one leg becoming caught behind the other.

One month. The legs are less flexed and therefore they do not tuck under the chest as much as when in the prone position.

Two months. When prone the child may now raise himself onto the forearms and may extend the head to look forwards.

Three months. The hips are now extended in prone lying so that the pelvis can now lie flat on the supporting surface. The pelvis also lies flat when the child is supine. The child's heel can rest on the surface for the first time.

Four months. The head is now vertical when the child lies prone with forearm support. The child begins to roll and to flex and to extend the limbs when supine.

Five months. The child may now take a major proportion of the body weight when he is supported in standing. This may be said to be the first time, albeit passively, that dorsiflexion has occurred. The infant can also extend the upper limbs in prone.

Six months. The child can support himself on his hands when lying prone. He begins to grab hold of his toes and to bounce up and down in supporting standing. This is brought about by reciprocal contraction of the flexors and extensor muscles of the lower limb. Rolling from prone to supine is now possible.

Seven months. The child can sit unsupported but he requires to keep the body weight well forward in order to prevent himself from toppling. The toes now reach the mouth and may be sucked. Rolling back to prone is now possible.

Eight months. Sitting posture is now much more stable. He can move from prone lying into prone kneeling with his hands and feet in contact with the floor.

Nine months. The child begins to crawl and can stand momentarily after having raised himself up on nearby furniture.

Ten months. Crawling and standing and holding on to furniture become easier.

Eleven months. The child can walk on hands and feet and in an upright position when he is held by both arms.

One year. Supported walking progresses to the child being able to walk supported by one hand. He can squat with a wide base of support.

Fifteen months. The child can walk, kneel and stand up unaided. He can climb stairs on all fours.

Two years. The child can climb stairs without help; two feet per step, and he can run and jump.

Three years. The child can now run and hop and he falls over less frequently.

Four years. The child can walk downstairs one foot per step.

Five years. He is now able to skip on both feet.

Appendix VII
Abbreviations Used in Text

Ach	Acetylcholine
ACTH	Adrenocorticotrophic hormone
ADP	Adenosine diphosphate
AFO	Ankle–foot orthosis
AIDS	Acquired immune deficiency syndrome
AMG	Adult myasthenia gravis
ANA	Antinuclear antibody
AP	Anteroposterior
ATP	Adenosine triphosphate
AV	Arteriovenous
AZT	Azidothymidine
BDA	British Diabetic Association
CAMBA	Calcaneal axis 1st metatarsal base angle
CAT	Computer aided axial tomography
CDH	Congenital dislocation of the hip
CMG	Congenital myasthenia gravis
CNS	Central nervous system
CP	Cerebral palsy
CPK	Creatine phosphokinase
CRS	Counter rotational system
CSF	Cerebral spinal fluid
CT	Computerised tomography
CTEV	Congenital talipes equinovarus
CVT	Congenital vertical talus
DA	Dopamine
DDVAP	1 Desamino-8-D-arginine vasopressin (analogue of vasopressin – antidiuretic hormone – ADH)
DKA	Diabetic keto-acidosis
DLA	Discoid lupus erythematosus
DMARD	Disease modifying anti-rheumatic drugs
DMD	Duchenne muscular dystrophy
DNA	Deoxyribonucleic acid
DQV	Digiti quinti varus
ECG	Electrocardiograph
EMG	Electromyograph
ESR	Erythrocyte sedimentation rate
FHL	Flexor hallucis longus
GABA	Gamma-aminobutyric acid
HAV	Hallux abductovalgus
HB Alc	Glycosylated haemoglobin
HIV	Human immunodeficiency virus
HLA	Human leucocyte antigen
HMSN	Hereditary motor sensory neuropathies

HPV	Human papilloma virus
HTLVI	Human T cell leukaemia virus
IDDM	Insulin-dependent diabetes mellitus
Ig	Immunoglobulin
IPJ	Interphalangeal joint
ITP	Idiopathic thrombocytopenic purpura
IUGR	Intrauterine growth retardation
IVH	Intraventricular haemorrhage
JCA	Juvenile chronic arthritis
JCP	Juvenile chronic polyarthritis
JMG	Juvenile myasthenia gravis
KOH	Potassium hydroxide
LE	Lupus erythematosus
LMN	Lower motor neuron
MDP	Methylene diphosphonate
MG	Myasthenia gravis
MODM	Maturity onset diabetes mellitus
MPJ	Metatarsophalangeal joint
MRI	Magnetic resonance imaging
MTJ	Midtarsal joint
NBT	Nitroblue tetrazolium
NCS	Nerve conduction system
NLD	Necrobiosis lipoidica diabeticorum
NMG	Neonatal myasthenia gravis
NMR	Nuclear magnetic resonance
NSAID	Non-steroidal anti-inflammatory drugs
PAS	Periodic acid–Schiff
PI	Pressure index
PNF	Proprioceptive neuromuscular facilitation
PNS	Peripheral nervous system
P-UVA	Psoralen + UVA
PV	Papilloma virus
PVC	Polyvinyl chloride
SCAT	Sheep red cell agglutination test
SF	Synovial fluid
SLE	Systemic lupus erythematosus
SM	Synovial membrane
SS	Systemic sclerosis
STJ	Subtalar joint
TA	Tendo Achillis
TAMBA	Talar axis 1st metatarsal base angle
TCN	Talocalcaneonavicular
TCV	Talipes calcaneovalgus

TEV	Talipes equinovarus	UCBL	University of California Biomechanical Laboratory
TSH	Thyroid stimulating hormone	UMN	Upper motor neuron
Tc 99	Technetium 99	UVA	Ultraviolet light

Index

P